The Herbst Appliance
Research-based Clinical Management

The Herbst Appliance
Research-based Clinical Management

Hans Pancherz
Sabine Ruf

Quintessence Publishing Co Ltd
Berlin, Chicago, London, Tokyo, Barcelona, Beijing, Istanbul, Milan,
Moscow, New Delhi, Paris, Prague, Sao Paulo, Seoul and Warsaw

British Library Cataloguing in Publication Data

Pancherz, Hans
The Herbst appliance : research-based clinical management
1. Malocclusion - Treatment
I. Title II. Ruf, Sabine
617.6'430592

ISBN-13: 9781850971696

Quintessence Publishing Co, Ltd
Grafton Road, New Malden, Surrey KT3 3AB,
Great Britain

www.quintpub.co.uk

Printed in Germany

Preface

After Emil Herbst introduced his bite jumping mechanism in 1909, it achieved some initial popularity, but from 1934 onwards there were very few references to the treatment method in literature until its reintroduction in 1979 by Pancherz. Due to the many clinically oriented research papers of Pancherz and co-workers (1979 onwards) and of other authors (1981 onwards), the appliance has become very popular all over the world.

The intention of this book is to present research-based clinical use of the Herbst appliance in the management of Class II malocclusions. Therefore, in the various chapters, different clinical problems and questions are addressed in light of the existing research. Most of the relevant scientific investigations referred to are those performed in Malmö, Sweden (1979 - 1985), and in Giessen, Germany (1985 onwards). Over a period of almost 30 years, the research activities in these two institutions have resulted in 75 publications, 22 doctoral and 3 PhD theses. Thus, in contrast to many other Class II treatment alternatives, the Herbst appliance approach is essentially based on scientific evidence.

Acknowledgement

We would like to express our warmest and most sincere thanks to Mr. Hartmut Meyer, our photographer at the Department of Orthodontics.

Without his knowledge of desktop publishing and his commitment and effort in performing the graphic design and chapter layout, this book would not have been what it is. Hartmut, you did a wonderful job.

Hans Pancherz
Sabine Ruf

About the authors

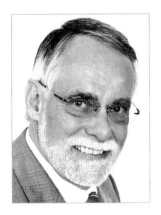

Hans Pancherz, DDS, Odont. Dr. (PhD), received his dental and orthodontic education at the School of Dentistry, University of Lund in Malmö, Sweden. He became a certified specialist in Orthodontics in 1974. In 1976 he finished his PhD thesis on "Long-term effects of activator (Andresen appliance) treatment". From 1975 to 1985 he was Associate Professor at the Orthodontic Department, University of Lund. In 1985 he was appointed Chair Professor at the University of Giessen, Germany, where he served from 1985 until 2005.

Professor Pancherz has published 140 scientific articles, 72 of which deal with the Herbst appliance. He has been invited as lecturer at more than 200 national and international conferences all over the world and has received numerous awards and honors. At the Dental Faculty in Hong Kong, Professor Pancherz served as Honorary Professor in 1996 and 1997 and as Visiting Professor in 2007. He was Keith Godfrey Visiting Professor in Sydney in 1997. Furthermore, he acted as External Examiner for the Masters in Orthodontics in Hong-Kong in 1996 and 1997 and in Sydney in 1997 and 2006. Moreover, he is Editorial Board Member of several orthodontic journals. Professor Pancherz is particularly interested in clinical research, focusing on functional appliances and their effects on growth, electromyography of the masticatory muscles and long-term evaluation of dentofacial orthopedic interventions.

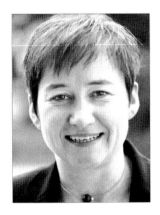

Sabine Ruf, DDS, Dr. med. dent. habil. (PhD) received her dental, orthodontic and scientific degrees from the School of Dentistry, Justus-Liebig-University of Giessen, Germany. In 1994 she obtained her Dr. med. dent. with the thesis entitled: "Facial morphology, size and activity of the masseter muscle". She became a certified specialist in Orthodontics in 1995. Thereafter, in 2001 she was granted the degree of Dr. med. dent. habil. (PhD) with the thesis entitled "Influence of the Herbst appliance on mandibular growth and TMJ function". From 2002 to 2005 she served as Professor and Chair of Orthodontics at the School of Dentistry at the University of Berne, Switzerland. Since October 2005 she has been Professor and Chair of the Department of Orthodontics at the Justus-Liebig-University of Giessen.

Professor Ruf has published 50 articles, 20 of which deal with the Herbst appliance. She has been an invited lecturer at 50 national and international conferences and has received several awards and honors. Additionally, she was active as Visiting Professor at the Dental Faculty at Hong Kong University in 1997, were she also served as External Examiner for the Masters in Orthodontics in 2005. Furthermore, she is Editorial Board Member of several orthodontic journals and was Meeting President of the German Orthodontic Society in 2007. Professor Ruf is especially interested in clinical research, focusing on functional appliances and their effect on masticatory muscle and TMJ function.

Contents

Chapter 1

Historical background

In two beautifully written theses by Herbeck (1991) and Geiss (1992) different aspects of Herbst´s personal and professional life are presented. Herbst was a remarkable man, far ahead of his time. Much of what we know about orthodontic appliances today was already described by him more than 90 years ago (Herbst 1910).

Emil Herbst was born in Bremen / Germany in 1872 and died in the same town in 1940. He graduated in dentistry from the University of Leipzig in 1894. Thereafter he went to the United States and studied at the Dental Colleges in Buffalo, NY, and Philadelphia / PA. Herbst got his American DDS in 1895 (Fig.1-1). After returning to Germany he worked for several years as a general practitioner, first in Berlin and later in his father´s dental office in Bremen. However, Herbst became more and more interested in orthodontics and he took his German doctor degree in 1921. In 1923 he defended his PhD thesis: "Die Bedeutung des Zwischenkiefers für die Missbildungen und Anomalien des menschlichen Gebisses". In 1930 Herbst was appointed professor in orthodontics at the University of Bremen. This made him the first acting orthodontic professor and chairman in Germany.

Herbst´s main contribution to modern orthodontics was the development of the Okklusionsscharnier or Retentionsscharnier (Herbst appliance) (Fig.1-2). Scharnier means joint, and the word retention was added because the maxillary part of the appliance served as a retainer for an expanded dental arch by the incorporation of a circumferential palatal arch wire. The appliance is a fixed "bite-jumping" (Kingsley 1877, in Weinberger 1926) device aimed at stimulate mandibular growth in the treatment of skeletal Class II malocclusions (Herbst 1934). The appliance can be compared with an artificial joint working between the maxilla and mandible. A bilateral telescope mechanism keeps the mandible in an anterior forced position during all mandibular functions such as speech, chewing, biting and swallowing. In the original design, the telescope mechanism (tube and plunger) was attached to bands or crowns / caps of German silver or gold. The tube was positioned in the maxillary first molar region and the plunger in the mandibular first premolar or canine region. In the earlier designs, the telescoping parts were curved (Fig.1-3) conforming to the Curve of Spee. The later designs were, however, straight as they are today. Until 1934, Herbst made the telescopes of German silver but recommended gold in cases in which the appliance had to be worn more than 6 months.

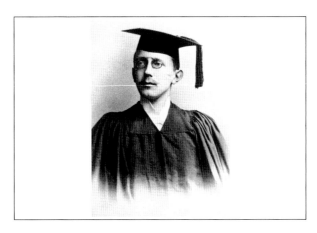

Fig.1-1 Emil Herbst appointed "Doctor of Dental Surgery" (DDS) in 1895 *(From Geiss 1992).*

1

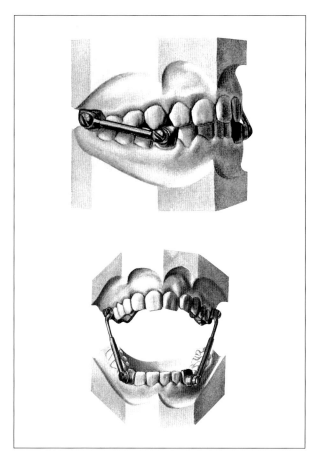

Herbst introduced his appliance to the orthodontic community at the 5th International Dental Congress in Berlin in 1909. He wrote extensively about it in his book from 1910. In 1934 Herbst presented 3 articles in Zahnärztliche Rundschau on his positive long-term experiences with the appliance. At the same time, Martin Schwarz (1934) from Vienna wrote two more or less critical articles about the treatment method in the same journal. Schwarz claimed that the Herbst appliance could result in an overload of the anchorage teeth with periodontal damage as a consequence. This claim, however, has been disproven in later research (see Chapter 20: Effects on anchorage teeth and tooth-supporting structures). After 1934 very little was published about the subject and the Herbst appliance was more or less forgotten until it was rediscovered by Hans Pancherz in 1979, who in the beginning primarily used it as a scientific tool in clinical research. Since 1979 the Herbst appliance has gained increasing interest and has grown to be one of the most popular functional appliances for the therapy of Class II malocclusions.

Fig.1-2 The original Herbst appliance (from Herbst 1910). Note the upside down position of the telescopes (the plunger attached to the maxillary molar crown and the tube on the mandibular canine crown). Furthermore, the tube had no open end, thus not allowing the plunger to extend behind the tube as was the case in later designs.

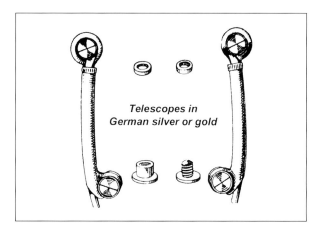

Telescopes in German silver or gold

Fig.1-3 Curved telescopes used in the earlier designs of the Herbst appliance *(From Herbst 1934)*.

References

Geiss E-M. Emil Herbst (1872 – 1940): Sein Leben, Werk und Einfluss auf die heutige Kieferorthopädie. Diss. Dr. med. dent. (Thesis), Giessen 1992.

Herbeck E. Emil Herbst: Einer der frühen Pioniere der deutschen Orthodontie. Diss. Dr. med. dent. (Thesis), Bonn 1991.

Herbst E. Atlas und Grundriss der Zahnärztlichen Orthopädie. München: J. F. Lehmann´s Verlag 1910.

Herbst E. Dreißigjährige Erfahrungen mit dem Retentions-Scharnier. Zahnärztl Rundschau 1934;43:1515-1524, 1563-1568, 1611-1616.

Pancherz H. Treatment of Class II malocclusions by jumping the bite with the Herbst appliance. Am J Orthod 1979;76:423-442.

Schwarz M. Erfahrungen mit dem Herbstschen Scharnier zur Behandlung des Distalbisses. Zahnärztl Rundschau 1934;43:47-54, 91-100.

Weinberger WW. Orthodontics. A historical review of its origin and evolution. Vol II. Chicago: The Mosby Company 1926.

Chapter 2

Dentoskeletal characteristics of Class II malocclusions

Research

In dentofacial orthopedics a thorough knowledge of dentoskeletofacial morphology and growth is essential for the diagnosis, treatment planning and evaluation of the treatment results.

The cephalometric characteristics of Class II malocclusions have been analyzed in a number of investigations (Henry 1957, Sassouni 1970, Harris et al. 1972, Hitchkock 1973, Moyers et al. 1980, McNamara 1981, Karlsen 1994, Rosenblom 1995). The value of these studies is limited, however, due to several factors. (1) No clear definition of Class II malocclusion with no demarcation between Class II and Class I, especially in the mixed dentition. (2) No differentiation between Class II:1 and Class II:2 cases; a differentiation is certainly most important as Class II:2 subjects may have a specific craniofacial morphology (Korkhaus 1953, Schwarz 1956, Smeets 1962, Wallis 1963, Houston 1967, Sassouni 1969, Ingervall and Lennartsson 1973, Droschel 1974, Maj and Lucchese 1982, Pancherz and Zieber 1998). (3) Insufficient sample size, which is especially true when evaluating Class II:2 malocclusions. (4) The influence of maturation (age) on the skeletofacial morphology has been neglected in most studies; age may have a decisive bearing on the choice of therapeutic approach in dentofacial orthopedics of Class II malocclusions, e.g. removable or fixed functional appliances, non-extraction or extraction therapy.

In the study of Pancherz et al (1997) assessing the dentoskeletal characteristics of Class II malocclusions by means of lateral head films, large samples of well-defined Class II:1 and Class II:2 subjects in two age groups were compared. The scientific evidence of this investigation will be scrutinized.

Cephalometric characteristics of Class II, division 1 and Class II, division 2 malocclusions: A comparative study in children (Pancherz et al. 1997)

The patient files of three university orthodontic departments (Giessen and Marburg in Germany and Malmö in Sweden), as well as two private orthodontic practices (Wiesbaden and Frankfurt in Germany) were screened. All those 347 (172 males and 175 females) Class II:1 and 156 (87 males and 69 females) Class II:2 subjects aged 8 to 13 years fulfilling the following requirements were selected: (1) Bilateral distal molar relationships > ½ cusp width, when the deciduous mandibular second molars were still present. (2) Bilateral distal molar and canine relationships ≥ ½ cusp width, when the permanent teeth in the lateral segments had erupted. (3) Proclination of the maxillary incisors with an overjet > 5 mm (Class II:1 only). (4) Retroclination of at least the two maxillary central incisors and a deep bite (Class II:2 only). While subject selection was based on the analysis of pretreatment dental casts, dentoskeletal morphology was assessed on pretreatment lateral head films. The subjects were divided into two age groups: 8-10 years (roughly corresponding to the early mixed dentition) and 11-13 years (roughly corresponding to the late mixed dentition).

In the evaluation of the dentoskeletal morphology in the two malocclusion samples, reference data from two cephalometric standards, representing the "normal" population, were used for comparison: the Michigan data (Riolo et al. 1974) and the London data (Bathia and Leighton 1993).

In the head film analysis all linear measures were corrected for radiographic enlargement ranging from 7% to 11%. The reference points and lines used are shown in Fig. 2-1.

When comparing males and females in the two malocclusion samples as well as the two age groups, no statistically significant differences existed. Therefore, with respect to gender, the samples were pooled.

Sagittal maxillary position – SNA (Fig. 2-2)

A normal maxillary position dominated in both malocclusion samples and age groups (73% to 77% of the cases). The frequency of cases with maxillary retrusion was higher in the Class II:2 sample (19% to 23%) than in the Class II:1 sample (13% to 15%).

Sagittal mandibular position – SNB (Fig. 2-2)

In the Class II:1 sample mandibular retrusion was seen in almost half (48%) of the younger and in one third (29%) of the older subjects. In the Class II:2 sample the frequency of subjects with mandibular retrusion was equally large in both age groups (48% and 49%, respectively).

Sagittal mandibular position – SNPg (Fig. 2-2)

When using the SNPg angle to evaluate sagittal mandibular position, a similar pattern was found as for the SNB angle.

Sagittal maxillary / mandibular relationship – ANB (Fig. 2-3)

In the Class II:1 sample a skeletal Class II relationship (ANB ≥ 5°) was seen in three quarters (76%) of the younger and in half (53%) of the older subjects. In the Class II:2 sample, in both age groups about half of the subjects (54% and 56%, respectively) had a skeletal Class II relationship.

Sagittal maxillary / mandibular relationship – ANPg (Fig. 2-3)

When using the ANPg angle to evaluate the maxillary / mandibular relationship, a pattern similar to that of the ANB was found.

Mandibular plane angle – ML/NSL (Fig. 2-3)

A balanced mandibular plane angle dominated in both the Class II:1 and Class II:2 malocclusion samples. The frequency of subjects with a normal ML/NSL (27.5° to 39.5°) was larger in the

younger (82% and 85%, respectively) than in the older (77% and 73%, respectively) subjects. However, both low-angle and high-angle cases existed in the two malocclusion samples and their frequency increased with age (not for high-angle cases in the Class II:1 sample).

Facial height index – (Sp´- Gn/N - Gn) x 100 (Fig. 2-4)

A short lower face existed in all Class II:1 (100%) and almost all Class II:2 (99% in the younger and 97% in the older) subjects. A long lower face was not seen in any of the subjects in either of the malocclusion samples.

Upper incisor position – U1/NL (Fig. 2-4)

Due to the method of case selection it was natural that, in comparison to the Michigan and London refrence data, the U1/NL angle was, on average, larger in the Class II:1 sample and smaller in the Class II:2 sample. However, in the Class II:1 sample, only 18% of the younger and 20% of the older subjects exhibited proclined upper incisors in accordance with the cephalometric definition used. In the Class II:2 sample, on the other hand, 100% of the older and 99% of the younger subjects showed retroclined incisors in accordance with the cephalometric definition.

Lower incisor position – L1/ML (Fig. 2-4)

In the Class II:1 sample, incisor proclination was present in about 50% of the subjects in each age group while incisor retroclination was seen in very few of the cases (0% to 3%). In the Class II:2 sample, incisor proclination and retroclination occurred at about the same frequency (6% to 11%) in the two age groups.

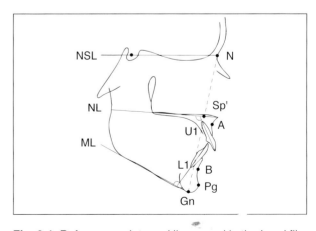

Fig. 2-1 Reference points and lines used in the head film analysis. (*Revised from Pancherz et al. 1997*)

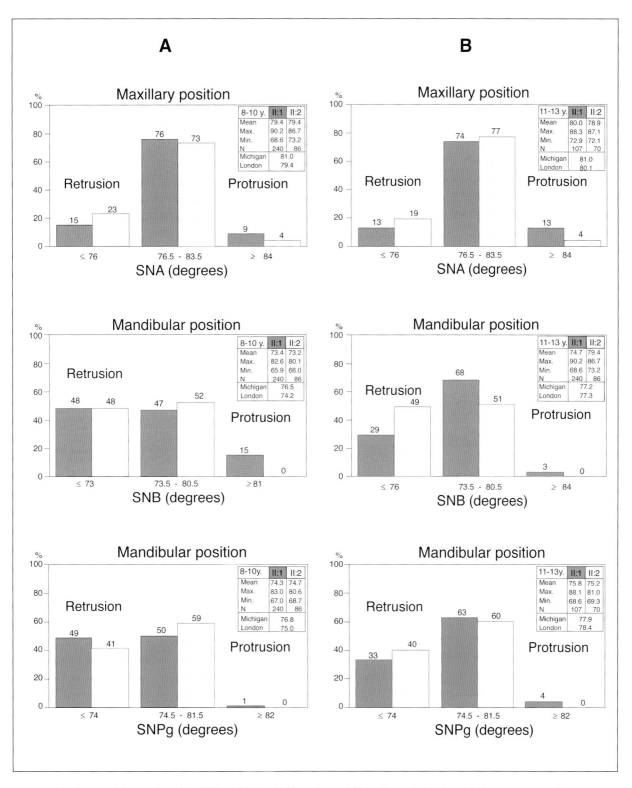

Fig. 2-2 Distribution of the angles SNA, SNB and SNPg in Class II:1 and Class II:2 malocclusions. **A**: Age 8-10 years. **B**: Age 11-13 years. (*Revised from Pancherz et al. 1997*)

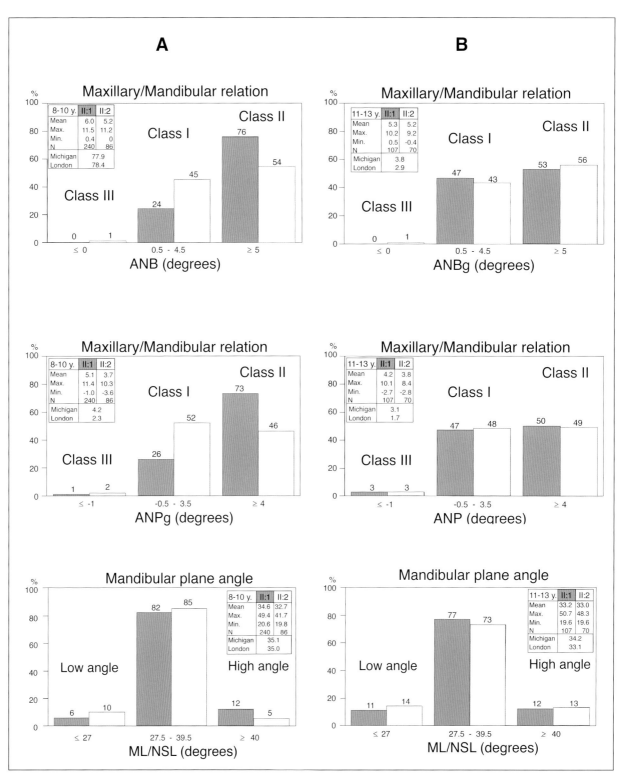

Fig.2-3 Distribution of the angles ANB, ANPg and ML/NSL in Class II:1 and Class II:2 malocclusions. **A**: Age 8-10 years. **B**: Age 11-13 years. (*Revised from Pancherz et al. 1997*)

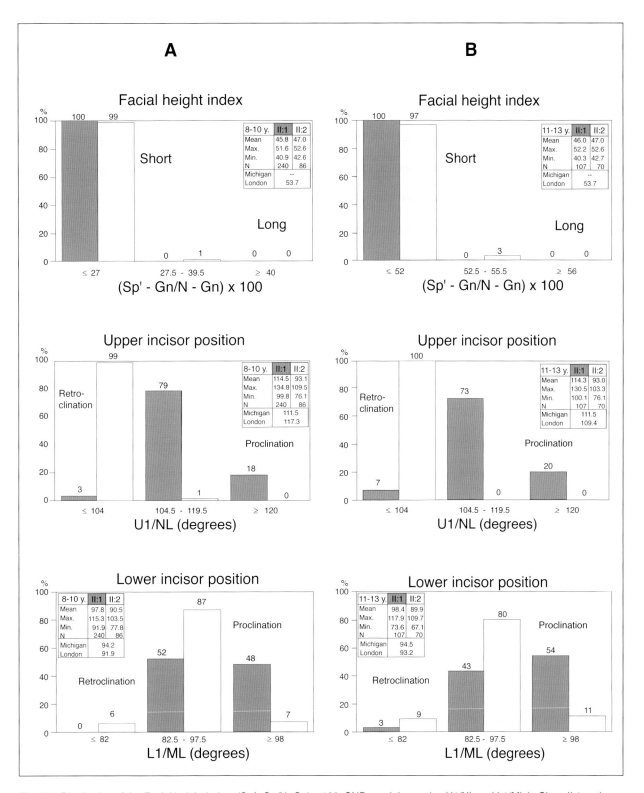

Fig. 2-4 Distribution of the Facial height index: (Sp´- Gn/N- Gn) x 100 SNPg and the angles U1/NL and L1/ML in Class II:1 and Class II:2 malocclusions. **A**: Age 8-10 years. **B**: Age 11-13 years. (*Revised from Pancherz et al. 1997*)

Interpretation of the results

Irrespective of the age of the subjects, a broad variation in dentoskeletal morphology existed in the two Class II malocclusion samples.

Considering mandibular position (SNB, SNPg), mandibular retrusion was a common characteristic of both Class II:1 and Class II:2 samples (Korkhaus 1953, Hauser 1953, Henry 1957, Harris et al. 1972, Hitchcock 1973, Moyers et al. 1980, McNamara 1981, Karlsen 1994, Rosenblom 1995, Carter 1987, Pancherz and Zieber 1998). Due to normal growth and development (Riolo et al. 1974, Bathia and Leighton 1993), the frequency of mandibular retrusion was expected to become lower with age. This was, however, only true for the Class II:1 sample. Possibly, mandibular growth was restricted in the Class II:2 subjects due to the retroclined maxillary incisors combined with the deep bite. This assumption is confirmed by the observation that in these cases dentoalveolar development (SNB) was restrained more than basal development (SNPg) (Korkhaus 1953, Hauser 1953, Arvystas 1990).

Mainly as a result of the high frequency of subjects with mandibular retrusion in the two malocclusion samples, a skeletal Class II jaw base relationship (large ANB and ANPg angles) was found in a large percentage of cases (46% - 76%). However, as mentioned earler, due to the possible restriction of mandibular growth in Class II:2 subjects the decrease in frequency of skeletal Class II cases with age was seen only in Class II:1 subjects. This was, because the proclined maxillary incisors in these cases did not hinder sagittal mandibular growth development. The average reduction of the ML/NSL angle (Class II:1) and the increase of low angle cases (Class II:1 and Class II:2) with age may be due to an anterior mandibular growth rotation (Karlsen 1994, Björk 1969, Björk and Skieller 1972), which is thought to occur especially in cases with insufficient incisal support (Björk 1969, Backlund 1958).

A short lower face height was a consistent finding in both malocclusion samples (97% - 100%). Similar results were found in other Class II:1 (Carter 1987, Karlsen 1994), and Class II:2 (Korkhaus 1953, Hauser 1953, Smeets 1962, Maj and Lucchese 1982, Pancherz and Zieber 1997) studies. In contrast, ex cessive vertical development of the lower face was found in the Class II:1 studies of Henry (1957), Hunter (1967) and McNamara (1981).

The mandibular incisor inclination (L1/ML) differed between the two malocclusion samples. The teeth were relatively more often proclined in the Class II:1 group and relatively more often retroclined in the Class II:2 group. This was thought to result mainly from dentoalveolar compensation (Solow 1980) in response to mandibular retrusion (Class II:1) and maxillary incisor retroclination (Class II:2). However, marked mandibular incisor retroclination in the Class II:2 malocclusions was found in only 6% - 9% of the subjects.

Conclusions and clinical implications

Neither Class II:1 nor Class II:2 malocclusions at the ages of 8-10 years and 11-13 years were single clinical entities and, with the exception of maxillary incisor position, no basic morphological differences existed between the two malocclusions.

- Mandibular retrusion and skeletal Class II jaw relationships were frequent findings .
- In Class II:1 malocclusions at the age of 8-10 years, a retrusive mandible and a skeletal Class II were seen more frequently than a normal mandible and a skeletal Class I, respectively. At the age of 11-13 years the frequency of cases with normal and retrusive mandibles as well as the frequency of skeletal Class I and II were comparable.
- In Class II:2 malocclusions at the ages of 8-10 years and 11-13 years, normal and retrusive mandibles as well as skeletal Class I and Class II were seen equally often.
- Skeletal Class III as well as high and low mandibular plane angles were seen to a small percentage in both malocclusion samples.
- Short lower face height was a consistent finding in both types of malocclusions.
- Proclined mandibular incisors in Class II:1 and normal mandibular incisor inclination in Class II:2 subjects were common findings.

References

Arvystas MG. Nonextraction treatment of severe Class II division 2 malocclusions. Part 1. Am J Orthod Dentofac Orthop 1990;97:510-521.

Backlund E. Overbite and incisor angle. Trans Eur Orthod Soc 1958;34:277-286.

Bathia SN, Leighton BC. A manual of facial growth: a computer analysis of longitudinal cephalometric growth data. Oxford: Oxford University Press, 1993:337.

Björk A. Prediction of mandibular growth rotation. Am J Orthod 1969;55:585-599.

Björk A, Skieller V. Facial development and tooth eruption. An implant study at the age of puberty. Am J Orthod 1972;62:339-383.

Carter NE. Dentofacial changes in untreated Class II, division 1 subjects. Br J Orthod 1987;14:225-234.

Droschl H. Die Morphologie des Deckbisses. Fortschr Kieferorthop 1974;35:209-220.

Harris JE, Kowalski CJ, Walker GF. Discrimination between normal and Class II individuals using Steiner´s analysis. Angle Orthod 1972;42:212-220.

Hauser E. Zur Ätiologie und Genese des Deckbisses. Fortschr Kieferorthop 1953;14:154-161.

Henry RG. A classification of Class II division 1 malocclusion. Angle Orthod 1957;27:83-92.

Hitchcock HP. A cephalometric description of Class II division 1 malocclusions. Am J Orthod 1973;63:414-423.

Houston WJB. A cephalometric analysis of Angle Class II division 2 malocclusion in the mixed dentition. Dental Pract 1967;17:372-376.

Hunter WS. The vertical dimension of the face and skeletodental retrognathism. Am J Orthod 1967;53:586-595.

Ingervall B, Lennartsson B. Cranial morphology and dental arch dimensions in children with Angle Class II division 2 malocclusion. Odont Revy 1973;24:149-160.

Karlsen AT. Craniofacial morphology in children with Angle Class II division 1 malocclusion with and without deep bite. Angle Orthod 1994;64:437-446.

Korkhaus G. Über den Aufbau des Gesichtsschädels beim Deckbiss. Fortschr Kieferorthop 1953;14:162-171.

Maj G, Lucchese FP. The mandible in Class II division 2. Angle Orthod 1982;52:288-292.

McNamara JA. Components of Class II malocclusion in children 8 -10 years of age. Angle Orthod 1981;51:177-202.

Moyers RE, Riolo ML, Guire KE, Wainright RL, Bookstein FL. Differential diagnosis of Class II malocclusions: Part I - Facial types associated with Class II malocclusions. Am J Orthod 1980;78:477-494.

Pancherz H, Zieber K. Dentoskeletal morphology in children with Deckbiss. J Orofac Orthop 1998;59:274-285.

Pancherz H, Zieber K, Hoyer B. Cephalometric characteristics of Class II, division 1 and Class II, division 2 malocclusions: a comparative study in children. Angle Orthod 1997;67:111-120.

Riolo M, Moyers RE, McNamara JA, Hunter SW. An atlas of craniofacial growth. Cephalometric standards from the University School Growth Study, The University of Michigan. Monograph No 2, Craniofacial Growth Series. Center of Human Growth and Development, University of Michigan. Ann Arbor, Michigan 1974.

Rosenblum RE. Class II malocclusion: mandibular retrusion or maxillary protrusion? Angle Orthod 1995;65:49-62.

Sassouni V. A classification of skeletal facial types. Am J Orthod 1969;55:109-123.

Sassouni V. The Class II syndrome: a differential diagnosis and treatment. Angle Orthod 1970;40:334-341.

Schwarz M. Der Deckbiss (Steilbiss) im Fernröntgenbild. Fortschr Kieferorthop 1956;17:89-103, 186-196, 258-282.

Smeets HJL. A roentgenocephalometric study of the skeletal morphology of Class II division 1 malocclusion in adult cases. Trans Eur Orthod Soc 1962;38:247-259.

Solow B. The dentoalveolar compensatory mechanism: background and clinical implications. Br J Orthod 1980;7:145-161.

Wallis SF: Integrations of certain variants of the facial skeleton in Class II, division 2 malocclusion. Angle Orthod 1963;33:60-67.

Chapter 3

Design, construction and clinical management of the Herbst appliance

With respect to the design and construction of the Herbst appliance there are two important factors to be considered: anchorage control and appliance durability. In modern times, however, instead of paying attention to these things, emphasis has frequently been placed on making the appliance simpler and less expensive.

In order to make the clinician aware of the above factors and to help him to avoid unwanted (uncontrolled) tooth movements and appliance breakages/dislodgements this chapter will deal with different designs of the Herbst appliance, their construction and clinical management.

Appliance design in the past

The standard anchorage form used by Herbst (1910, 1934) is shown in Fig. 3-1. Crowns or caps were placed on the maxillary permanent first molars and mandibular first premolars (or canines). The crowns or caps were connected by wires along the palatal surfaces of the maxillary teeth and the lingual surfaces of the mandibular teeth to distal of the mandibular molars.

In cases in which the maxillary second permanent molars were not erupted, Herbst found it advisable to anchor the appliance more firmly by placing bands also on the maxillary canines, which were soldered to the palatal arch wire as were the maxillary molars (Fig. 3-2). Alternative to bands on the maxillary canines, a thin gold wire on the labial surfaces of the maxillary incisors, also soldered to the palatal arch wire, was utilized (Fig. 3-3).

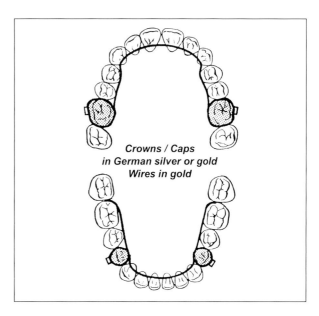

Fig. 3-1 Herbst´s standard anchorage system. (*Revised from Herbst 1934*)

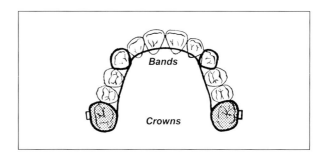

Fig. 3-2 Herbst´s maxillary anchorage system when the second permanent molars were not erupted - bands on canines. (*Revised from Herbst 1934*)

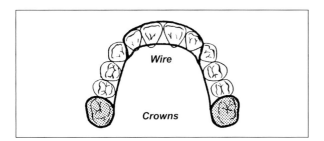

Fig. 3-3 Herbst´s maxillary anchorage system when the second permanent molars were not erupted - wires on the front teeth. (*Revised from Herbst 1934*)

When using the Herbst appliance in the early mixed dentition (after eruption of the permanent incisors and first molars), Herbst had the following solution: in the maxilla the permanent central incisors were used for anchorage instead of the canines (Fig. 3-4), and in the mandible, crowns were placed on the permanent first molars and bands on the four permanent incisors (Fig. 3-4). A thick (1.2 mm) gold wire was used to join the mandibular incisors and molars on their labial surfaces. The telescopic axles were soldered directly onto this wire in the region of the first deciduous molars.

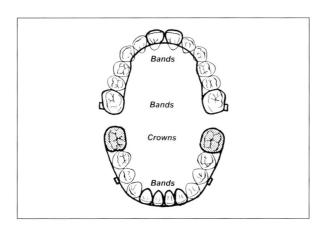

Fig. 3.4 Herbst´s early mixed dentition anchorage system. (*Revised from Herbst 1934*)

In the late mixed dentition when the permanent canines had erupted but the mandibular permanent premolars were still missing, the design of the appliance was modified by using the canines as anchorage teeth instead of the incisors (Fig. 3-5). The

necessity to incorporate as many teeth as possible in order to avoid unwanted side effects was realized early by Herbst and others. The solution offered by Schwarz (1934) is shown in Figs. 3-6 and 3-7.Most teeth in the maxilla and mandible were interconnected by labial as well as lingual arch wires (block anchorage).

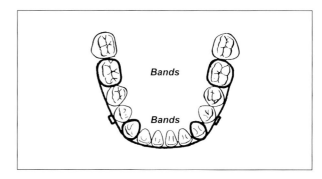

Fig. 3-5 Herbst´s late mixed dentition anchorage system. (*Revised from Herbst 1934*)

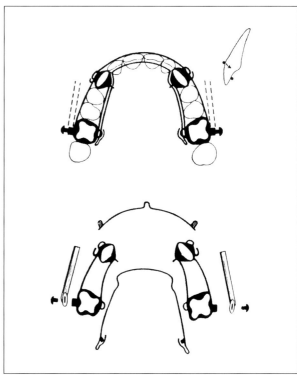

Fig. 3-6 Schwarz´s maxillary block anchorage system. (*From Schwarz 1934*)

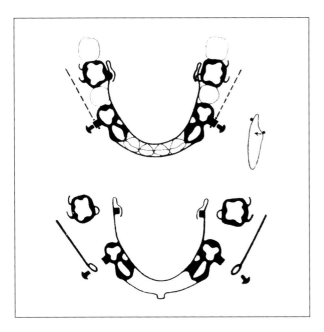

Fig. 3-7 Schwarz´s mandibular block anchorage system. (*From Schwarz 1934*)

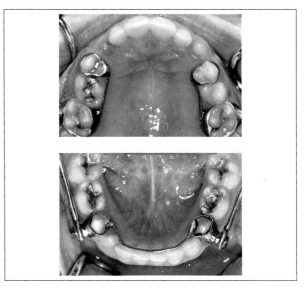

Fig. 3-8 Pancherz´s partial anchorage system with bands.

Pancherz (1979) originally used a banded type of Herbst appliance with a simple anchorage system (*partial anchorage*) resembling that used by Herbst (1910, 1934) (Fig. 3-8). Individually made stainless steel bands were used. An indirect fabrication of the bands using an extra thick band material (0.15 - 0.18 mm) was utilized to prevent breakage (splitting). In the maxilla, the bands were placed on the first permanent molars and first premolars. On each side, the bands were connected by half-round (1.5 x 0.75 mm) or round (1.0 mm) sectional arch wires. In the mandible, bands were placed on the first premolars and connected by a palatal half-round (1.5 x 0.75 mm) or round (1.0 mm) sectional lingual arch wire. After having used this partial anchorage system for a couple of years Pancherz found several unwanted side effects that could not be controlled. The maxillary side effects included space opening distal to the canines, buccal flaring and tipping of the premolars, excessive intrusion and mesiobuccal rotation of the molars. The mandibular side effects comprised of excessive intrusion of the mandibular premolars and proclination of the incisors. Therefore, anchorage was increased by incorporating the maxillary and mandibular front teeth in the anchorage system (labial sectional arch wires connected to the premolar bands), and by extending the mandibular lingual arch wire to the first permanent molars which also were banded (*total anchorage*) (Fig. 3-9).

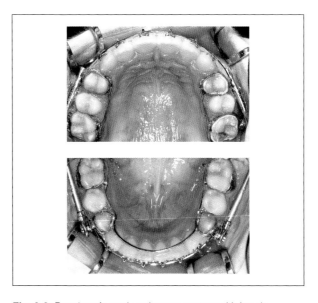

Fig. 3-9 Pancherz´s total anchorage system with bands.

Current appliance design

In spite of the use of individually made bands, band splitting was an unsolved problem (Sanden et al. 2004). Therefore, since 1995, instead of bands, cast cobalt-chromium splints are used routinely at our Department. The splints cover the buccal teeth in the maxillary and mandibular dental arches as well as the mandibular canines (Fig. 3-10). This design of the appliance is very hygienic and has a low breakage prevalence (Sanden et al. 2004).

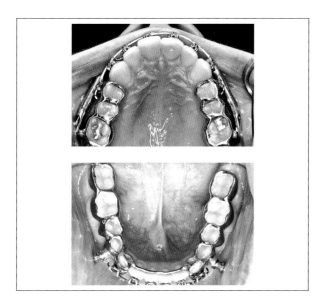

Fig.3-10   Pancherz´s total anchorage system with cast cobalt-chronium splints.

Since the reintroduction of the Herbst appliance in 1979 (Pancherz 1979), the Herbst appliance has become very popular in both Europe and the United States. Parallel to the design evolution by Pancherz, clinicians began using stainless steel crowns instead of bands (Langford 1982, Goodman and McKenna 1985, Dischinger 1989) (Fig. 3-11) to avoid the problem of band breakages. Other attempts to make bands stronger were to solder a reinforcing wire to the occlusal margin of the bands (Fig. 3-12) or to use double bands which were laser welded one into the other.

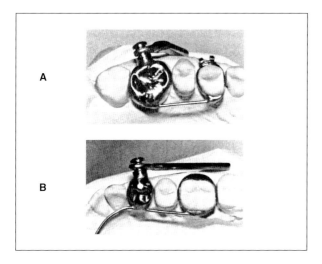

Fig. 3-11   Langford´s Herbst appliance design using steel crowns on the maxillary permanent first molars (**A**) and mandibular first premolars (**B**). (*From Langford 1982*)

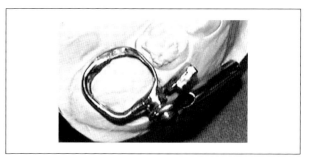

Fig. 3-12   Reinforcing arch wire soldered to the edge of the maxillary molar bands.

Howe (1982) Howe and McNamara (1983) developed the acrylic splint Herbst appliance (Fig. 3-13), which to begin with was used fixed (bonded to the teeth) and later removable to facilitate oral hygiene and to reduce the incidence of caries. However, the use of the Herbst appliance as a removable device is not recommended because the main advantage of a fixed Herbst appliance is that it works continuously 24 hours a day without dependence on patient cooperation.

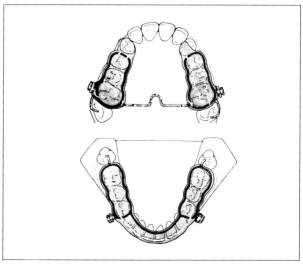

Fig. 3-13   The acrylic splint Herbst appliance of Howe (1982) and Howe and McNamara (1983). (*From McNamara and Brudon 2001*)

A variant of the stainless steel crown Herbst appliance that has become popular is the so-called cantilever Herbst appliance (Dischinger 1989, Mayes 1994) (Figs. 3-14 and 3-15). This design was originally meant to be used in the early mixed dentition before the eruption of the mandibular permanent canines and first premolars). Nowadays, however, orthodontists also use it in the late mixed and permanent dentitions. In constructing the appliance, heavy metal extension arms are soldered buccallly to the mandibular permanent molar crowns. The arms terminate in the premolar region where the telescoping axles are placed. Occlusal rests on the first or second primary molars or premolars attached to the cantilever arms, are essiental (Fig. 3-16). Without these rests (Figs, 3-14 and 3-15), the vertical force vector of the telescopes acting on the lever arms will result in mesial tipping of the molars. The anchorage control of the mandibular permanent molars with the cantilever design of the Herbst appliance (even when using occlusal rests on the teeth anterior to the molars) is rather questionable.

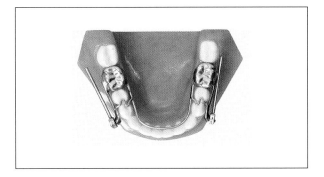

Fig. 3-16 Cantilever Herbst appliance with crowns on the mandibular molars, and lingual arch with occlusal stops on the premolars as anchorage.

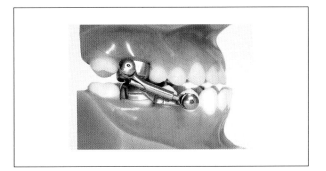

Fig. 3-14 Cantilever Herbst appliance with only crowns on the mandibular molars as anchorage.

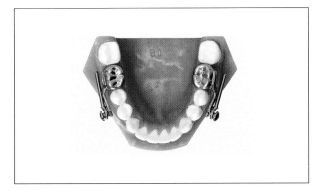

Fig. 3-15 Cantilever Herbst appliance with only crowns on the mandibular molars as anchorage.

In order to secure lateral movements of the mandible, different solutions have been presented. Enlargement of the tube and plunger pivot openings is the standard procedure (see below: Construction of the banded Herbst appliance). Attempts have, however, been made by Pancherz to enlarge the mandibular lateral movement range by the use of a "double pivot" for the tube part of the telescope mechanism (Fig. 3-17). This construction was utilized in only a restricted number of patients and never appeared on the market. Other constructions such as the Flip-Lock Herbst (Miller 1996), Herbst Type IV appliance from Dentaurum Inc. (Pfortzheim, Germany) and Hanks´ telescoping Herbst appliance (Hanks 2003) have incorporated ball-and-socket joints to improve the range of lateral motion. An own prototype of the ball head Herbst appliance is shown in Fig. 3-18.

Attempts have also been made to incorporate the Herbst appliance as an adjunct to a multibracket appliance treatment procedure. Thereby, the telescopic parts are either attached directly to the maxillary and mandibular arch wires (Fig. 3-19) or to the headgear tube and an auxillary mandibular arch wire (Fig. 3-20). By these variants of the Herbst appliance, however, maxillary molar and mandibular arch wire breakages and bracket loss were frequent findings.

In summary, when considering both anchorage control and appliance durability the cast splint Herbst appliance has to be recommended, despite the fact that the costs of this appliance design are higher than for the banded and crown types of Herbst appliances.

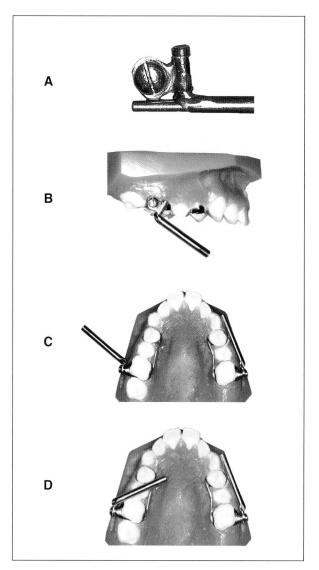

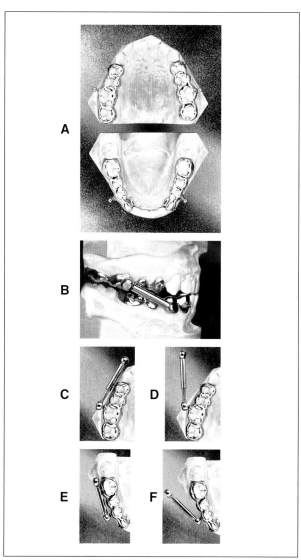

Fig. 3-17 (A-D) Double pivot Herbst telescope mechanism allowing a large lateral movement range. The mechanism is not offered on the market.

Fig. 3-18 (A-F) Ball head Herbst appliance allowing a large mandibular movement range. This construction is not offered on the market.

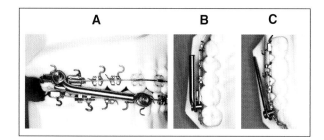

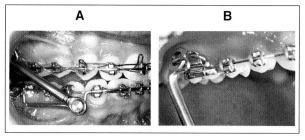

Fig. 3-19 (A-C) Integrated Herbst appliance. The telescope mechanism is attached to maxillary and mandibular arch wires.

Fig. 3-20 (A and B) Integrated Herbst appliance according to Hägglund and Segerdahl (1997). The telescope mechanism is attached to the maxillary headgear tube and to an auxillary heavy (0.8-1.0 mm) mandibular arch wire.

Construction of the Herbst appliance

The procedure for fabricating the banded and cast splint Herbst appliances is shown in Fig. 3-21 [1-63].

Banded Herbst appliance

In order to avoid problems with broken bands it is most important to form the bands individually using orthodontic band material of at least 0.15 mm in thickness. Prefabricated bands are too weak. They will break (split) under the strains placed on them during treatment.

In constructing the banded type of Herbst appliance (Fig. 3-21 [1-46]), three clinical and two laboratory sessions are necessary.

First clinical session
Standard alginate impressions for plaster casts (in super hard stone) of the upper and lower dental arches are made and sent to the laboratory. Tooth separators (elastomerics) are placed mesially and distally to the teeth which are to be banded.

First laboratory session
At the laboratory, bands for the maxillary permanent first molars and maxillary and mandibular premolars are made on the plaster models using 0.15 mm thick orthodontic band material (Fig. 3-21 [4-20]). The finished bands are sent back to the orthodontist.

Second clinical session
The laboratory made bands together with prefabricated mandibular permanent first molar bands are seated on the teeth (tight band fitting is important) (Fig. 3-21 [21]) and a construction bite is taken (Figs. 3-21 [22, 23]) with the mandible advanced to usually an incisal edge to edge relationship. While the bands are still seated, alginate impressions are taken. The impressions, bands and bite registration wax are sent to the laboratory (Fig. 3-21 [24]). New separators are placed.

Second laboratory session
The bands are waxed into the impressions and the impressions are poured. The models (with the bands on the teeth) are oriented to each other with help of the bite registration wax and mounted in any simple hinge articulator (Fig. 3-21 [25]). Lingual stainless steel arch wires (1.5 x 0.75 mm half-round or 1.0 mm round) and pivots (axles) for the telescope mechanism are soldered to the bands (Fig. 3-21 [26-28]). The use of a jig will facilitate orienting and soldering the pivots to the bands (Fig. 3-21 [29-33]).

When a jig is not available the procedure recommended by Langford (1981) may be helpful: "Take the tube with the screw and pivot assembled, and hold the pivot base alongside of the upper molar band, with the opposite end of the tube about 2 mm from the buccal surface of the lower first premolar band. This is the working position in which the pivot must be soldered to the molar band (the tubes come in rights and lefts with pivot ends angulated to allow for the mesiodistal angulation of the upper first molar buccal surface). Disassemble screw, pivot and tube. To solder pivot to the upper molar band hold pivot with college pliers….Solder pivot to the lower premolar band so that its axis is roughly parallel to that of the upper pivot. There is enough play in the assembly to allow for some variability."

The length of the tube and plunger are adjusted to fit the inter-pivot distance (Fig. 3-21 [34-38]). Then the tube and plunger pivot openings are enlarged to provide a loose fit of the telescoping parts, thus increasing the lateral movement capacity of the lower jaw (Fig. 3-21 [39-44]). With an increased lateral movement range, the load on the anchorage teeth (and bands) during mandibular lateral excursions will be reduced. The finished appliance is sent back to the orthodontist.

Third clinical session
All bands are cemented (glass ionomer cement) and the telescope mechanism is attached to the bands with help of the locking screws. A screwdriver that firmly grips the screws (Fig. 3-21 [47-57]) makes the procedure easy. With respect to the tubes, it could be advantageous to attach them to the upper axles before the cementation of the bands, as it is often difficult to get access to the screw holes in the maxillary molar region, especially if the patient has tight cheeks. Furthermore, in order to avoid loose molar screws during treatment, it may be advisable to secure them by cementing. This can be done without any disadvantage as a removal of the tube during treatment, for possible adjustments, is hardly ever necessary.

After band cementation, the telescoping plungers are placed to the pivots, but first without screws. The plungers are held in place using the fingers and the following considerations are checked. (1) Proper length of the plunger. If the plunger is too long (in most patients this will be the case if it stands out of the tube more than 3 mm) and impinges on the buccal mucosa distal to the maxillary molar upon mouth closure, it is shortened. (2) Opening, closing and lateral jaw movements. The patient must be able to open and close without interference of the mechanism. In addition there should be at least 4-5 mm of lateral freedom in each direction (Fig. 3-21 [58-60]). Otherwise the amount of lateral movement can be increased by further enlargement of the pivot openings of the plunger. (3) Midline. Correction is accomplished by adding preformed advancement shims on the plunger unilaterally. If everything is in order, the screws are placed to lock the plungers to the axles.

Cast splint Herbst appliance

In comparison to the banded Herbst appliance, the clinical work for the orthodontist in constructing the cast splint Herbst appliance (Fig. 3-21 [61]) is much easier and chair time is shortened to a great extend. The laboratory work, on the other hand, is more time-consuming and the appliance will be more expensive.

In constructing the cast splint type of Herbst appliance, two clinical and one laboratory sessions are necessary.

First clinical session
Alginate impressions for maxillary and mandibular plaster casts (in super hard stone) are made and a construction bite is taken. The impressions and the wax bite are sent to the laboratory. No separators are needed.

Laboratory session
Maxillary and mandibular splints are cast from cobalt cromium alloy (Fig. 3-21 [62]) The lower lingual arch wire and the pivots for the plunger and tube are soldered to the splints. The length of the telescoping tube and plunger are adjusted and their pivot openings are widened. The same procedure is used as for the banded Herbst appliance. The appliance is finished completely (Fig. 3-21 [63]) and sent back to the orthodontist.

Second clinical session
The splints are checked with respect to their fitting accuracy on the teeth and are then cemented using a regular glass ionomer cement. The telescope mechanism is attached to the splints. The procedure is the same as for the banded Herbst appliance.

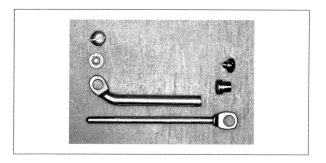

Fig. 3-21[1]: The different components of the Herbst telescope mechanism. The telescopes are available in pairs (right and left side) and of a standard length. The design shown is from Dentaurum Inc.

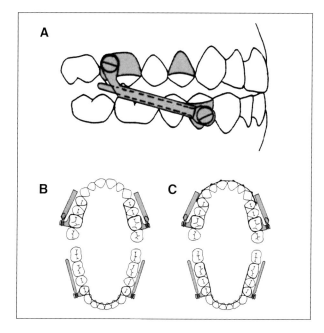

Fig. 3-21[2]: The banded Herbst appliance. **A**: Working position with the appliance in place. **B**: Partial maxillary and mandibular anchorage. **C**: Total maxillary and mandibular anchorage. Note the distal pivot position on the maxillary molar band and mesial pivot position on the mandibular premolar band to maximize the interpivot distance for preventing a plunger and tub disengagement on mouth opening (**see Fig. 3-21 [3]**).

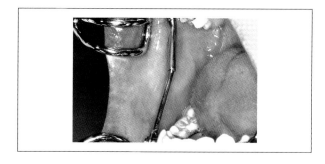

Fig. 3-21[3]: Disengagement of the plunger from the tube on wide mouth opening.

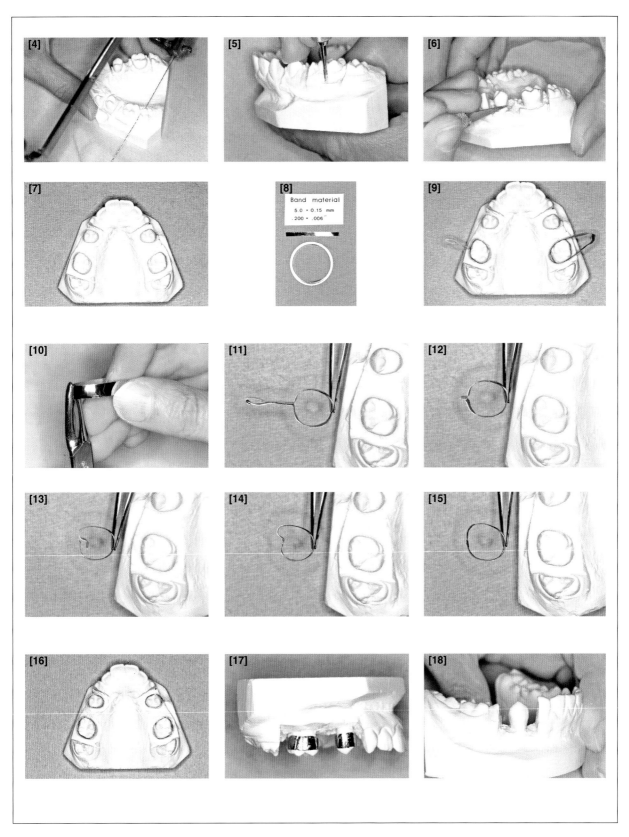

Fig. 3-21 [4-18]: Fabrication of the banded Herbst appliance.

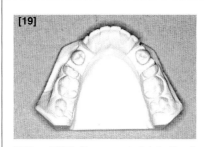

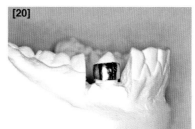

[19] and [20]: Sequency in fabricating the bands for the Herbst appliance.

[21] Bands seated on the teeth.

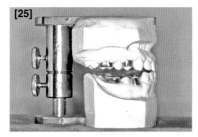

[22] Construction bite - lateral view.

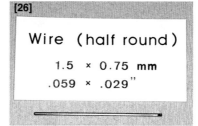

[23] Construction bite - frontal view.

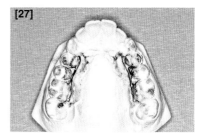

[24] Impressions with bands and construction bite.

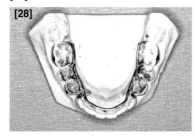

[25] Mounted dental casts.

Wire (half round)

1.5 × 0.75 mm

.059 × .029"

[26] to [28]: Soldering maxillary and mandibular lingual arch wires to the bands.

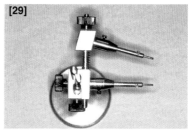

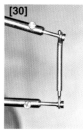

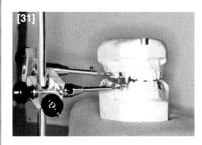

[29] to [31]: Jig for the orientation of the telescoping pivots to the bands. (The orientation jig is not offered on the market.)

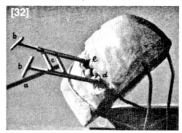

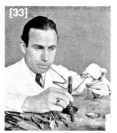

[32] and [33]: The original orientation jig of Emil Herbst and his soldering procedure (Herbst 1934).

Fig. 3-21 [19-33]: Fabrication of the banded Herbst appliance.

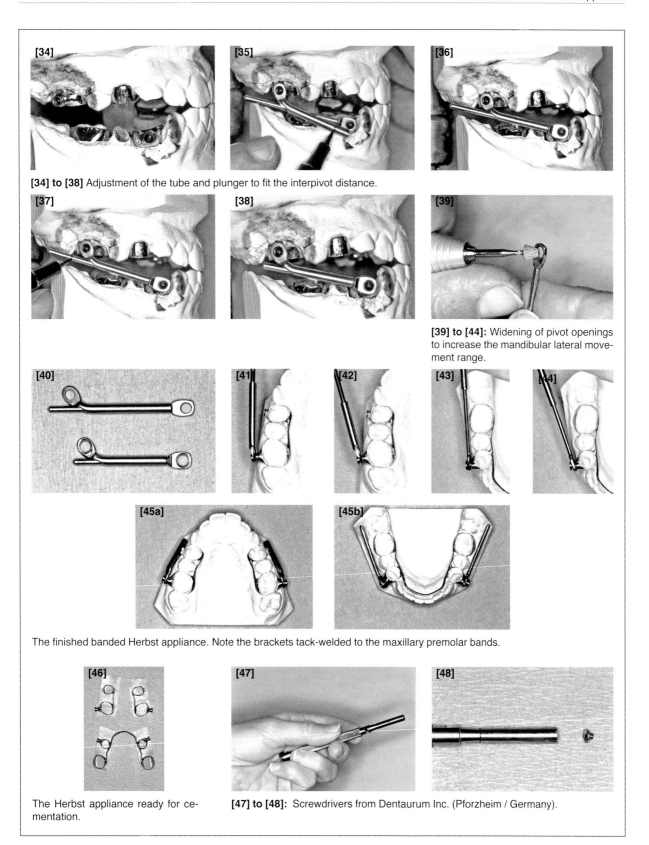

[34] to [38] Adjustment of the tube and plunger to fit the interpivot distance.

[39] to [44]: Widening of pivot openings to increase the mandibular lateral movement range.

The finished banded Herbst appliance. Note the brackets tack-welded to the maxillary premolar bands.

The Herbst appliance ready for cementation.

[47] to [48]: Screwdrivers from Dentaurum Inc. (Pforzheim / Germany).

Fig. 3-21 [34-48]: Fabrication of the banded Herbst appliance.

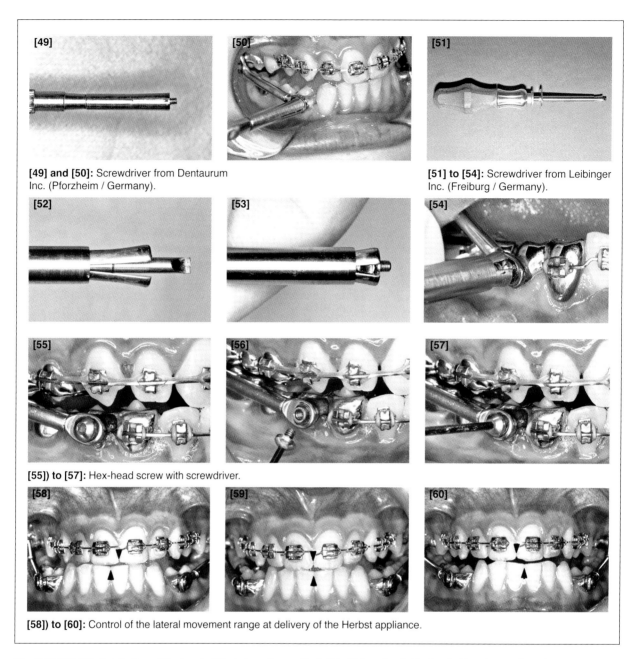

[49] and [50]: Screwdriver from Dentaurum Inc. (Pforzheim / Germany).

[51] to [54]: Screwdriver from Leibinger Inc. (Freiburg / Germany).

[55]) to [57]: Hex-head screw with screwdriver.

[58]) to [60]: Control of the lateral movement range at delivery of the Herbst appliance.

Fig. 3-21 [49-60]: Fabrication of the banded Herbst appliance. (In [54] to [57] cast splint instead of bands are shown)

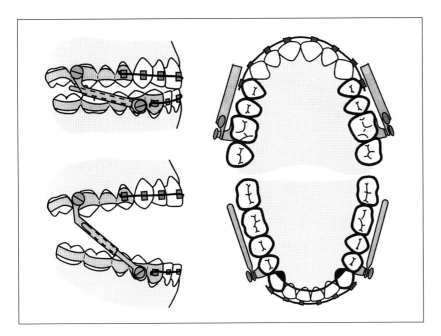

Fig. 3-21 [61]: The cast splint Herbst appliance.

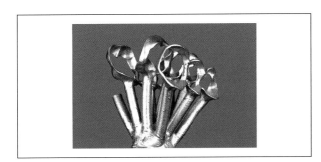

Fig. 3-21 [62]: Castings of the splints.

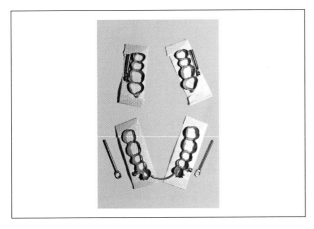

Fig. 3-21 [63]: The splints ready for cementation. Note that the tubes are attached to the splints while the plungers are removed.

Clinical management of the Herbst appliance

After delivery of the Herbst appliance, before dismissing the patient home, information about the function of the Herbst appliance must be given. The patient may suffer from some muscle discomfort and eating difficulties during the first week. After that time, however, adaptation to the appliance will usually have taken place and no discomfort is felt by the patient. Furthermore, the patient is instructed to avoid hard and sticky food that may dislodge the appliance. If the telescoping elements come apart on opening the mouth wide, the patient will quickly learn to reinsert the lower plunger into the upper tube. If soft tissue ulcerations occur (too long plunger impinging on the mucosa), the patient must be seen immediately. The cure is simple, the plunger should be shortened.

In cases with crowding of the maxillary incisors or canines, brackets on the front teeth are first placed when space has been created by distalizing the teeth in the maxillary lateral segments (Fig. 3-22) due to the headgear effect of the Herbst appliance (see Chapter 9: The headgear effect of the Herbst appliance).

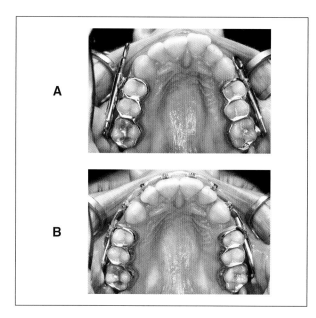

Fig. 3-22 Maxillary part of the cast splint Herbst appliance. **A**: Due to incisor crowding no brackets on the front teeth. **B**: After 3 months of treatment, when anterior space was created, the front teeth were furnished with brackets and an arch wire for tooth alignment.

In cases in which maxillary lateral expansion is needed, the Herbst appliance is combined with a quad helix (Fig. 3-23) or a rapid maxillary expansion (RME) device (Fig. 3-24) soldered to the bands or splints. Expansion is performed before adapting the telescope mechanism when a large maxillary / mandibular transverse discrepancy is present, otherwise it is done simultaneously with the mandibular advancement procedure. After the transverse problem is solved, the expansion appliances are left in place (the quad helix not always, the RME always) until the end of Herbst treatment.

Normally, the first control visit takes place 7-10 days after appliance delivery, when the patient has got used to the appliance and the initial chewing problems have subsided. An earlier first-visit is not recommended because the patient still will be uncomfortable with the new situation and nothing can really be done to help him. Future control visits usually take place at an interval of 6 -10 weeks. During these visits the following check-ups are made:

- Control that the appliance has not loosened from the teeth. Such a complication is not always observed by the patient.
- Control of the amount of mandibular advancement. Usually, the mandible is kept in an incisal edge-to-edge position throughout treatment. This

will most of the time require a reactivation of the appliance every other appointment by adding 1-2 mm shims (sleeves of tubing) on the mandibular plunger (Fig. 3-25). The shim can be crimped on the plunger with a heavy-duty wire cutter or can be tack-welded in place.
- Control of the midline. Correction is made by adding unilateral plunger shims.
- Control of the treatment progress. This is done by measuring the overjet with the mandible in a "manually forced" retruded position (RP) after the two plungers have temporarily been removed from the appliance. In the RP the condyles will be in a "centered" glenoid fossa position (see Chapter 16: Effects on TMJ function). The overjet measurement should not be done until after about 5-6 months of treatment. Earlier registrations are experienced as very uncomfortable (painful) by the patient. A normal or overcorrected normal overjet in the RP indicates that treatment could be finished. Treatment with the Herbst appliance usually takes 6-8 months in preadolescent / adolescent patients and 8 -12 months in postadolescent / young adult patients.

Removal of the banded Herbst appliance after treatment is generally no problem. Removal of the cast splint Herbst appliance can, however, be difficult. It is sometimes necessary to split the splints to facilitate the removal (see Chapter 24: Complications).

As our patients are almost exclusively treated in the permanent dentition, after removal of the Herbst appliance, they usually proceed directly into a multibracket appliance treatment phase for final tooth alignment and active Class I settling of the occlusion (see Chapter 21: Treatment indications).

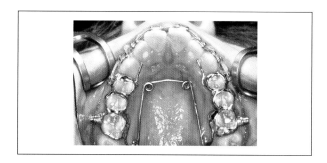

Fig. 3-23 Herbst appliance with quad helix for maxillary expansion.

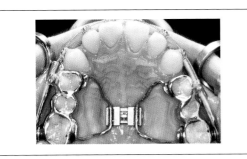

Fig. 3-24 Herbst appliance with RME for maxillary expansion.

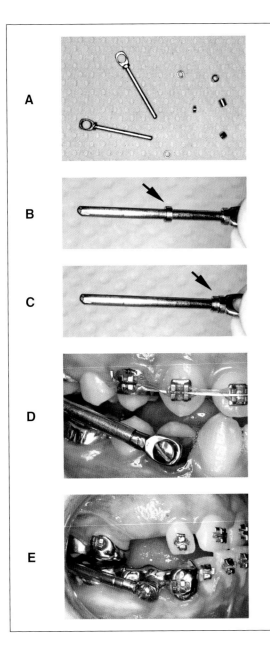

References

Dischinger TG. Edgewise bioprogressive Herbst appliance. J Clin Orthod 1989;23:608-612.

Goodman P, McKenna P. Modified Herbst appliance for the mixed dentition. J Clin Orthod 1985;19:811-814.

Hägglund P, Segerdahl S. The Swedish-style integrated Herbst appliance. J Clin Orthod 1997;31:378-390.

Hanks SD. A new Herbst appliance. J Clin Orthod 2003;37:376-379.

Herbst E. Atlas und Grundriss der Zahnärztlichen Orthopädie. München: J. F. Lehmann´s Verlag 1910.

Herbst E. Dreissigjährige Erfahrungen mit dem Retentions-Scharnier. Zahnärztl Rundschau 1934;43:1515-1524, 1563-1568, 1611-1616.

Howe RP. The bonded Herbst appliance. J Clin Orthod 1982;16:663-667.

Howe RP, McNamara JA. Clinical management of the bonded Herbst appliance. J Clin Orthod 1983;17:456-463.

Langford NM. The Herbst appliance. J Clin Orthod 1981;15:558-561.

Langford NM. Updating fabrication of the Herbst appliance. J Clin Orthod 1982;16:173-174.

McNamara JA, Brudon WL. Orthodontics and Dentofacial Orthopedics. Ann Arbor, MI: Needham Press, 2001: 304

Mayes JH. Improving appliance efficiency with a cantilever Herbst – A new answer to old problems. Clin Impressions 1994;3:2-5, 17-19.

Miller AM. The Flip-Lock Herbst appliance. J Clin Orthhod 1996;30:552-558.

Pancherz H. Treatment of Class II malocclusions by jumping the bite with the Herbst appliance. Am J Orthod 1979;76:423-442.

Sanden E, Pancherz H, Hansen K. Complications during Herbst treatment. J Clin Orthod 2004;38:130-133.

Schwarz M. Erfahrungen mit dem Herbstschen Scharnier zur Behandlung des Distalbisses. Zahnärztl Rundschau 1934;43:47-54, 91-100.

Fig. 3-25 Mandibular advancement shims. **A-C**: Shims placed on the plunger. **D**: Single activation with a 2 mm shim. **E**: Triple activation with one 1 mm and two 2 mm shims.

Chapter 4

Derivates of the Herbst appliance

Since the reintroduction of the Herbst appliance in the field of orthodontics (Pancherz 1979), a large number of modifications or derivates of the telescope mechanism have appeared on the market. Many of the derivates exhibit a close resemblance with the original Herbst design but are presented as new "inventions" using names like: Mandibular Anterior Repositioning Splint (MARS), Cantilever Bite-Jumper (CBJ), Universal Bite Jumper (UBJ), Mandibular Locking Unit (MALU), Ventral Telescope, Ritto Appliance, Standard Bite Jumping Appliance, Integrated Snoring Therapy (IST).

In a survey of 789 orthodontists in the United States (Keim et al. 2002a), the Herbst appliance was shown to be the most frequently used functional appliance (35% in 2002) of all removable and functional appliances utilized routinely in orthodontic practices. The most common design was the "Crown"-Herbst followed by the "Banded"-, "Bonded"-, "Removable"- and "Fixed/Removable"-Herbst (Keim et al 2002b).

In an another survey among leading orthodontic manufacturers and laboratories (Rogers 2006; unpublished material), the Herbst appliance was found to be the leading appliance for Class II correction: 74% in the year 2004 and 81% in the year 2005. The "Crown" design was used about twice as much as the "Band" design.

Using Pubmed, orthodontic journals, and catalogues/homepages from different orthodontic manufactures, a search was recently made at the Orthodontic Department in Giessen (Schrodt et al. 2006) concerning the existence of various fixed bite jumping appliances and the scientific evidence on their mode of action.

Fifty-three different fixed bite jumping appliances were identified (the original Herbst appliance and 52 derivates or hybrids). The 53 appliances could be assigned to four groups: rigid appliances (n=32), flexible appliances (n=14), oblique bite planes (n=3) and tension springs (n=4). The different appliances and their manufacturers are listed below.

I. Rigid appliances	Manufacturer
Single telescopes	
1. Herbst (Original type)	Dentaurum Inc.
2. Herbst (Type II)	Dentaurum Inc.
3. Herbst (Type IV)	Dentaurum Inc.
4. Ormco Bite Jumping Appliance	Ormco Corp.
5. Flip Lock Herbst	TP Orthodontics Inc.
6. MALU (Mandibular Locking Unit)	Saga Dental
7. Swedish Style Integrated Herbst (based on MALU)	Saga Dental
8. MARS (Mandibular Advancement Repositioning Splint)	Dentaurum
9. Standard Bite Jumping Appliance	Ormco Corp.
10. CBJ (Cantilever Bite-Jumper)	Ormco Corp.
11. Intrusion Herbst	Ormco Corp.
12. Ritto Appliance	Ritto
13. Ventral Telescope	Profess. Positioners Inc.
14. UBJ (Universal Bite Jumper)	---
15. IST (Integrated Snoring Therapy)	Sheu Dental GmbH
16. HUPS	---
17. OPM	Sheu Dental GmbH

I. Rigid appliances (cont.)   Manufacturer

18. Magnethic Telescopic Device Ritto
19. BioPedic Appliance   GAC Internatio-
                                 nal Inc.
20. Smith Type I Herbst   Ormco Corp.
21. Smith Type II Herbst   Ormco Corp.
22. Smith Type III Herbst   Ormco Corp.
23. MPA (Mandibular Protraction ---
    Appliance)
24. MCA (Mandibular Corrector   Cormar Inc.
    Appliance)
25. Magnusson Herbst   Dentaurum Inc.

Multi telescopes
26. Eureka Spring   Eureka Ortho-
                                 dontics
27. Elasto Harmonizer   Bredent
28. Hanks Telescoping Herbst   American Ortho-
                                 dontics
29. Herbst TS (TeleScoping)   Dentaurum Inc.
    (*New*)
30. MiniScope (*New*)   American Ortho-
                                 dontics
31. SUS (Sabbagh Universal   Dentaurum Inc.
    Spring)
32. Twin Force Bite Corrector   Ortho Organi-
                                 zers Inc.

II. Flexible appliances

1. Jasper Jumper   American Ortho-
                                 dontics
2. JAR (Jasper Jumper   ---
   Anterior Reposition Splint)
3. Gentle Jumper   American Ortho-
                                 dontics
4. Millenium Distal Mover   American Ortho-
                                 dontics
5. Forsus Nitinol Flat Spring   3M Unitec
6. Forsus Fatigue Resistant   3M Unitec
   Device
7. Bite Fixer   Ormco Corp.
8. Scandee Tubular Jumper   Saga Dental
9. Flex Developer   Adenta
10. Klapper SUPERspring   ORTHOdesign
11. Adjustable Bite Corrector   Ortho Plus Inc.
12. Amoric Torsion Coils   ---
13. Churro Jumper   ---
14. ABC (Adjustable Bite Cor-   Orth Plus Inc.
    rector)

III. Oblique bite plane

1. MARA (Mandibular Anterior   AOA Laborato-
   Repositioning Appliance)   ries
2. FMA (Functional Mandibular   Forestadent Inc.
   Advancer)
3. Bite Ramps   UP Dental/Ultra-
                                 dent Products

IV. Tension springs

1. Safe Springs   Pacific Coast
                                 Manufacturing
2. Perm-A-Force   Masel
3. Calibrated Force Module   Cormar Inc.
4. Alpern Class II Closers   GAC Internatio-
                                 nal Inc.

Out of the 53 fixed bite jumping appliances, only 6 (11%) were tested scientifically with respect to their skeletal and dental effects: Herbst (in over 50 publications; see references in this book), Jasper Jumper (Cope et al. 1994, Weiland et al. 1997, Stucki and Ingervall 1998, Covell et al. 1999, Nalbantgil et al. 2005, Karacay et al. 2006), Forsus Nitinol Flat Spring (Heinig and Göz 2001, Karacay et al. 2006), Eureka Spring (Strohmeyer et al. 2002), MARA (Pangrazio-Kulbersh et al. 2003) and FMA (Kinzinger and Diedrich 2005). The 6 scientifically tested appliances are shown in Fig. 4-1.

Eighteen (34%) of the 53 appliances were described in case reports. For the remaining 29 (55%) appliances only unproven statements from the manufacturers about their mode of action were available.

Concerning the Herbst appliance and the 5 scientifically analyzed Herbst derivates and hybrids, the skeletal and dental contribution to Class II correction was assessed, thus making it possible to compare the applications with each other. The results of this comparison (Fig. 4-2) revealed a large inter-appliance variation in skeletal (7% to 47%) and dental (53% to 93%) components contributing to Class II molar correction.

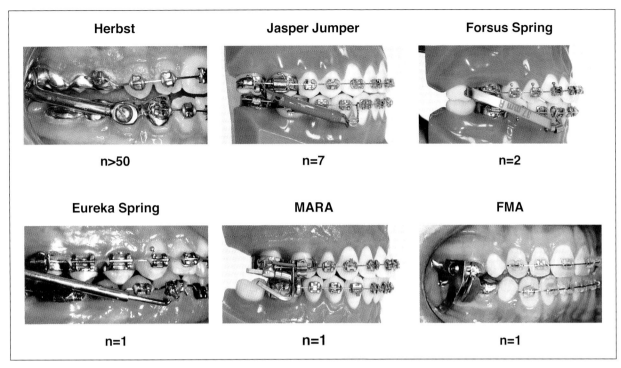

Fig. 4-1 The Herbst appliance, three of its derivates and two hybrids which have been analyzed scientifically with respect to skeletal and dental changes: Jasper Jumper, Forsus Spring, Eureka Spring, MARA (Mandibular Anterior Repositioning Appliance), FMA (Functional Mandibular Advancer). The number of publications is given.

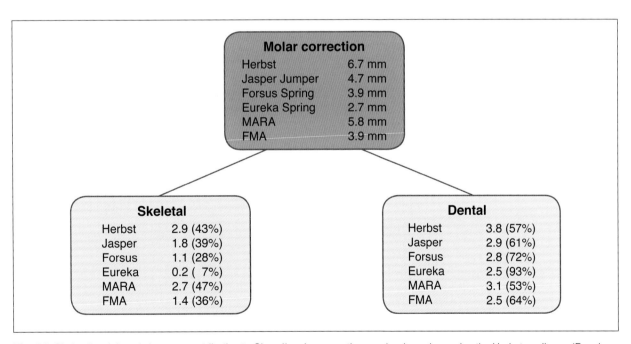

Fig. 4-2 Skeletal and dental changes contributing to Class II molar correction mechanism when using the Herbst appliance (Pancherz 1982) the Jasper Jumper (Weiland et al. 1997), Forsus Spring (Heinig and Göz 2001), Eureka Spring (Stromeyer et al. 2002), MARA (Pangrazio-Kulbersch et al. 2003), FMA (Kinzinger and Diedrich 2005).

Conclusion

There exists a large number of derivates and hybrids of the Herbst appliance on the market. In 2006, 52 Herbst modifications were found. Scientific evidence of their mode of action existed for only five.

References

Cope JB, Buschang PH, Cope DD, Parker J, Blackwood HO. Quantitative evaluation of craniofacial changes with Jasper Jumper therapy. Angle Orthod 1994;64:113-122.

Covell DA, Trammell DW, Boero RP, West R. A cephalometric study of Class II; Division 1 malocclusions treated with the Jasper Jumper appliance. Angle Orthod 1999;69:311-320.

Heinig N, Göz G. Clinical application and effects of the Forsus Spring. J Orofac Orthop 2001;62:436-450.

Karacay S, Akin E, Olmez H, Gurton AU, Sagdic D. Forsus Nitinol Flat Spring and Jasper Jumper corrections of Class II division 1 malocclusions. Angle Orthod 2006;76:666-672.

Keim RG, Gottlieb EL, Nelson AH, Vogels DS. 2002 JCO study of orthodontic diagnosis and treatment procedures. Part 1: Results and trends. J Clin Orthod 2002a;36:553-568.

Keim RG, Gottlieb EL, Nelson AH, Vogels DS. 2002 JCO study of orthodontic diagnosis and treatment procedures. Part 3: More breakdowns of selected variables. J Clin Orthod 2002b;36:690-699.

Kinzinger G, Diedrich P. Skeletal effects in Class II treatment with the Functional Mandibular Advancer (FMA)? J Orofac Orthop 2005;66:469-490.

Nalbantgil D, Arun T, Sayinsu K, Isik F. Skeletal, dental and soft-tissue changes induced by the Jasper Jumper appliance in late adolescence. Angle Orthod 2005;75:382-392.

Pancherz H. Treatment of Class II malocclusions by jumping the bite with the Herbst appliance. Am J Orthod 1979;76:423-442.

Pancherz H. The mechanism of Class II correction in Herbst appliance treatment. A cephalometric investigation. Am J Orthod 1982;82:104-113

Pangrazio-Kulbersch V, Berger JL, Chermak DS, Kacynski R, Simon RS. Treatment effects of the mandibular anterior repositioning appliance on patients with Class II malocclusion. Am J Orthod Dentofac Orthop 2003;123:286-295.

Rogers MB. Advances in Class II correction with the Herbst appliance (Lecture). American Association of Orthodontists Annual Session in Las Vegas 2006.

Schrodt C, Pancherz H, Ruf S. Fixed bite jumping appliances and their scientific evidence. Manuscript in preparation 2006.

Stromeyer EL, Caruso JM, DeVincenco JP. A cephalometric study of the Class II correction effects of the Eureka spring. Angle Orthod 2002;72:203-210.

Stucki N, Ingervall, B. The use of the Jasper Jumper for the correction of Class II malocclusion in the young permanent dentition. Eur J Orthod 1998;20:271-281.

Weiland FJ, Ingervall B, Bantleon HP, Droschl H. Initial effects of treatment of Class II malocclusion with the Herren activator, activator-headgar combination and Jasper Jumper. Am J Orthod Dentofac Orthop 1997;112:19-27.

Chapter 5

Experimental studies on bite jumping

Carl Breitner (1930) was the first to study the effects of experimental mandibular protrusion ("jumping the bite") on temporomandibular joint (TMJ) growth in a young rhesus monkey using maxillary and mandibular splints furnished with inclined planes, which forced the mandible forward when biting the teeth together. Looking at the TMJ histologically, after an experimental period of 46 days, Breitner could verify modeling processes at the condylar head and glenoid fossa.

Studies on functional bite jumping with splints

Since Breitner, bite jumping experiments in primates and rats, using maxillary and mandibular splints, have been performed repeatedly over the last 75 years. For the assessment of TMJ growth adaptation, histological studies have been carried out in both *growing monkeys* (Derichsweiler 1958, Baume and Derichsweiler 1961, Joho 1968, Stöckli and Willert 1971, Elgoyen et al. 1972, McNamara 1973, 1980, McNamara et al.1975, McNamara and Carlson 1979, McNamara and Bryan 1987) and *adult monkeys* (Häupl and Psansky 1939, Hiniker and Ramfjord 1966, Ramfjord and Enlow 1971, McNamara 1973, McNamara et al. 1982, Hinton and McNamara 1984a) as well as in *growing rats* (Charlier and Petrovic 1967, Charlier et al. 1969, Petrovic 1972, Petrovic et al. 1975, 1981, Rabie et al. 2001, 2002a,b, 2003a,b,c,d,e,f, Chayanupatkul et al. 2003) and *adult rats* (Rabie et al. 2004, Xiong et al. 2004, 2005a,b).
Furthermore, in monkeys, electromyographic (EMG) analyses of the muscles of mastication were undertaken in order to correlate adaptations in TMJ growth and in the activity of the muscles (McNamara 1973, 1975, 1980).

Splint appliance design
The mandibular protrusion splints in the monkeys were cast in gold or cobalt cromium alloy and were cemented on the maxillary and mandibular teeth. The upper and lower splints were constructed in such a manner as to force the mandible into a protruded position when the lower canines came in contact with the mesial surfaces of the upper canines (Fig. 5-1). In the rats, the mandible was put in hyperpropulsion by a splint device attached to the upper teeth, keeping the lower incisors ahead of the upper incisors when the mouth was closed. In the experiments, the hyperpropulser was either fixed to the snout by a strip (Petrovic et al. 1975) and used 12 hours a day or the device was cemented on the teeth (Rabie et al. 2001) (Fig. 5-2) and used 24 hours a day. In the monkeys the experimental periods varied in length from 2 to 96 weeks, corresponding to a human equivalent period (HEP) of 1.5 months to 6.2 years (Luder 1996). In the rats the experimental period lasted between 3 to 60 days. This corresponds to a HEP of 3.5 months to 5.8 years (Luder 1996).

Studies on forced bite jumping with the Herbst appliance

In primates, a few histologic studies have been carried out using the Herbst bite jumping mechanism for the assessment of TMJ growth adaptation. Both juvenile (Woodside et al. 1983, Peterson and McNamara 2003, Voudouris et al. 2003a,b) and adult (Woodside et al. 1987, McNamara et al, 2003) monkeys were analyzed. The influence of the Herbst appliance on EMG muscle activity has been considered in two primate studies (Sessle et al.1990, Voudouris et al. 2003 a,b).

A
B

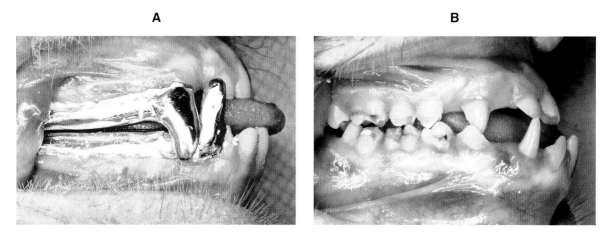

Fig. 5-1 A: Cemented maxillary and mandibular bite jumping splints in a rhesus monkey *(Macaca mulatta).* **B**: Situation after the appliance has been removed at the end of the experimental period. Note the Class III molar and cuspid relationship. *(From McNamara 1975)*

A
B

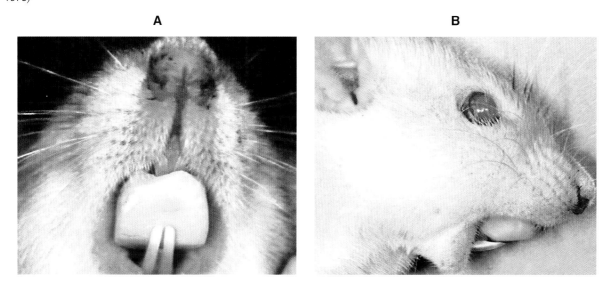

Fig. 5-2 Cemented maxillary bite jumping splint in a rat. **A**: Frontal view. **B**: Lateral view. *(From Rabie with kind permission)*

Herbst appliance design

The Herbst bite jumping mechanism was connected to either cemented maxillary and mandibular cast-metal splints (Sessle et al. 1990, Voudouris et al. 2003a) or bonded acrylic splints (Peterson and McNamara 2003) (Fig. 5-3). Mandibular advancement was performed either in one step (Peterson and McNamara 2003, McNamara et al. 2003) or progressively in several steps (Woodside et al. 1987, Sessle et al. 1990). The experimental period varied between 3 and 24 weeks (61 weeks in the study of Woodside et al. 1983). This corresponds to a HEP of 2 to 19 months (48 months).

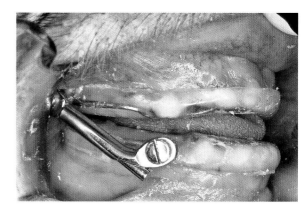

Fig. 5-3 Bonded acrylic splint Herbst appliance in a rhesus monkey *(Macaca mulatta).* The Herbst bite jumping mechanism is reversed to avoid ramal impingement posteriorly. *(From Peterson and McNamara 2003)*

Findings from the experimental studies

As Class II malocclusions do not exist in monkeys and rats it was characteristic in all the functional as well as forced animal bite jumping studies that there was an occlusal alteration from a normal occlusion to a Class III relationship (Fig. 5-1). This was mainly accomplished by adaptations in the TMJ and dentoalveolar structures. TMJ growth adaptation was more obvious in growing, than in adult animals, in which the adaptation was dentoalveolar in nature to a large extent.

Functional bite jumping studies
Growing animals
Independent of the species (monkeys or rats), adaptation to functional bite jumping was found in the condyle and in the glenoid fossa (Fig. 5-4).

A

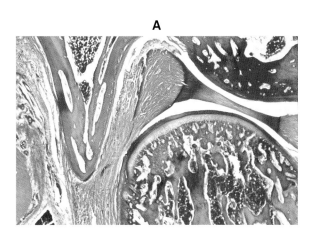

B

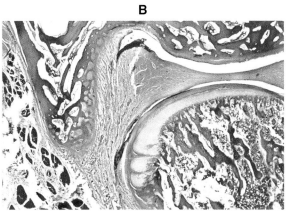

Fig. 5-4 Condylar and glenoid fossa adaptation in a juvenile rhesus monkey *(Macaca mulatta)* treated with functional bite jumping splints. **A**: Control animal. **B**: Experimental animal at 2 weeks. Note the increase in thickness in the prechondroblastic and chondroblastic layers of the condylar cartilage and deposition of new bone along the anterior surface of the postglenoid spine. *(From McNamara et al. 1975)*

Condylar adaptation. Especially in the posterior-superior part of the condyle, forward mandibular positioning accelerated and enhanced the prechondroblast/chondroblast activity, chondrocyte differentiation and cartilage matrix formation followed by increased bone apposition (Stöckli and Willert 1971, McNamara 1973, McNamara et al. 1975, Charlier et al. 1969, Petrovic 1972, Petrovic et al. 1975, Rabie et al. 2002b, 2003a,b,c,d), which finally resulted in an increased mandibular length. It was demonstrated that the final length of the mandible was significantly increased and greater than that of controls when the mandibular protrusion appliances were worn from juvenile age to adulthood (Petrovic et al. 1981, McNamara and Bryan 1987). However, if the appliance was removed before the end of the growth, the results were contradictory. Some investigators showed that early removal of the bite jumping splints resulted in subnormal posttreatment growth of the posterior condyle (but not of the glenoid fossa) (Chayanupatkul et al. 2003). Others demonstrated that the enhancement of condylar growth did not result in a subsequent pattern of subnormal growth after the removal of the splints (Petrovic et al. 1981, Rabie et al. 2003a).

In the monkey, proliferation of the condylar cartilage was observed as early as 2 weeks (HEP = 1.6 months) after appliance placement, and maximum cartilage proliferation occurred after 6 weeks (HEP = 4.6 months). Thereafter, a gradual return of condylar morphology to that observed in untreated control animals was noted (McNamara and Carlson 1979) (Fig. 5-5). In the rat, the earliest sign of condylar modeling was seen 3 days (HEP = 3.5 months) after appliance placement and the largest cellular activity (the thickest chondroblastic layer) was noted after 7 days (HEP = 8.1 months) of treatment (Fig. 5-6).

Glenoid fossa adaptation. In addition to the condylar response, significant adaptive changes occurred in the temporal component of the TMJ. In monkeys, bone deposition was seen along the anterior surface of the postglenoid spine (Stöckli and Willert 1971, McNamara 1973, McNamara and Carlson 1979, Hinton and McNamara 1984 a) (Fig. 5-4). In rats, an increased bone formation was noted in the posterior region of the glenoid fossa, with a growth peak at day 21 (HEP = 24 months) (Rabie et al. 2001, 2002a, 2003b) (Fig. 5-7).

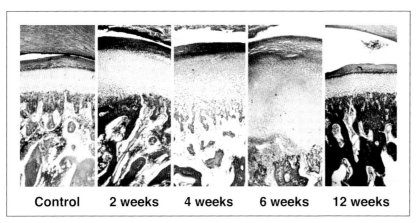

Fig. 5-5 Condylar adaptation in juvenile rhesus monkeys *(Macaca mulatta)* treated with functional bite jumping splints. Sagittal sections through the posterior portion of the condylar head. Comparison of the thickness of the condylar cartilage in a control animal and four experimental animals at 2, 4, 6 and 12 weeks, respectively. Note increased cartilage proliferation at 2 weeks with a maximum at 6 weeks. By 12 weeks, the proliferation of condylar cartilage has returned to a level similar to that of the control animal and most bony remodeling has been completed. *(From McNamara 1975)*

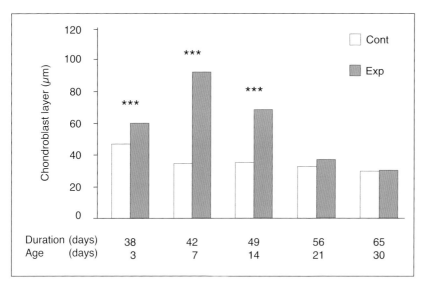

Fig. 5-6 Condylar adaptation in growing rats treated with functional bite jumping splints. Thickness (mean values) of the chondroblastic layer in control animals (Cont) and experimental animals (Exp). Significant differences between control and experimental animals are marked with asterisks (***$p < 0.001$). *(Revised from Rabie et al. 2003d)*

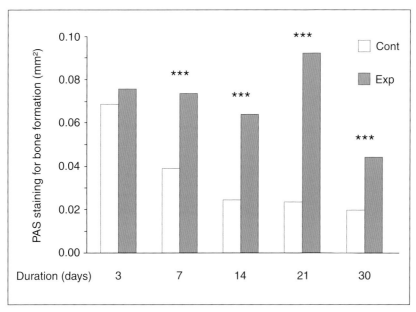

Fig. 5-7 Glenoid fossa adaptation in growing rats treated with functional bite jumping splints. Amount of new bone formation in the posterior region of the glenoid fossa in control animals (Cont) and experimental animals (Exp). Significant differences between control and experimental animals are marked with asterisks (***$p < 0.001$). *(Revised from Rabie et al. 2001)*

Muscle adaptation. Electromyography (EMG) of the masticatory muscles may help us to understand more precisely what takes place in the mandibular condyle and glenoid fossa, both when analyzing experimental animals and clinical patients.

Studies in monkeys have revealed that during the course of bite jumping, functional adaptation occurred simultaneously with structural adaptation (McNamara 1973, 1975, 1980). An increase in lateral pterygoid muscle EMG activity was associated with anterior positioning of the mandible. At the end of the experimental period there was a return towards the pre-appliance level of muscle activity and this change was correlated in time with the TMJ growth adaptations observed. In contrast, Sessle and Gurza (1982) showed that lateral pterygoid activity is depressed for up to 18 weeks by the placement of functional appliances. Based on lateral pterygoid muscle resection studies in rats, Petrovic et al. (1975) claimed that increased lateral pterygoid activity stimulates increased proliferation of condylar tissue. Whetten and Johnston (1985) were, however, unable to demonstrate this increased response.

Adult animals

Studies in adult rhesus monkeys have shown conflicting results with respect to structural changes in the temporomandibular joint (condyle and glenoid fossa) as a response to functional bite jumping. Hiniker and Ramfjord (1966) observed only insignificant adaptation in the TMJ and occasional pathological changes have been reported by Colico (1958).

McNamara et al. (1982) found that the TMJ response in young adult monkeys was qualitatively comparable to that of juvenile animals but that the response magnitude was reduced. In ranking the above young adult animals by age, Hinton and McNamara (1984b) supported the view that, although the adaptive potential of the TMJ may diminish with age, the ability to adapt to altered function will persist in some younger adult animals. This view is supported by a histomorphometric and scanning electron microscopy study of human condylar cartilage (Paulsen et al. 1999) demonstrating condylar growth potential up to the age of 30. Furthermore, independent of any treatment, Suzuki et al. (2004) found that local injection of IGF-I (insuline-like growth factor I) stimulated the growth of mandibular condyle in adult rats.

Functional bite jumping studies in adult rats (Rabie et al. 2004, Xiong et al. 2004, 2005b) revealed that forward mandibular positioning caused changes in the biophysical environment of the TMJ which led to neovascularization and osteogenesis resulting in adaptive condylar growth. It was shown that the proliferative cartilage layer at the posterior condyle became continuously thicker and reached a maximum at day 21 (HEP = 24 months) (Xiong et al. 2005b) (Figs. 5-8 and 5-9), and new bone formation at the posterior condyle reached a maximum at day 30 (HEP = 34 months) (Rabie et al. 2004) (Fig 5-10,). Due to the new bone formation, the condylar process as well as the mandibular length were significantly increased (Xiong et al. 2004).

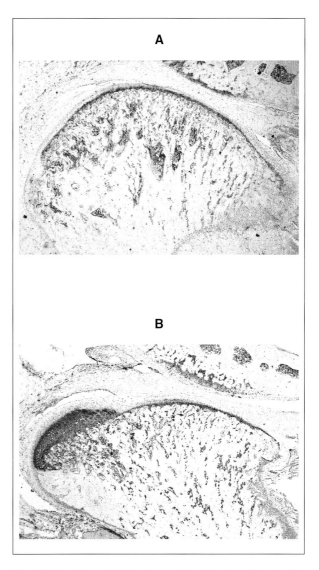

Fig. 5-8 Condylar adaptation in an adult rat treated with a functional bite jumping splint. **A**: Control animal. **B**: Experimental animal after 21 days. Note the increased thickness of the proliferative cartilage layer in the posterior condyle. *(From Rabie et al. 2004)*

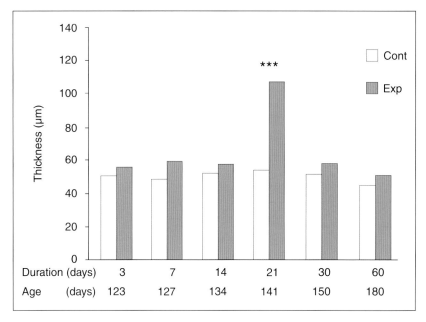

Fig. 5-9 Condylar adaptation in adult rats treated with functional bite jumping splints. Thickness (mean values) of the proliferative cartilage layer in the posterior condyle in control animals (Cont) and experimental animals (Exp). Significant differences between control and experimental animals are marked with asterisks (***p<0.001). *(Revised from Xiong et al. 2005b)*

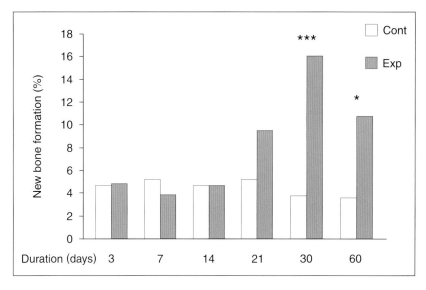

Fig. 5-10 Condylar adaptation in adult rats treated by functional bite jumping splints. Amount (mean values) of new bone formation at the posterior condyle in control animals (Cont) and experimental animals (Exp). Significant differences between control and experimental animals are marked with asterisks (***p<0.001, *p<0.05). *(Revised from Rabie et al. 2004)*

Forced bite jumping studies

Growing animals

Although only a few experimental studies on forced bite jumping using the Herbst appliance have been performed, the findings on condylar and glenoid fossa adaptation were basically the same as for functional bite jumping as presented above.

After placement of a Herbst bite jumping mechanism in a juvenile monkey *(Macaca fascicularis)* for a 13-week experimental period, Woodside et al. (1983) found small amounts of modeling in the superior part of the condyle and extensive modeling in the posterior region of the glenoid fossa.

In a large-scale Herbst bite jumping study using 20 juvenile monkeys *(Macaca mulatta)* with experimental periods ranging from 3 to 24 weeks (HEP = 2 to 19 months), Peterson and McNamara (2003) observed the following adaptations (Fig. 5-11): (1) Increased proliferation of the condylar cartilage, primarily in the posterior and posterosuperior regions of the condyle. (2) Significant deposition of new bone on the anterior surface of the postglenoid spine, indicating an anterior repositioning of the glenoid fossa (also suggested by Breitner 1940, Häupl and Psansky 1939, Woodside et al. 1987). (3) Significant apposition of bone on the posterior border of the mandibular ramus.(4) No evidence of pathological changes in the TMJ.

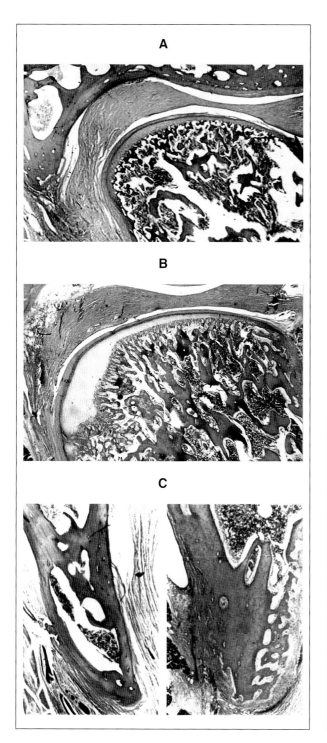

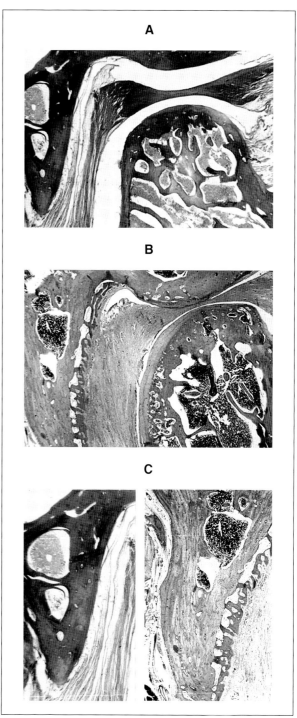

Fig. 5-11 TMJ growth adaptation in juvenile monkeys *(Mucaca mulatta)* treated by forced bite jumping with the Herbst appliance. **A**: Condyle of a control animal. **B**: Condyle of an experimental animal at 12 weeks. Note the increased proliferation of the posterior condylar cartilage. **C**: Postglenoid spine of a control animal (left) and an experimental animal at 3 weeks (right). Note the deposition of new bone at the anterior surface of the postglenoid spine. *(From Peterson and McNamara 2003)*

Fig. 5-12 TMJ growth adaptation in adult monkeys *(Mucaca mulatta)* treated by forced bite jumping with the Herbst appliance. **A**: Condyle of a control animal. **B**: Condyle of an experimental animal at 12 weeks. Note the increased proliferation of the posterior condylar cartilage. **C**: Postglenoid spine of a control animal (left) and an experimental animal at 12 weeks (right). Note the deposition of new bone at the anterior surface of the postglenoid spine. *(From McNamara et al. 2003)*

With respect to muscle adaptation in response to forced bite jumping with the Herbst appliance, experimental EMG studies are sparse.

The study of Sessle et al. (1990) included two juvenile monkeys *(Macaca fascicularis)* in which the postural EMG activity from the superior and inferior heads of the lateral pterygoid, superficial masseter and anterior digastric muscles was monitored with permanent surgically implanted EMG electrodes. A stepwise bite jumping procedure with the Herbst appliance was used. Comparisons were made between pre- and post-appliance EMG levels and with EMG levels in untreated controls. The results of the investigation revealed the following. (1) Decrease in postural EMG activity in all muscles upon insertion of the appliance. (2) After 6 weeks a gradual return of postural EMG activity to pre-appliance levels. (3) Progressive (stepwise) bite jumping (1.5 mm to 2 mm every 10 to 15 days) did not prevent a decrease in postural EMG activity.

In the study of Voudouris et al. (2003a,b) muscle-bone interactions were analyzed in the two monkeys from the previous Herbst study (Sessle et al. 1990). The results revealed that new bone formation at the condyle and the glenoid fossa was associated with decreased postural EMG activity in the four muscles analyzed in the above study (Sessle et al.1990). The results support a nonmuscular etiology for condylar and glenoid fossa growth modification.

Adult animals

To this date only two studies exist with respect to experimental forced bite jumping with the Herbst appliance in adult monkeys. The results were as conflicting as those from the adult primate and rat studies using functional bite jumping appliances.

Performing progressive (stepwise) bite jumping with the Herbst appliance in one adult monkey *(Macaca fasicularis)*, Woodside et al. (1987) found the following adaptive changes. (1) Extensive modeling of the glenoid fossa (especially at the postglenoid spine). The fossa modeling was supposed to contribute to the anterior mandibular positioning and altered jaw relationships (Class III) seen. (2) No condylar response. (3) Proliferation of the posterior part of the fibrous articular disk to fill the space created by the condylar displacement. The authors suggested that the overgrowth of the fibrous tissue was the reason why the mandible could not be manipulated posteriorly. Furthermore, it was speculated that it could be possible that the fibrous tissue resorbs after the stimulus is removed and the mandible returns partially toward its original position, resulting in a relapse in sagittal occlusion (Voudouris and Kuftinek 2000).

In an extensive study, screening 14 adult monkeys *(Macaca mulatta)* with experimental periods of 3 to 24 weeks (HEP = 2 to 19 months), McNamara et al. (2003) found the following adaptive changes in the TMJ in response to bite jumping with the Herbst appliance (Fig. 5-12). (1) Increased proliferation of the condylar cartilage. The thickness of the cartilage increased with treatment time. (2) Minimal adaptations along the anterior surface of the postglenoid spine. (3) No evidence of bone apposition or resorption on the posterior border of the ramus. (4) No evidence of TMJ pathology in any of the joints examined.

Stepwise bite jumping

Clinical investigations have indicated that stepwise mandibular advancement in the treatment of Class II malocclusions elicits a more favorable response in the mandible than a one-step approach (Pancherz et al. 1989, Du et al. 2002).

Experimental work of Petrovic et al. (1981) in the growing rat revealed that optimal functional bite jumping involved periodic mandibular advancements and that this was the best procedure to produce mandibular overlengthening orthopedically.

When comparing experimental mandibular stepwise advancement with one-step advancement it was shown that during the first advancement (in the stepwise procedure), the number of replicating mesenchymal cells in the glenoid fossa (Rabie et al. 2003f) and bone formation in the condyle and glenoid fossa (Rabie et al. 2003e,g, Leung et al. 2004) were less than in one-step advancement. However, in response to the second advancement (in the stepwise procedure), new bone formation was significantly higher in comparison to the one-step procedure Figs. 5-13A and B). Thus, the stepwise advancement was thought to deliver mechanical stimuli that produced a series of tissue responses that lead to increased vascularization and bone formation (Shum et al. 2004). However, a minimum threshold of strain must first be exceeded before the mesenchymal cells can differentiate to ultimately form new bone (Rabie et al. 2003f).

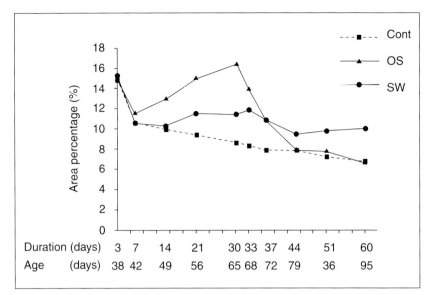

Fig. 5-13A Condylar adaptation in growing rats treated with functional bite jumping splints. Amount of bone formation at the posterior condyle in control animals (Cont) and experimental animals using one-step (OS) and stepwise (SW) mandibular advancement. The second SW-step was instituted on day 30. *(Revised from Rabie et al. 2003g)*

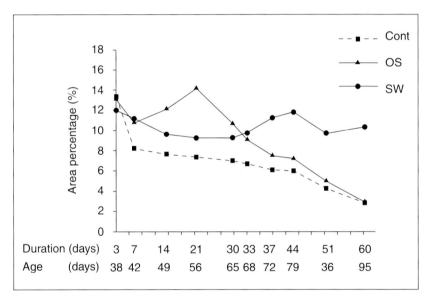

Fig. 5-13B Glenoid fossa adaptation in growing rats treated with functional bite jumping splints. Amount of bone formation at the posterior glenoid fossa in control animals (Cont) and experimental animals using one-step (OS) and stepwise (SW) mandibular advancement. The second SW-step was instituted on day 30. *(Revised from Rabie et al. 2003f)*

Conclusion and clinical implications

Experimental functional and forced bite jumping in animals (monkeys and rats) revealed the following adaptations in the TMJ and masticatory muscles:

- In young growing animals, cartilage / bone growth at the posterior condyle and new bone deposition at the anterior surface of the postglenoid spine is accelerated and enhanced.
- Due to increased bone formation at the posterior condyle, mandibular length is increased.

- In adult animals the ability of the TMJ to adapt to bite jumping persists. Qualitatively, the adaptive processes in the condyle and glenoid fossa are similar but quantitatively, they are reduced in comparison to those of growing animals.
- Due to deposition of new bone on the anterior surface of the postglenoid spine, the glenoid fossa is likely to be repositioned anteriorly in relation to the skull.
- There is no evidence of pathologic changes in the TMJ in either growing or adult animals.

- In comparison to one-step bite jumping, stepwise bite jumping results in less bone formation in the condyle and glenoid fossa in the first advancement step but in larger bone formation in the second advancement step. Thus, it seems as if bite jumping must exceed a minimum threshold value before the mesenchymal cells differentiate to form new bone.
- The nature of muscle – bone interactions is obscure and needs further investigation.

The evidence on adaptation of TMJ growth and masticatory muscle activity that has been collected in the experimental animal bite jumping studies is of importance for:
- the successful clinical use of the Herbst appliance in the treatment of Class II malocclusions, and
- the understanding and the interpretation of the findings from the clinical Herbst research reported in this book.

References

Baume LJ, Derichsweiler H. Is the condylar growth center responsive to orthodontic therapy? An experimental study in *Macaca mulatta*. Oral Surg Oral Med Oral Pathol 1961;14:347-362.

Breitner C. Experimentelle Veränderungen der mesiodistalen Beziehungen der oberen und unteren Zahnreihen. II. Teil. Jumping the bite. Zeitschr Stomatol 1930;28:620-635. (Translated to English: Breitner C. Bone changes resulting from experimental orthodontic treatment. Am J Orthod Oral Surg 1940;26:521-547.)

Charlier JP, Petrovic AG. Recherches sur la mandibule de la rat en culture d'organs: Le cartilage condylien a-t-il un potentiel de croissance independent? Orthod Franc 1967;38:165-175.

Charlier JP, Petrovitc AG, Hermann-Stutzmann J. Effects of mandibular hyperpropulsion on the prechondroblastic zone of young rat condyle. Am J Orthod 1969;55:71-74.

Chayanupatkul A, Rabie ABM, Hägg U. Temporomandibular response to early and late removal of bite jumping devices. Eur J Orthod 2003;25:465-470.

Derichsweiler H. Experimentelle Tieruntersuchungen über Veränderungen der Kieferelenke bei Bisslageveränderungen. Fortschr Kieferorthop 1958;19:30-44.

Du X, Hägg U, Rabie ABM. Effects of headgear Herbst and mandibular step-by-step advancement vs conventional Herbst appliance and maximal bite jumping of the mandible. Eur J Orthod 2002;24:167-174.

Elgoyen JC, Moyers, RE, McNamara JA, Riolo ML. Craniofacial adaptation of protrusive function in young rhesus monkeys. Am J Orthod 1972;62:469-480.

Häupl K, Psansky R. Experimentelle Untersuchungen über Gelenktransformation bei Verwendung der Methoden der Funktionskieferorthopädie. Dtsch Zahn Mund Kieferheilkd 1939;6:439-448.

Hinton RJ, McNamara JA. Temporal bone adaptation in response to protrusive function in juvenile and young adult rhesus monkeys *(Macaca mulatta)*. Eur J Orthod 1984a;6:155-174.

Hinton RJ, McNamara JA. Effect on age on the adaptive response of the adult temporomandibular joint. A study of induced protrusion in *Macaca mulatta*. Angle Orthod 1984b;54:154-162.

Hiniker J, Ramfjord S. Anterior displacement of the mandible in adult rhesus monkey. J Prosthet Dent 1966;16:503-512.

Joho J-P. Changes in form and size of the mandible in the orthopeadically treated *Macacus Irius*: an experimental study. Trans Eur Orthod Soc 1968;44:161-173.

Leung FYC, Rabie ABM, Hägg U. Neovascularization and bone formation in the condyle during stepwise mandibular advancement. Eur J Orthod 2004;26:137-141.

Luder H-L. Postnatal development, aging and degeneration of the temporomandibular joint in humans, monkeys and rats. Chapter 4: Comparative skeletal maturation, somatic growth and aging. Craniofacial Growth Series, Volume 32, Center of Human Growth and Development, The University of Michigan, Ann Arbor 1996:111-132.

McNamara JA. Neuromuscular and skeletal adaptations to altered function in the orofacial region. Am J Orthod 1973;64:578-606.

McNamara JA. Functional adaptation in the temporomandibular joint. Dent Clin North Am 1975;19:457-471.

McNamara JA, Conelly TG, McBride MC: Histologic studies of the temporomandibular joint adaptations. In: McNamara JA, ed. Determinants of mandibular form and growth. Monograph 4, Craniofacial Growth Series, Center of Human Growth and Development, The University of Michigan, Ann Arbor, 1975:209-227.

McNamara JA, Carlson DS. Quantitative analysis of temporomandibular joint adaptations to protrusive function. Am J Orthod 1979;76:593-611.

McNamara JA. Functional determinants of craniofacial size and shape. Eur J Orthod 1980;2:131-159.

McNamara JA, Hinton RJ, Hoffman DL. Histologic analysis of temporomandibular joint adaptation to protrusive function in young adult rhesus monkeys *(Macaca mulatta)*. Am J Orthod 1982;82:288-298.

McNamara JA, Bryan FA. Long-term mandibular adaptations to protrusive function: An experimental study in *Macaca mulatta*. Am J Orthod Dentofac Orthop 1987;92:98-108.

McNamara JA, Peterson JE, Pancherz H. Histologic changes associated with the Herbst appliance in adult rhesus monkeys *(Macaca mulatta)*. Semin Orthod 2003;9:26-40.

Pancherz H, Malmgren O, Hägg U, Ömblus J, Hansen K. Class II correction in Herbst and Bass therapy. Eur J Orthod 1989;11:17-30.

Paulsen HU, Thomsen JS, Hougen HP, Moskilde L. A histomorphometric and scanning electron microscopy study of human condylar cartilage and bone tissue changes in relation to age. Clin Orthod Res 1999;2:67-78.

Peterson JE, McNamara JA. Temporomandibular joint adaptations associated with Herbst appliance treatment in juvenile rhesus monkeys *(Macaca mulatta)*. Semin Orthod 2003;9:12-25.

Petrovic AG. Mechanisms and regulation of mandibular condylar growth. Acta Morphol Neerln Scand 1972;10:25-34.

Petrovic AG, Stutzmann JJ, Oudet CL. Control processes in the postnatal growth of the condylar cartilage of the mandible. In: McNamara JA, ed. Determinants of mandibular form an growth. Monograph 4, Craniofacial Growth Series, Center of Human Growth and Development, The University of Michigan, Ann Arbor, 1975:101-153.

Petrovic AG, Stutzmann JJ, Gasson N. The final length of the mandible: Is it genetically determined? In: Carlson DS, ed. Craniofacial biology. Monograph 10, Craniofacial Growth Series, Center of Human Growth and Development, The University of Michigan, Ann Arbor, 1981: 105-126.

Rabie ABM, Zhao Z, Shen S, Hägg U, Robinson W. Osteogenesis in the glenoid fossa in response to mandibular advancement. Am J Orthod Dentofac Orthop 2001;119:390-400.

Rabie ABM, Shum L, Chayanupatkul A. VEGF and bone formation in the glenoid fossa during forward mandibular positioning. Am J Orthod Dentofac Orthop 2002a;122:202-209.

Rabie ABM, Leung FYC, Chayanupatkul A, Hägg U. The correlation between neovascularization and bone formation in the condyle during forward mandibular positioning. Angle Orthod 2002b;72: 431-438.

Rabie ABM, She TT, Hägg U. Functional appliance therapy accelerates and enhances condylar growth. Am J Orthod Dentofac Orthop 2003a;123:40-48.

Rabie ABM, Wong L, Tsai M. Replicating mesenchymal cells in the condyle and the glenoid fossa during mandibular forward positioning. Am J Orthod Dentofac Orthop 2003b;123:49-57.

Rabie ABM, She TT, Harley VR: Forward mandibular positioning up-regulates SOX9 and Type II collagen expression in the glenoid fossa. J Dent Res 2003c;82:725-730.

Rabie ABM, Tang GH, Xiong H, Hägg H. PTHrP regulates chondrocyte maturation in condylar cartilage. J Dent Res 2003d;8:627-631.

Rabie ABM, Chayanupatkul A, Hägg U. Stepwise advancement using fixed functional appliances: experimental perspective. Semin Orthod 2003e;9:41-46.

Rabie ABM, Wong LW, Hägg U. Correlation of replicating cells and osteogenesis in the glenoid fossa during stepwise advancement. Am J Orthod Dentofac Orthop 2003f;123:521-526.

Rabie ABM, Tsai M-LM, Hägg U, Du X, Chou B-W. The correlation of replicating cells and osteogenesis in the condyle during stepwise advancement. Angle Orthod 2003g;73:457-465.

Rabie ABM, Xiong H, Hägg U. Forward mandibular positioning enhances condylar adaptation in adult rats. Eur J Orthod 2004;26:353-358.

Ramfjord S, Enlow,R. Anterior displacement of the mandible in adult rhesus monkeys: Long-term observations. J Prosthet Dent 1971:26:517-531.

Shum L, Rabie ABM, Hägg U. Vascular endothelial growth factor expression and bone formation in posterior glenoid fossa during stepwise mandibular advancement. Am J Orthod Dentofac Orthop 2004;125:185-190.

Sessle BJ, Gurza SC. Jaw movement-related activity and reflexly induced changes in lateral pterygoid muscle of the monkey *Macaca fascicularis*. Arch Oral Biol 1982;27:163-173

Sessle BJ, Woodside P, Borque P, Gurza S, Powell J, Voudouris J, Metaxas A, Altuna G. Effect of functional appliances on jaw muscle activity. Am J Orthod Dentofac Orthop 1990;98:220-230.

Stöckli PW, Willert HG. Tissue reactions in the temporomandibular joint resulting from anterior displacement of the mandible in the monkey. Am J Orthod 1971;60:142-155.

Suzuki S, Itoh K, Ohyoma K. Local administration of IGF-I stimulates the growth of the mandible in mature rats. J Orthod 2004;31:138-143.

Voudouris JC, Kuftinek MM. Improved clinical use of Twin-block and Herbst as a result of radiating viscoelastic tissue forces on the condyle and fossa in treatment and long-term re tention: Growth relativity. Am J Orthod Dentofac Orthop 2000;117:247-266.

Voudouris JC, Woodside DG, Altuna G, Kuftinek MM, Angelopoulos G, Borque PJ. Condyle-fossa modifications and muscle interactions during Herbst treatrnent, Part 1. New technological methods. Am J Orthod Dentofac Orthop 2003a;123:604-613.

Voudouris JC, Woodside DG, Altuna G, Angelopoulos G, Borque PJ. Lacouture CY, Kuftinek MM. Condyle-fossa modifications and muscle interactions during Herbst treatment, Part 2. Results and conclusions. Am J Orthod Dentofac Orthop 2003b;124:13-29.

Whetten LL, Johnston LE. The control of condylar growth: an experimental evaluation of the role of the lateral pterygoid muscle. Am J Orthod 1985;88:181-190.

Woodside DG, Altuna G, Harvold E, Herbert M, Metaxas A. Primate experiments in malocclusion and bone induction. Am J Orthod 1983;83:460-468.

Woodside DG, Metaxas A, Altuna G. The influence of functional appliance therapy on glenoid fossa remodeling. Am J Orthod Dentofac Orthop 1987;92:181-198.

Xiong H, Hägg U, Tang G-H, Rabie ABM, Robinson W. The effect of continuous bite-jumping in adult rats: a morphologic study. Angle Orthod 2004;74:86-92.

Xiong H, Rabie ABM, Hägg U. Mechanical strain leads to condylar growth in adult rats. Frontiers Bioscience 2005a;10:65-73.

Xiong H, Rabie ABM, Hägg U. Neovascularization and mandibular condylar bone remodeling in adult rats under mechanical strain. Frontiers Bioscience 2005b;10:74-82.

Chapter 6

Herbst research - subjects and methods

A. Subjects investigated

Herbst subjects

The scientific evidence of the clinical-experimental research presented in this book is to the most part based on prospective studies. In total 366 consecutively Class II malocclusions treated with the Herbst appliance over a period of 28 years, from 1977 to 2005 were evaluted. In 134 subjects the banded type of Herbst appliance and in 232 subjects the cast splint Herbst appliance was used. As there was continuous research during this period, the publications over the years comprised varying numbers of subjects.

The Herbst patients were treated at three Orthodontic University Departments, either by the two authors of this book, the senior department staff or by the postgraduate students under the guidance of the authors: University of Lund, Sweden (Pancherz), University of Giessen, Germany (Pancherz and Ruf), University of Berne, Switzerland (Ruf). The Swedish patients were treated between 1977 and 1985, the German patients since 1985 and the Swiss patients between 2002 and 2005.

Approximately 80% of the patients had a Class II:1 malocclusion and 20% a Class II:2 malocclusion. In the subjects from earlier years, Herbst treatment was performed in the mixed/early permanent dentition, before or at the pubertal peak of growth, while in later years, treatment almost exclusively was conducted in the permanent dentition, primarily after the peak of pubertal growth (see Chapter 22: Treatment timing). Since 1995 the number of adults treated with the Herbst appliance has increased steadily (see Chapter 23: Treatment of adults – an alternative to orthognathic surgery).

Control subjects

In a large number of the presented investigations, matched untreated Class II subjects were available. However, in the long-term evaluation studies, for ethical reasons, it was difficult to maintain longitudinal data of untreated Class II controls.

Therefore, when no untreated Class II controls were at hand, the so called "Bolton Standards" (Broadbent et al. 1975) were used for comparison. The Standards consist of longitudinal growth data and annual composite lateral head film tracings from 32 untreated subjects (16 males and 16 females) with ideal occlusion followed from 6 years to 18 years of age.

In comparative studies analyzing various Herbst subgroups, which differed in: (1) age, (2) maturation, (3) morphology, (4) growth pattern, (5) treatment approach, and (6) appliance design, the presence of untreated control subjects was not considered mandatory for the performance of evidence based research.

B. Analyzing methods

The methods used in the scientific evaluation of the Herbst subjects is presented below.

1. Standard cephalometry

In the analysis of lateral head films a large number of different "standard" methods have been presented in the literature. The reference points and their abbreviations vary and are sometimes obscure. Therefore, the specific reference points, angular and linear variables of our "Standard analysis" are presented in the corresponding book chapters.

2. Superimposition of lateral head films

In the assessment of treatment and growth changes, lateral head films were superimposed using reference points and structures that were not affected by growth or at least affected as little as possible, thus representing "fixed" reference points and structures.

Three lateral head film superimposition techniques were used:

(1) Cranial base superimposition, using the *anatomic reference points nasion and sella*. This superimposition technique was predominantly used in the short-term evaluation of growth and treatment changes (less than 2 years between the registrations) or in the evaluation of non-growing patients.

(2) Cranial base superimposition using the *stable bone structures in the anterior cranial base* (Björk and Skieller 1983): (a) the contour of the anterior wall of the sella turcica, (b) the anterior contours of the middle cranial fossa, (c) the contour of the cribiform plate, (d) the contours of the bilateral fronto-ethmoidal crests and (e) the cerebral surfaces of the orbital roofs. This superimposition technique was mainly used in the long-term evaluation of growth and treatment changes (more than 2 years between the registrations).

The reason for using the anatomic point method in the short-term evaluations and the stable bone structure method in the long-term evaluations was that, in a short-term perspective, the method error for head film orientation is larger when using stable bone structures than when using anatomic points (Pancherz and Hansen 1984). In the long-term perspective, on the other hand, the opposite is true as the vertical growth of nasion causes an increasing inaccuracy in head film orientation upon superimposition of the films on the NSL (Pancherz and Hansen 1984).

(3) Mandibular superimposition using the *mandibular stable structures* for orientation (Björk and Skieller 1983): (a) the anterior contour of the bony chin, (b) the inner contour of the bony plate at the lower border of the symphysis, (c) any distinct trabecular structure in the

symphysis, (d) the contour of the mandibular canal, (e) the lower contour of a mineralized molar germ before root development begins.

3. SO-Analysis (Analysis of changes in sagittal occlusion)

With the SO-Analysis (Pancherz 1982) it is possible to relate alterations in sagittal occlusion (overjet, molar relationship) to skeletal and dental components in the maxilla and mandible. The analysis is performed on lateral head films in habitual (centric) occlusion. The method can be used in any Class II orthodontic, orthopedic and/or surgical treatment procedure involving fixed or removable appliances with and without extractions of teeth.

An important factor to consider in the SO-analysis is to choose a reference plane close to the occlusal plane, as changes in sagittal occlusion occur along this plane. It is, however, up to the orthodontist to use an occlusal plane of his preference as the outcome of the analysis is only marginally affected by different occlusal planes (functional, maxillary, mandibular or average) (Birkenkamp 2004). In the Herbst studies presented in this book the maxillary occlusal plane was the most frequently used reference plane.

The decisive factor for the SO-Analysis to be valid, is to use the *original* occlusal plane for all measurements on all head films (Birkenkamp 2004). Therefore, a reference grid (Fig. 6-1) comprising an occlusal reference line (RL) and a line perpendicular to that through sella (RLp) is *defined on the first head film* and than transferred to the after treatment as well as the follow-up head films by superimposition of the films on either the nasion-sella line (NSL) with sella (s) as common registration point or on the stable anterior cranial base bone structures (see above).

The SO-Analysis comprises 8 linear measurements that are all performed parallel with RL to RLp (Fig. 6-1):

1. is/RLp minus ii/RLp – Overjet.
2. ms/RLp minus mi/RLP – Molar relation
3. ss/RLp – Position of the maxillary base
4. pg/RLp – Position of the mandibular base
5. is/RLp – Position of the maxillary central incisor
6. ii/RLp – Position of the mandibular central incisor
7. ms/RLp – Position of the maxillary permanent first molar
8. mi/RLp – Position of the mandibular permanent first molar

Changes of the different measuring points in relation to RLp during different examination periods are registered by calculating the difference (d) in landmark position. Changes of the variables 1 and 2 represent changes in the occlusion, changes of the variables 3 and 4 represent skeletal changes, while changes of the variables 5 to 8 represent a composite picture of skeletal and dental changes. Variables for dental changes within the maxilla and mandible are obtained by the following calculations:

9. is/RLp (d) minus ss/RLp (d) – Change in position of the maxillary central incisor within the maxilla.
10. ii/Rlp (d) minus pg/RLp (d) – Change in position of the mandibular central incisor within the mandible.
11. ms/RLp (d) minus ss/RLp (d) – Change in position of the maxillary permanent first molar within the maxilla.
12. mi/RLp (d) minus pg/RLp (d) – Change in position of the mandibular permanent first molar within the mandible.

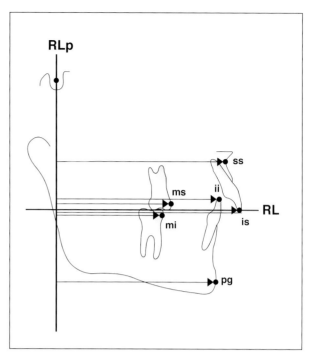

Fig. 6-1 Analysis of changes in sagittal occlusion (SO-Analysis).

The RL/RLp reference system has the following advantages in the evaluation of a Class II treatment procedure. (1) The system is close to the problem area. (2) The system is consistent. The main reference point sella (s) is relatively stable (Björk 1968). This is of utmost importance for a correct transformation of the RLp reference line from the first head film to the other head films in a series. Furthermore, by the use of the original RL and RLp lines for both before and after treatment measurements, any tipping of the occlusal plane (RL line) will not influence the reference system and thus bias the measurements (Birkenkamp 2004). (3) All registrations are performed to the same reference line (RLp). This makes it possible to assess the mechanism of changes in sagittal occusion (overjet, molar relationship) and to quantify the interrelationship between the skeletal and dental changes in and between the jaws (Figs. 6-2 and 6-3).

The SO-Analysis is used in a number of publications presented in this book. References will be made at the appropriate places.

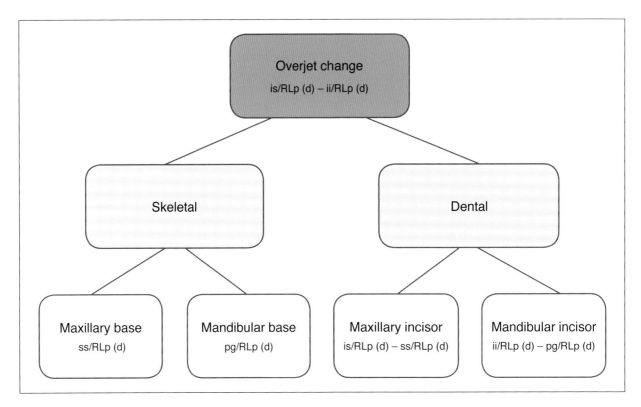

Fig. 6-2 Measurements used in the assessment of the mechanism of Overjet changes (SO-Analysis).

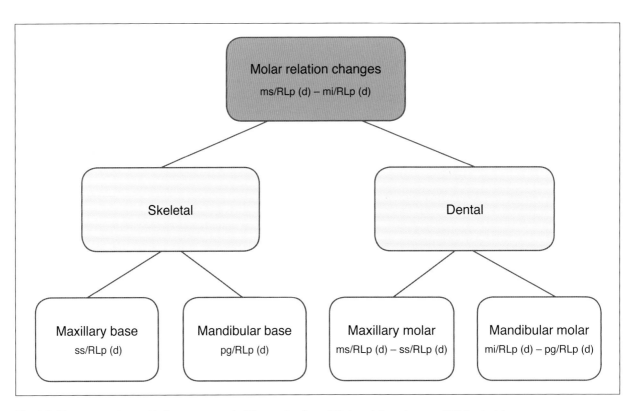

Fig. 6-3 Measurements used in the assessment of the mechanism of Molar relation changes (SO-Analysis).

4. Somatic maturity

Somatic maturity assessment by means of velocity growth curves of standing height is a reliable method in clinical orthodontics (Björk 1972).

From all Herbst patients treated in Sweden, longitudinal growth records of standing body height over 5- to 10-years were available. The growth records were obtained from the childrens´ school clinics and from the Orthodontic University Department. At the University, the body height measurements were made to the nearest 1 mm with registrations performed about every month. At the school clinics, body height measurements were made to the nearest 0.5 cm and registrations were done every year or every second year from 7 years of age onward. Data from the school clinics were included for the assessment of somatic maturity only when they covered a period before the subject was registered at the Orthodontic Department.

By means of a computer program, individual distance and velocity curves of standing height were constructed. The velocity curves were smoothed by spline function (Largo et al. 1978). By visual inspection the peak height velocity was identified on the velocity curves and different growth periods were established (Pancherz and Hägg 1985 = 3 growth periods, Hägg and Pancherz 1988 = 7 growth periods). The examination period in each subject was assigned to one of the growth periods. If the examination period coincided with more than one growth period, the subject was assigned to the growth period that covered most of the examination period.

5. Skeletal maturity

The use of growth curves for the assessment of somatic maturity is generally useful for retrospective but not for prospective studies. For prospective use, the somatic maturity level of subjects at the time of examination can be assessed indirectly by means of various skeletal developmental stages of the hand and wrist (hand radiographic analysis) or of the cervical vertebrae (lateral head film analysis).

Development of hand-wrist bones and cervical vertebrae

At the Department in Giessen skeletal maturity of our patients is assessed in two ways:
  (1) Judging the skeletal development of the middle phalanx of the third finger and the distal epiphysis of the radius on hand radiographs using the method of Hägg and Taranger (1980) as well as of Hägg and Pancherz (1988). Nine epiphysial stages are used in the evaluation (Fig. 6-4): 6 stages of the middle phalanx of the third finger (MP3) and 3 stages of the distal epiphysis of the radius (R).
  (2) Judging the skeletal development of the cervical vertebrae on lateral head films using the method of Hassel and Farman (1995). Six developmental stages of the cervical (C3) vertebra are used in the evaluation (Fig. 6-5).

In the Herbst subjects treated in Sweden, hand radiographs and lateral head films were taken before and after Herbst therapy and then annually to the end of growth. In the subjects from Germany and/or Switzerland, hand radiographs and lateral head films were available before and after Herbst treatment as well as after multibracket appliance treatment and at follow-up.

In a longitudinal study (Pancherz and Szyska 2000) analyzing 401 hand-wrist radiographs and 401 lateral head films as well as individual velocity growth curves of standing height from 48 subjects followed over a period of 16 years (from 8 to 22 years of age) a close interrelation between skeletal and somatic maturation was found:
  (1) The combined hand-wrist stages MP3-E and -F coincided with the Prepeak growth period in 78%, the combined stages MP3-FG and -G with the Peak period in 62% and the combined stages MP3-H and -I as well as the R-stages with the Postpeak period in 92% of the registrations.
  (2) The combined vertebrae stages S1 and S2 coincided with the Prepeak growth period in 83%, the combined stages S3 and S4 with the Peak period and the combined stages S5 and S6 with the Postpeak period in 85% of the registrations.

In conclusion, it can be said that somatic maturity can be reliable assessed by skeletal maturity measures. In orthodontic patients, the C3-vertebra analysis has a comparable high validity as the hand-wrist analysis for the identification of the Prepeak and Peak growth periods (Pancherz ans Szyska 2000). However, when it comes to the question whether growth has finished or not, the cervical vertebra stages S5 and/or S6 can not replace the hand-wrist R-stages (I, IJ and J). This is due to the fact that the C3 stages S5 and S6 (1) cover too large a time span at the end of the growth period and (2) are difficult to differentiate from each other.

Somatic and skeletal maturity assessments have been used in a number of Herbst publications. References will be made at the appropriate places in this book.

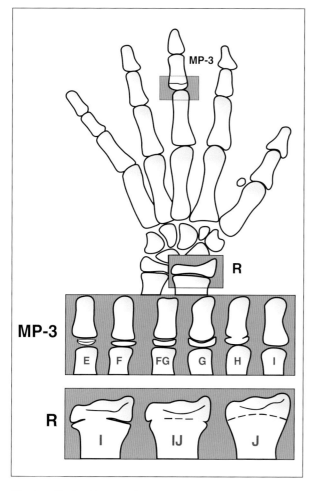

Fig. 6-4 *Six developmental stages of the middle phalanx epiphysis of the third finger (MP3).* **E** - The width of the epiphysis is less than that of the metaphysis. **F** - The epiphysis is as wide as the metaphysis. **FG** - The epiphysis is as wide as the metaphysis and there is a distinct medial and/or lateral border of the epiphysis forming a line of demarcation at right angles to the metaphysis side. **G** - The epiphysis is wider than the metaphysis and also caps it. **H** - Fusion of the epiphysis and metaphysis has begun. **I** - The fusion of the epiphysis and metaphysis is complete.
Three developmental stages of the distal epiphysis of the radius (R). **I** - Fusion of the epiphysis and metaphysis has begun. **IJ** - Fusion of the epiphysis and metaphysis is almost completed but there is still a small gap at one or both margins. **J** - Fusion of the epiphysis and metaphysis is complete. (*Revised from Hägg and Taranger 1980*)

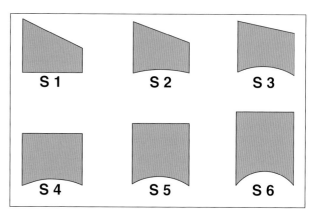

Fig. 6-5 *Six developmental stages of the C3-vertebra.* **S1** - The inferior border is flat. The vertebra is wedge shaped, and the superior border tapered from posterior to anterior. **S2** - An inferior border concavity is developing. **S3** - The inferior border shows a more pronounced cavity. The body is approaching a rectangular shape. **S4** - The inferior border shows a more distinct cavity. The body has become more square in shape. **S5** - The inferior border cavity is more accentuated. The body is nearly completely square. **S6** - The lower border cavity has become deep. The body is square and greater in vertical than in horizontal dimension.

6. Condylar growth changes

Four methods were used in the assessment of condylar growth changes during Herbst treatment:

(1) Mandibular length measurements on mouth open lateral lateral head films (Pancherz 1979, 1982, Pancherz and Hägg 1985, Hägg and Pancherz 1988).

(2) Condylar growth measurements on superimposed mandibles of mouth open lateral head films (Pancherz and Littmann 1988, 1989).

(3) Condylar modeling on magnetic resonance imaging (MRI) of the TMJ (Ruf and Pancherz 1998a,b, 1999).

7. Glenoid fossa growth changes

Two methods were used in the evaluation of glenoid fossa growth changes during Herbst treatment:

(1) Glenoid fossa modeling as seen on MRIs of the TMJ (Ruf and Pancherz 1998a, 1999)

(2) Glenoid fossa displacement assessed by the method of Buschang and Santos-Pinto (1998): lateral habitual (centric) occlusion head films were superimposed on the stable bone structures of the cranial base (Björk and Skieller 1983). The change of an anatomic condylar (Co) point (defined on corresponding mouth open lateral head films and transferred to the occlusion head films) in relation to its pretreatment position represents the fossa displacement (Fig. 6-6). It must be pointed out

that the validity of the method is dependent on an unchanged condyle-fossa relationship at all times of registration. This approach has been used in two Herbst studies (Pancherz and Fischer 2003, Pancherz and Michaelidou 2004).

8. Condylar position changes within the fossa

Three methods were used in the evaluation of condylar position changes during and after Herbst therapy:

(1) Assessment on lateral head films in habitual (centric) occlusion. To visualize the condylar head, mandibular tracings (with the condyle) from mouth open head films were superimposed on the habitual occlusion head films. Condylar changes were measured in relation to a reference grid which comprised the nasion-sella line (NSL) and its perpendicular line, NSLp, through sella (s). This approach was used in one long-term Herbst study (Pancherz and Stickel 1989).

(2) Assessment of lateral tomograms using a subjective grading method (Hansen et al. 1990).

(3) Assessment of parasagittal MRIs of the TMJ by measuring the anterior and posterior joint spaces and by calculating a joint space index. The method of Kamelchuk et al. (1996) was used in two Herbst studies (Ruf and Pancherz 1998a,b) and the method of Mavreas and Athanasiou (1992) in one Herbst study (Ruf and Pancherz 2000).

9. "Effective TMJ growth", chin position changes and mandibular rotation

In dentofacial orthopedics the position of the chin is affected by the following mechanisms: (1) mandibular condylar modeling, (2) glenoid fossa modeling, (3) condylar position changes within the fossa and (4) mandibular rotation. The three TMJ changes have been analyzed in several Herbst studies as single factors (see above). This, however, will not answer the question how and to what extent the position of the chin is affected by TMJ changes. In using the method of Creekmore (1967) it is, however, possible to overcome this problem. With his approach the "effective TMJ growth" is assessed, which is a summation of the above three TMJ changes: (1) condylar modeling, (2) fossa modeling and (3) condylar position changes. All measurements are performed on lateral head films using an arbitrary condylar point.

The methods for the assessment of "effective TMJ growth", chin position change and mandibular rotation are shown in Fig. 6-7. The following reference points were used:

- The point CoA (arbitrary condylar point) was used as reference for "effective TMJ growth". The point was defined on the first head film and transferred to the other head films in a series after superimposition of the head films on the stable bone structures of the cranial base (Björk and Skieller 1983).

- The point Pg (pogonion) was used as reference for chin position changes. The point was defined on the first head film and transferred to the other head films in a series after superimposition of the films on the mandibular stable structures (Björk and Skieller 1983).

- The line RL was used as reference for mandibular rotation. The line was defined on the first head film by the incisal edge of the most prominent central mandibular incisor and the distobuccal cusp tip of the first permanent mandibular molar. The line was transferred from the first head film to the other films in a series by superimposition of the films on the mandibular stable structures (Björk and Skieller 1983). The line thus represents an artifical implant line (Björk and Skieller 1983). The angular change of the RL represents the true rotation of the mandible not masked by remodeling processes at the mandibular lower corpus border (Björk and Skieller 1972).

The treatment and posttreatment changes of the reference points (CoA and Pg) and line (RL) were related to a reference grid (RL/RLp) defined on the first head film and transferred to the other films in a series by superimposition of the films on stable bone structures of the cranial base (Björk and Skieller 1983). The line RL of the RL/RLP reference grid corresponds to the X-axis of the grid. The RLp is a line perpendicular to RL through the midpoint of sella turcica and corresponds to the Y-axis of the grid. The above method analyzing TMJ growth, chin position changes and mandibular rotation has been applied in five Herbst studies (Pancherz et al. 1998, Ruf and Pancherz 1998a, Pancherz and Fischer 2003, Pancherz and Michaelidou 2004, Marku 2006).

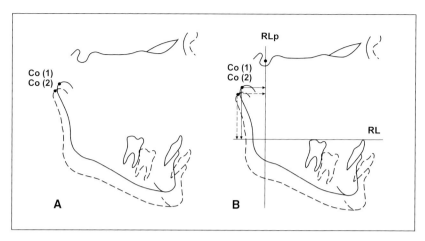

Fig. 6-6 Method for the assessment of glenoid fossa displacement (Co). **A**: Cranial base superimposition. **B**: Measurement of fossa displacement (Co point change) in relation to the RL/RLp reference grid.

10. Masticatory muscle activity (EMG)

In the short- and long-term evaluation of masseter and temporal muscle function in consecutively treated Herbst patients a standardized electromyographic (EMG) method was used:

- Bipolar hook electrodes (Ahlgren 1967) were placed bilaterally on the temporal and masseter muscles according to Fig. 6-8.
- Direct and integrated recordings were obtained with the aid of a Mingograph 800 (Elema-Schönander, Stockholm).
- An amplification of 500 μV was used.
- Paper speed was 50 mm per second.
- The integrators were constructed to integrate the EMG potentials during a fixed time period of 0.05 seconds (so-called époque integration). The relative value of the integral was calculated by measuring the height (mm) of the integrated signal from the base line. The absolute value of the integrated (peak-to-peak) activity was obtained by multiplying the height of the époque by a calibration factor of 50 μV.

The following registrations and measurements were made on the integrated EMG recordings:

- *Maximal biting in intercuspal position.* The patients were instructed to close their jaws in habitual occlusion as forcibly as possible for about 2 seconds. The maximal integrated activity of a biting cycle (the mean value of five consecutive biting cycles) was used for evaluation. For both the masseter and temporal muscles the mean value of right- and left-side measurements was used.
- *Chewing five peanuts.* No instructions were given to the patients except for eating the

peanuts. The maximal integrated activity during a chewing cycle (the mean value of ten consecutive cycles) was used for evaluation. For the temporal muscle the mean value of right- and left-side measurements were used. The same was done for the masseter muscle in case of a bilateral chewing pattern. In case of a unilateral chewing pattern the EMG measurements were made from the chewing side only.

This standardized EMG approach has been used in the analysis of children and adults with normal occlusion (Pancherz 1980a), in untreated Class II:1 malocclusions (Pancherz 1980b) and in Class II:1 malocclusions treated with the Herbst appliance on a short-term (Pancherz and Anehus-Pancherz 1980) and a long-term (Pancherz 1995) basis.

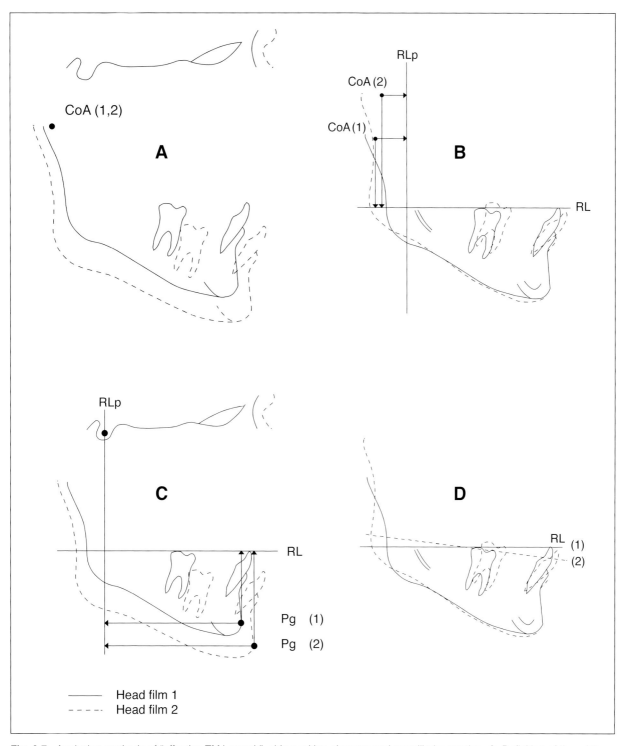

Fig. 6-7 Analyzing methods of "effective TMJ growth", chin position changes and mandibular rotation. **A**: Definition of the arbitrary condylar point (CoA). **B**: Measurements of "effective TMJ growth" (CoA point changes). **C**: Measurements of chin position changes (Pg changes). **D**: Measurements of mandibular rotation (RL inclination changes). In **A** to **D** the second head film (2) was superimposed on the the first head film (1) using stable anterior cranial base (**A** and **C**) or stable mandibular (**B** and **D**) structures for orientation. (*Revised from Pancherz et al. 1998*)

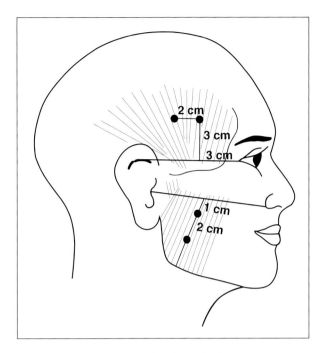

Fig. 6-8 Diagram demonstrating electrode placement on temporal and masseter muscles in the EMG analysis. (*From Pancherz 1980a*)

11. TMJ function

Four approaches were used in the evaluation of the short- and long-term effects of Herbst treatment on craniomandibular (TMJ) function:

(1) *Anamnesis* focusing on sounds and pain from the TMJ, pain from the jaw musculature, the incidence of head aches, parafunction, biting and chewing difficulties and restriction of jaw movements (Pancherz and Anehus-Pancherz 1982, Hansen et al. 1990, Ruf and Pancherz 1998b, 2000).

(2) *Clinical examination* using a conventional procedure (Pancherz and Anehus-Pancherz 1982, Hansen et al.1990) that involved an assessment of the range of mandibular motion, TMJ sounds, TMJ and muscle tenderness on palpation and the so called "Manual Functional Analysis" (MFA) (Ruf and Pancherz 1998b). The MFA according to Bumann (Bumann and Lotzmann 2000) included isometric contraction, passive jaw movements, joint play, and dynamic tests for the differentiation of clicking.

(3) *Magnetic resonance imaging (MRI)* assessing disk displacements (Foucart et al. 1998, Ruf and Pancherz 1998b, 2000, Pancherz et al. 1999) and structural TMJ bony changes (Ruf and Pancherz 1998b, 2000). The MRIs

were obtained by means of a Magnetom Expert® 1.0 Tesla (Siemens AG, Erlangen, Germany) equipped with TMJ coils for simultaneous imaging of the left and right joints. The MRI protocol included closed mouth proton density weighted spin echo sequences in parasagittal and coronal orientation, as well as mouth open parasagittal T-2 weighted sequences. All closed mouth images were taken with the teeth in habitual occlusion. Five slices of each joint were made. Slice thickness was 3 mm with no interslice gap. The parasagittal MRIs were taken perpendicular to and the coronal MRIs were taken parallel to the long axis of the condyle. The closed mouth parasagittal MRIs were analyzed visually and metrically whereas the coronal and mouth open images were analyzed only visually. In the analysis of the parasagittal MRIs, the lateral, central and medial slices of each joint were evaluated separately. For the metric analysis, all MRIs were traced and analyzed twice with a one week interval between the two registrations. In the final evaluation, the mean value of the duplicate registrations was used. In order to facilitate a comparison of the MRIs within a series and between individuals, all images were taken with the same magnification. Furthermore, to make the measuring procedure more simple and accurate, all tracings were magnified to 156% by a photocopying procedure.

(4) *Lateral tomography* assessing condylar position and structural bony changes in the TMJ (Hansen et al. 1990). Simultaneous tomography of the TMJ was performed with a Polytome U (Massiot-Philips, Paris, France) using a hypocycloidal motion pattern. A multisection cassette containing four pairs of rare earth screens and four films were used. Two exposures were made on each joint to cover the total medial-lateral width of the joints. The tomograms were made with the teeth in habitual occlusion. The tomographic sections were perpendicular to the long axis of the condyle.

12. Chewing efficiency

Masticatory performance during different phases of Herbst treatment (Pancherz and Anehus-Pancherz 1982) was evaluated by a masticatory efficiency test (Edlund and Lamm 1980). In this test the patients chewed five separate portions of a standardized test material (Optosil® Bayer, a silicon dental impression material) for 20 chews. Each of the samples of chewed material was fractioned in a system of sieves. A masticatory efficiency value (R) was calculated for each test portion (Edlund and Lamm 1980) and the mean of the best four R values out of five was used as the subject´s efficiency index (Ri).

References

Ahlgren J. An intracutaneous needle electrode for kinesiologic EMG studies. Acta Odont Scand 1967;25:15-19.

Birkenkamp T. Die Sagittale-Okklusions-Analyse (SO-Analyse) bei Verwendung verschiedener Bezugslinien. Diss. med. dent. (Thesis), Giessen 2004.

Björk A. The use of metallic implants in the study of facial growth in children: method and application. Am J Phys Anthropol 1968;29:243-254.

Björk A, Skieller V. Facial development and tooth eruption: an implant study at the age of puberty. Am J Orthod 1972;62:339-383.

Björk A, Skieller V. Normal and abnormal growth of the mandible. A synthesis of longitudinal cephalometric implant studies over a period of 25 years. Eur J Orthod 1983;5:1-46.

Broadbent BH, Broadbent BH Jr, Golden WH. Bolton Standards of dentofacial development. St. Louis: CV Mosby, 1975

Bumann A, Lotzmann U. Funktionsdiagnostik und Therapieprinzipien. Stuttgart: Thieme, 2000.

Buschang PH, Santos-Pinto A. Condylar growth and glenoid fossa displacement during childhood and adolescence. Am J Orthod Dentofac Orthop 1998;113:437-442.

Creekmore TD. Inhibition or stimulation of vertical growth of the facial complex: its significance to treatment. Angle Orthod 1967;37:285-297.

Edlund J, Lamm CJ. Masticatory efficiency. J Oral Rehab 1980;7:123-130.

Foucart JM, Pajoni D, Carpentier P, Pharaboz C. MRI study of temporomandibular joint disk behaviour in children with hyperpropulsion appliances. Orthod Fr 1998;69:79-91.

Hansen K, Pancherz H, Peterson A. Long-term effects of the Herbst appliance on the craniomandibular system with special reference to the TMJ. Eur J Orthod 1990;12:244-253.

Hassel B, Farman AG. Skeletal maturation evaluation using cervical vertebrae. Am J Orthod Dentofac Orthop 1995;107:58-66.

Hägg U, Taranger J. Skeletal stages of hand and wrist as indicators of the pubertal growth spurt. Acta Odont Scand 1980;38:187-200.

Hägg U, Pancherz H. Dentofacial orthopaedics in relation to chronological age, growth period and skeletal development. An analysis of 72 male patients with Class II division 1 malocclusion treated with the Herbst appliance. Eur J Orthod 1988;10:169-176.

Kamelchuk LS, Grace MGA, Major PW. Postimaging temporomandibular joint space analysis. J Craniomand Pract 1996;14-23-29.

Largo RH, Gaser T, Prader A, Stuetle W, Hiber PJ. Analysis of the adolescent spurt using smoothing spline function. Ann Hum Biol 1978;5:421-434.

Marku K. Die Klasse II/2 Behandlung bei Postadolescenten und jungen Erwachsenen mit der Herbst-/Multibracket-Apparatur. Eine röntgenkephalometrische Langzeituntersuchung. Diss. med. dent. (Thesis), Giessen 2006.

Mavreas D, Athanasiou AE: Tomograhic assessment of alterations of the temporomandibular joint after orthognathic surgery. Eur J Orthod 1992;14:3-15.

Pancherz H. Treatment of Class II malocclusions by jumping the bite with the Herbst appliance. A cephalometric investigation. Am J Orthod 1979;76:423-442.

Pancherz H. Temporal and masseter muscle activity in children and adults with normal occlusion. Acta Odont Scand 1980a;38:343-348.

Pancherz H. Activity of the temporal and masseter muscles in Class II, Division 1 malocclusions. Am J Orthod 1980b;77:679-688.

Pancherz H. The mechanism of Class II correction in Herbst appliance treatment. A cephalometric investigation. Am J Orthod 1982;82:104-113.

Pancherz H. The Herbst appliance. Sevilla: Editorial Aguiram, 1995.

Pancherz H, Anehus-Pancherz M. Muscle activity in Class II, Division 1 malocclusions treated with the Herbst appliance. Am J Orthod 1980;78:321-329.

Pancherz H, Anehus-Pancherz M. The effect of continuous bite jumping with the Herbst appliance on the masticatory system: a functional analysis of treated Class II malocclusions. Eur J Orthod 1982;4:37-44.

Pancherz H, Fischer S. Amount and direction of temporomandibular joint growth changes in Herbst treatment: a cephalometric long-term investigation. Angle Orthod 2003;73:493-501.

Pancherz H, Hansen K. The Nasion-Sella reference line in cephalometry. A methodological study. Am J Orthod 1984;86:427-434.

Pancherz H, Hägg U. Dentofacial orthopedics in relation to somatic maturation. An analysis of 70 consecutive cases treated with the Herbst appliance. Am J Orthod 1985;88:273-287.

Pancherz H, Littmann C. Somatische Reife und morphologische Veränderungen des Unterkiefers bei der Herbst Behandlung. Inf Orthod Kieferorthop 1988;20:455-470.

Pancherz H, Littmann C. Morphologie und Lage des Unterkiefers bei der Herbst-Behandlung. Eine kephalometrische Analyse der Veränderungen bis zum Wachstumsabschluss. Inf Orthod Kieferorthop 1989;21:493-513.

Pancherz H, Michaelidou C. Temporomandibular joint changes in hyperdivergent and hypodivergent Herbst subjects. A long-term roentgenographic cephalometric study. Am J Orthod Dentofac Orthop 2004;126:153-161.

Pancherz H, Szyska M. Analyse der Halswirbelkörper statt Handknochen zur Bestimmung der skelettalen und somatischen Reife. Eine Reliabilitäts- und Validitätsuntersuchung. Inf Orthod Kieferorthop 2000;32:151-161.

Pancherz H, Stickel A. Lageveränderungen des Condylus Mandibulae bei der Herbst-Behandlung. Inf Orthod Kieferorthop 1989;21:517-527.

Pancherz H, Ruf S, Kohlhas, P. "Effective condylar growth" and chin position changes in Herbst treatment: a cephalometric roentgenographic long-term study. Am J Orthod Dentofac Orthop 1998;114:437-446.

Pancherz H, Ruf S, Thomalske-Faubert C. Mandibular articular disk position changes during Herbst treatment: a prospective longitudinal MRI study. Am J Orthod Dentofac Orthop 1999;116:207-214.

Ruf S, Pancherz H. Temporomandibular joint adaptation in Herbst treatment: a prospective magnetic resonance imaging and cephalometric roentgenographic study. Eur J Orthod 1998a;20:375-388.

Ruf S, Pancherz H. Long-term TMJ effects of Herbst treatment: a clinical and MRI study. Am J Orthod Dentofac Orthop 1998b;114:475-483.

Ruf S, Pancherz H. Temporomandibular joint remodeling in adolescents and young adults during Herbst treatment: a prospective longitudinal magnetic resonance imaging and cephalometric radiographic investigation. Am J Orthod Dentofac Orthop 1999;115:607-618.

Ruf S, Pancherz H. Does bite-jumping damage the TMJ? A prospective longitudinal clinical and MRI study of Herbst patients. Angle Orthod 2000;70:183-199.

53

Chapter 7

Short-term effects on the dentoskeletal structures

Research

Since the reintroduction of the Herbst appliance into the orthodontic community in 1979 (Pancherz 1979), its effectiveness in the correction of sagittal and vertical (deep bite) discrepancies in Class II:1 and Class II:2 malocclusions has been documented in many investigations (Pancherz 1982a, 1982b, 1985, 1996, 1997, Wieslander 1984, 1993, Valant and Sinclair 1989, McNamara et al. 1990, Windmiller 1993, Sidhu et al. 1995, Konik et al. 1997, Obijou and Pancherz 1997, Wong et al.1997, Lai and McNamara 1998, Ruf and Pancherz 1999a, Franchi et al. 1999, Pancherz and Ruf 2000a, 2000b, Nelson et al. 2000, Hägg et al. 2002, Burkhardt et al. 2003, Schaefer et al. 2004, de Almeida et al. 2005). Originally, it was thought that Class II and deep bite correction were accomplished mainly by mandibular skeletal changes (Pancherz 1979). Later research, however, revealed that maxillary and mandibular dental components also contributed to the correction of the Class II dental arch relationship (Pancherz 1982a, Barnett et al. 2008) and the deep overbite (Pancherz 1982b).

The mechanism of Class II correction in Herbst appliance treatment. A cephalometric investigation (Pancherz, 1982a)

Sagittal skeletal and dental changes contributing to Class II correction in Herbst appliance treatment were evaluated quantitatively on lateral head films. The subject material comprised 42 Class II:1 malocclusions with a deep overbite. Twenty-two (mean age 12.1 years; SD = 0.9 years) were treated with the Herbst appliance for an average period of 6.2 months (SD = 14 days). The other 20 subjects (mean age 11.2 years; SD = 0.7 years) served as an untreated control group for an average period of 6.2 months (SD = 11 days). They had the same severity of malocclusion and skeletofacial morphology as the treated cases. In the treatment group, a banded Herbst appliance with a partial anchorage system (see Chapter 3: Design, construction and clinical management of the Herbst appliance) was used. In the Herbst group, lateral head films - one in habitual occlusion and one with the mouth wide open (for the identification of the condylar head) - were taken before treatment, at start of treatment when the appliance was placed and at the end of treatment, 6 months later. In the control group, habitual occlusion and mouth-open head films were taken before and after the observation period of 6 months.

Standard cephalometrics and the SO-Analysis (see Chapter 6: Herbst research - subjects and methods) were used in the evaluation of the head films. Angular measurements were made to the nearest 0.5 degrees and linear measurements to the nearest 0.5 mm. No correction was made for linear enlargement (approximately 7% in the median plane). The true treatment effects were calculated by taking the normal growth changes in the control group into account. In order to analyze possible changes in the position of the condylar head within the glenoid fossa, TMJ radiographs in centric occlusion were taken before and after treatment. An oblique lateral transcranial projection with individualized technique was used (Omnell and Petersson 1976).

After Herbst treatment all subjects attained a Class I occlusion with normal overjet and overbite. Considering the skeletal and dental changes in the control group, Herbst treatment resulted in an increase in mandibular length (Fig. 7-1) and SNB angle (Fig. 7-2). The effects of the Herbst appliance on the maxillary and mandibular jaw bases as well as on the dentition are shown in Figs. 7-3 and 7-4.

The improvement of the occlusion was about equally a result of skeletal and dental changes. Class II molar correction (Fig. 7-5) was mainly a result of an advancement of the mandible, and a posterior movement of the maxillary molars. Overjet correction (Fig. 7-6) was mainly a result of an advancement of the mandible and an anterior movement of the mandibular incisors. It should be noted, however, that there was large individual variation. When comparing the mandibular position (pogonion point), when the appliance was placed, with that after treatment, on average, 54% of the original amount of mandibular advancement recovered.

The TMJ radiographs revealed an unchanged condyle-fossa relationship in all subjects investigated.

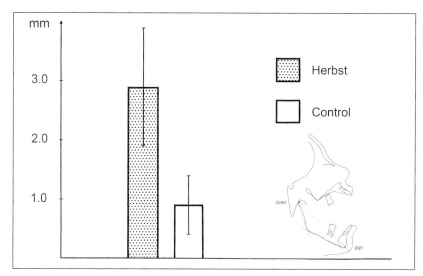

Fig. 7-1 Increase (Mean and SD) of mandibular length in Class II:1 malocclusions during 6 months: Herbst (n=22); Control (n=20).

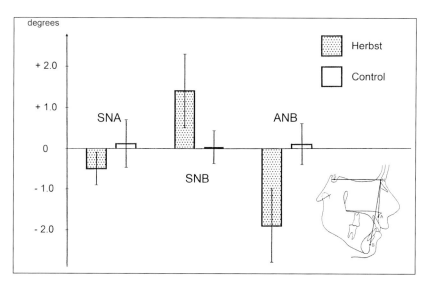

Fig. 7-2 Changes (Mean and SD) of angles SNA, SNB and ANB in Class II:1 malocclusions during 6 months: Herbst (n=22); Control (n=20).

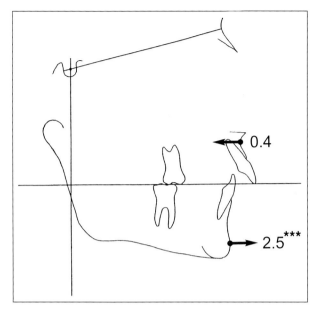

Fig. 7-3 Skeletal effects (Mean) of 6 months of Herbst treatment in 22 Class II:1 malocclusions considering normal growth changes in the control group. *** indicates significance at 0.1 % level.

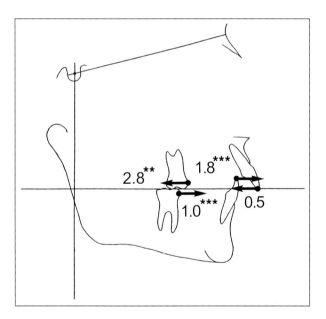

Fig. 7-4 Dental effects (Mean) of 6 months of Herbst treatment in 22 Class II:1 malocclusions considering normal growth changes in the control group. ** indicates significance at 1% level. *** indicates significance at 0.1 % level.

Interpretation of the results

The increase in mandibular prognathism (SNB angle) after Herbst treatment was mainly a result of an increase in mandibular length, which, in turn, was most likely due to condylar growth stimulation in response to bite jumping as has been verified by resonance imaging (MRI) of the TMJ in growing (Ruf and Pancherz 1998) as well as in adult (Ruf and Pancherz 1999b) Herbst subjects and by histological analysis of the TMJ in growing (Peterson and McNamara 2003) and non-growing (McNamara et al. 2003) monkeys treated with the Herbst appliance. The dental changes seen during therapy were basically a result of anchorage loss in the two dental arches (see Chapter 19: Anchorage problems). The telescope mechanism produced a posterior-directed force on the maxillary teeth and an anterior-directed force on the mandibular teeth. Clinically, anchorage loss was noted by developing spaces between the maxillary canines and first premolars and by proclination of the mandibular incisors (see Clinical examples: Figs. 7-10 and 7-11). The relative stability of the maxillary incisors was due to the fact that these teeth were not incorporated into the partial maxillary anchorage system used in these subjects.

As mentionend above, 54% of the original mandibular advancement recovered. This was the result of the dental anchorage loss. As the telescope mechanism pushed the maxillary first molars posteriorly and the mandibular first premolars anteriorly the telescopic inter-axis distance increased, thus allowing the mandible to slide backwards.

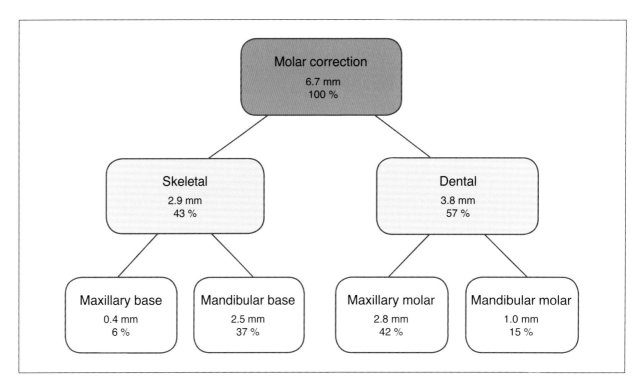

Fig. 7-5 The mechanism of Class II molar correction (Mean) in 22 Class II:1 malocclusions treated with the Herbst appliance for 6 months. In the evaluation, normal growth changes in the control group were considered. *(Revised from Pancherz 1982a)*

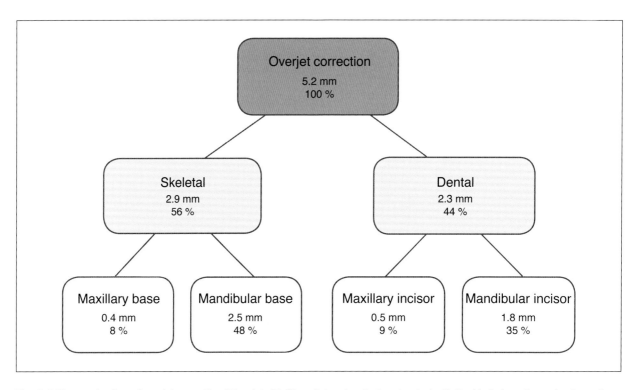

Fig. 7-6 The mechanism of overjet correction (Mean) in 22 Class II:1 malocclusions treated with the Herbst appliance for 6 months. In the evaluation, normal growth changes in the contol group were considered. *(Revised from Pancherz 1982a)*

Vertical dentofacial changes during Herbst appliance treatment. A cephalometric investigation (Pancherz 1982b)

The effect of Herbst treatment on the vertical dimensions of the dentofacial complex was analyzed in the same 42 Class II:1 deep bite malocclusions presented above. In the assessment of the vertical skeletal and dental changes, lateral head films in habitual occlusion were used.

When placing the Herbst appliance at the start of treatment, the maxillary and mandibular front teeth were placed in an incisal edge-to-edge position and the bite was opened (measured as the difference in overbite between before treatment and start of treatment) by an average of 5.5 mm. During treatment, while the appliance was in place, 2.7 mm (49%) of the initial bite opening recovered. Thus, the net overbite reduction was, on average, 2.8 mm which is 51% of the initial value (5.5 mm). Herbst treatment resulted in an increase in lower facial height, intrusion of the mandibular incisors and maxillary molars and enhanced vertical eruption of the mandibular molars (Fig. 7-7). Due to the vertical dental changes, the angulation of the maxillary and mandibular occlusal planes increased in relation to the NSL (Fig. 7-8). The Herbst appliance had only a limited effect on vertical maxillary and mandibular jaw positions, as expressed by the palatal plane angle (NL/NSL) and mandibular plane angle (ML/NSL), respectively (Fig. 7-8).

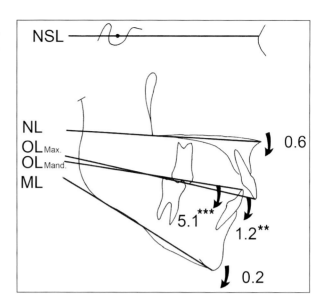

Fig. 7-8 Mean vertical angular effects (in degrees) in 22 Class II:1 malocclusions during 6 months of Herbst treatment considering normal growth changes in the control group. ** indicates significance at 1% level. *** indicates significance at 0.1% level.

Interpretations of the results

Overbite reduction at the end of Herbst treatment was mainly accomplished through an intrusion of the lower incisors and extrusion of the lower molars. It must be pointed out, however, that part of the registered changes in vertical mandibular incisor position resulted from a proclination of these teeth.

The overbite recovery of 49% during treatment, while the appliance was in place, can be explained by the sagittal maxillary and mandibular dental anchorage loss, allowing the mandible to slide backwards and the bite to close (Fig 7-9).

Furthermore, the Class II intermaxillary mechanism of the Herbst appliance produced an upward directed force on the maxillary molars and a downward directed force on the mandibular incisors resulting in an intrusion of these teeth. The extrusion of the lower molars seen can be explained by the lateral open bite existing during the first 3-4 months of treatment allowing the teeth to erupt freely. This was facilitated due to the fact that they were not included in the lower anchorage system .

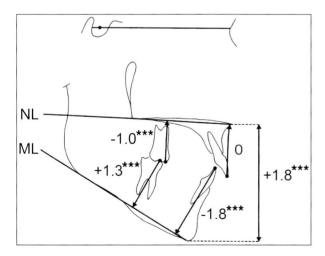

Fig. 7-7 Mean vertical linear effects (in mm) in 22 Class II:1 malocclusions during 6 months of Herbst treatment considering normal growth changes in the control group. *** indicates significance at 0.1% level.

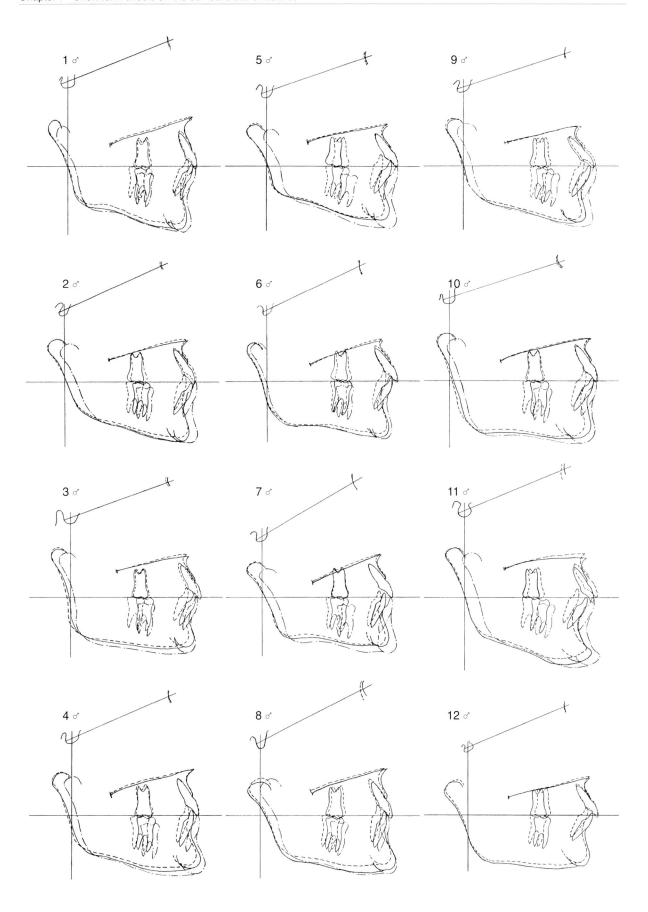

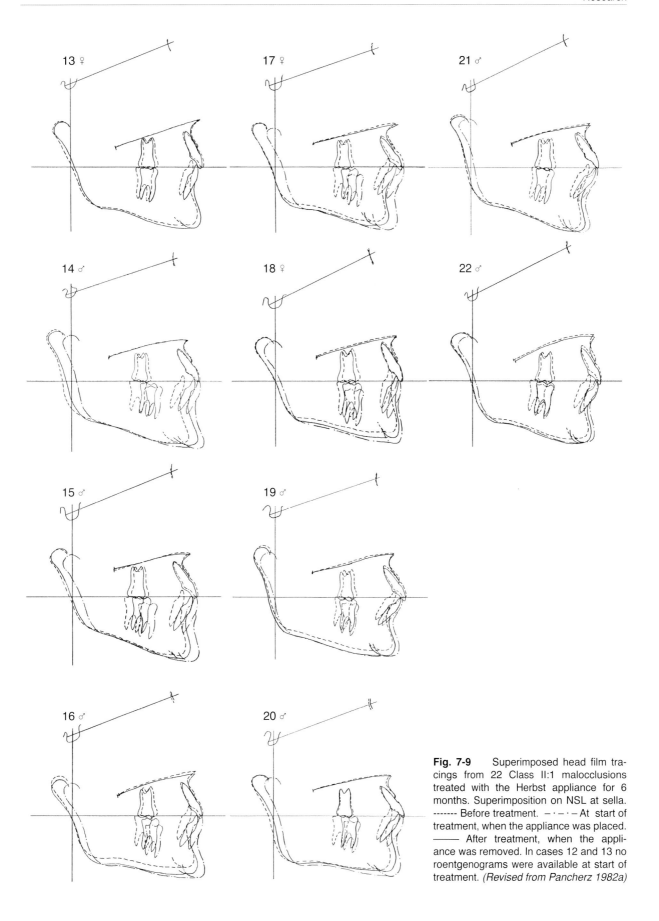

Fig. 7-9 Superimposed head film tracings from 22 Class II:1 malocclusions treated with the Herbst appliance for 6 months. Superimposition on NSL at sella. ------ Before treatment. − · − · − At start of treatment, when the appliance was placed. ——— After treatment, when the appliance was removed. In cases 12 and 13 no roentgenograms were available at start of treatment. *(Revised from Pancherz 1982a)*

Clinical examples

From the group of 22 Herbst patients, two subjects, No. 5 (Case 7-1) and No. 11 (Case 7-2) are presented. Treatment length in both cases was 6 months. A banded Herbst appliance with a partial anchorage system (see Chapter 3: Design, construction and clinical management of the Herbst appliance) was used in both subjects. No other treatment was performed. In both cases pronounced skeletal and dental treatment changes were seen.

Case 7-1 (Fig. 7-10)

11-year-old male. At pretreatment the overjet was 10.5 mm, the overbite 7.5 mm and the ANB angle 7.5 degrees. A full Class II molar relationship existed. After treatment the overjet and overbite were both reduced to 3.0 mm and the ANB angle to 5.5 degrees. The molars were in an overcorrected Class I relationship of one cusp width. Mandibular length (pgn – cond) had increased by 4.5 mm. Note the dental anchorage loss: the space appearing between the maxillary canine and first premolar and the proclination of the mandibular anterior teeth.

Case 7-2 (Fig. 7-11)

13-year-old male. At pretreatment the overjet was 12.5 mm, the overbite 6.5 mm and the ANB angle 8.0 degrees. A full Class II molar relationship was present. After treatment the overjet was reduced to 4.0 mm and the overbite to 3.0 mm. The ANB angle was reduced to 5.0 degrees. The molars were in an overcorrected Class I relationship of 1.5 cusp width. Mandibular length (pgn – cond) had increased by 5.0 mm. Note the dental anchorage loss: the space appearing between the maxillary canine and first premolar and the proclination of the mandibular anterior teeth.

Conclusions and clinical implications

In children with a Class II:1 malocclusion and a deep overbite, a Herbst treatment of 6 months generally results in Class I dental arch relationships, a normal overjet and normal overbite.

- The improvement of the occlusal relationships is a result of mandibular skeletal and maxillary and mandibular dental changes.
- Class II molar correction is mainly due to an increase in mandibular length and posterior movement of the maxillary molars.
- Overjet correction is mainly due to an increase in mandibular length and proclination of the mandibular incisors.
- Overbite correction is mainly due to an intrusion / proclination of the mandibular incisors and extrusion of the mandibular molars.

The clinician should be aware of the dental changes occurring during Herbst treatment and consider these changes when designing the treatment strategy and planing the posttreatment retention.

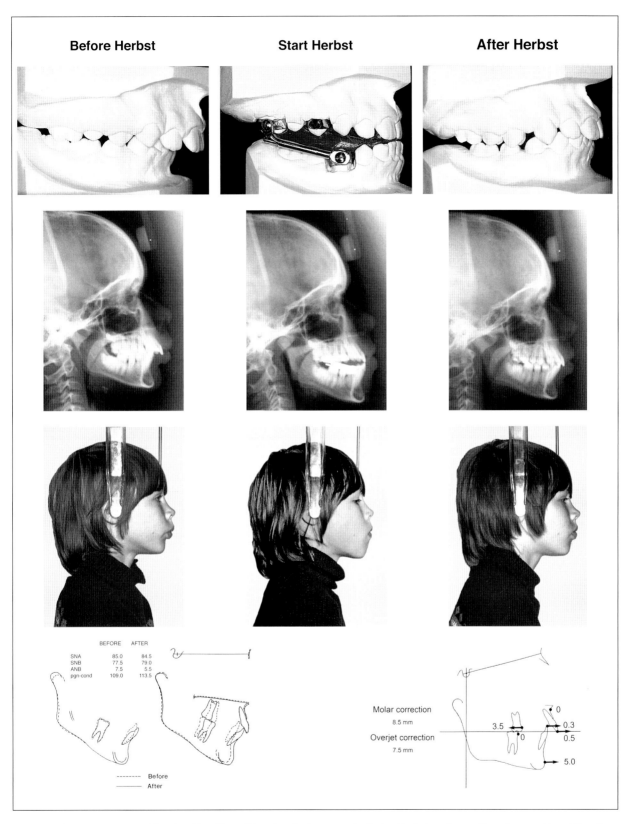

Before Herbst   **Start Herbst**   **After Herbst**

	BEFORE	AFTER
SNA	85.0	84.5
SNB	77.5	79.0
ANB	7.5	5.5
pgn-cond	109.0	113.5

-------- Before
——— After

Molar correction
8.5 mm

Overjet correction
7.5 mm

Fig. 7-10 Case 7-1. 11-year-old male with a Class II:1 malocclusion treated with the Herbst appliance. Superimposed head films from before and after treatment were analyzed by means of standard cephalometrics and the SO-Analysis (see Chapter 6: Herbst research - subjects and methods).

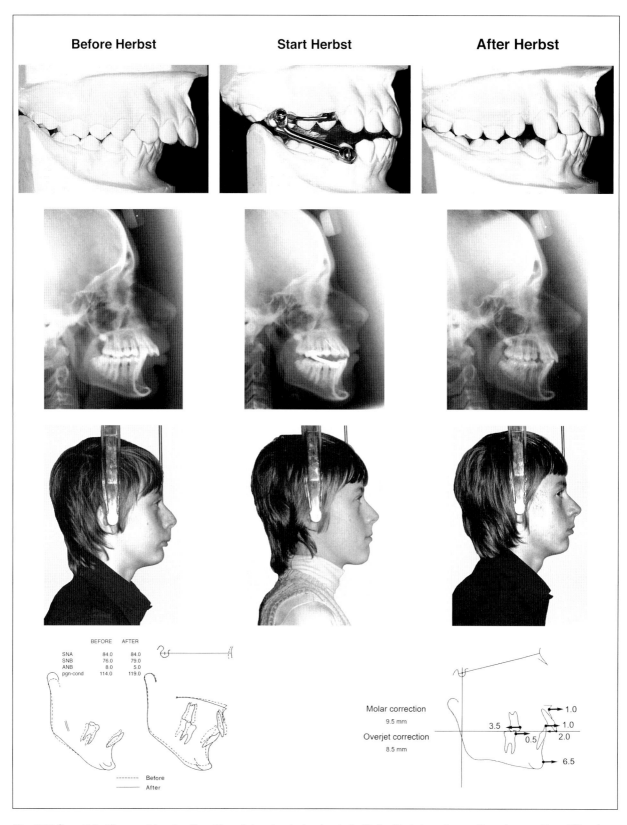

Fig. 7-11 Case 7-2. 13-year-old male with a Class II:1 malocclusion treated with the Herbst appliance. Superimposed head films from before and after treatment were analyzed by means of standard cephalometrics and the SO-Analysis (see Chapter 6: Herbst research - subjects and methods).

References

Barnett GA, Higgins DW, Major PW, Flores Mir C. Immediate skeletal and dentoalveolar effects of the crown- or banded type Herbst appliance on Class II division malocclusion. A systematic review. Angle Orthod 2008;2:361-369.

Burkhardt DR, McNamara JA, Baccetti T. Maxillary molar distalization or mandibular enhancement: a cephalometric comparison of comprehensive treatment including the pendulum and the Herbst appliance. Am J Orthod Dentofac Orthop 2003;123:108-116.

de Almeida MR, Henriques JFC, de Almeida PR, Ursi W, McNamara JA. Short-term treatment effects produced by the Herbst appliance in the mixed dentition. Angle Orthod 2005;75:540-547.

Franchi L, Baccetti T, McNamara JA. Treatment and posttreatment effects of acrylic splint Herbst appliance therapy. Am J Orthod Dentofac Orthop 1999;115:429-438.

Hägg U, Due X, Rabie AB. Initial and late treatment effects of headgear-Herbst appliance with mandibular step-by-step advancement. Am J Orthod Dentofac Orthop 2002;122:477-485.

Konik M, Pancherz H, Hansen K. The mechanism of Class II correction in late Herbst treatment. Am J Orthod Dentofac Orthop 1997;112:87-91.

Lai M, McNamara JA. An evaluation of two-phase treatment with the Herbst appliance and preadjusted edgewise therapy. Semin Orthod 1998;4:46-58.

McNamara JA, Howe RP, Dischinger TG. A comparison of the Herbst and the Fränkel appliances in the treatment of Class II malocclusions. Am J Orthod Dentofac Orthop 1990;98:134-144.

McNamara JA, Peterson JE, Pancherz H. Histologic changes associated with the Herbst appliance in adult rhesus monkeys (Macaca mulatta). Semin Orthod 2003;9:26-40.

Nelson B, Hansen K, Hägg U. Class II correction in patients treated with Class II elastics and with fixed functional appliances: a comparative study. Am J Orthod Dentfac Orthop 2000;118:142-149.

Obijou C, Pancherz H. Herbst appliance treatment of Class II, Division 2 malocclusions. Am J Orthod Dentofac Orthop 1997;112:287-291.

Omnell KA, Peterson A. Radiography of the temporomandibular joint utilizing oblique lateral transcranial projections. Odontol Revy 1976;27:77-92.

Pancherz H. Treatment of Class II malocclusions by jumping the bite with the Herbst appliance. A cephalometric investigation. Am J Orthod 1979;76:423-442.

Pancherz H. The mechanism of Class II correction in Herbst appliance treatment. A cephalometric investigation. Am J Orthod 1982a;82:104-113.

Pancherz H. Vertical dentofacial changes during Herbst appliance treatment. A cephalometric investigation. Swed Dent J 1982b;Suppl 15:189-196.

Pancherz H. The Herbst appliance - Its biologic effects and clinical use. Am J Orthod 1985;87:1-20.

Pancherz H. Herbst Apparatur. In: Kleines Lehrbuch der Angle-Klasse II,1 unter besonderer Berücksichtigung der Behandlung. Eds. RR Miethke, D Drescher. Berlin: Quintessenz, 1996:225-251.

Pancherz H. The modern Herbst appliance. In: Dentofacial Orthopedics with Functional Appliances. Chapter 16. Eds. TM Graber, T Rakosi, AG Petrovic. St. Louise: Mosby 1997:336-366.

Pancherz H, Ruf S. The Herbst appliance: Research based updated clinical possibilities. World J Orthod 2000a;1:17-31.

Pancherz H, Ruf S. Herbst Apparatur. In Kieferorthopädie II, Therapie. Praxis der Zahnheilkunde 11/II. Ed. P Dietrich. Urban & Fischer 2000b:282-297.

Peterson JE, McNamara JA. Temporomandibular joint adaptations associated with Herbst appliance treatment in juvenile rhesus monkeys (Macaca mulatta). Sem Orthod 2003;9:12-25.

Ruf S, Pancherz H. Dentoskeletal effects and facial profile changes in young adults treated with the Herbst appliance. Angle Orthod 1999a;69:239-246.

Ruf S, Pancherz H. Temporomandibular joint remodeling in adolescents and young adults during Herbst treatment: a prospective longitudinal magnetic resonance imaging and cephalometric radiographic investigation. Am J Orthod Dentofac Orthop 1999b;69:115:607-618.

Schaefer AT, McNamara JA, Franchi L. A cephalometric comparison of treatment with the Twin-block and stainlesss steel crown Herbst appliance followed by fixed appliance therapy. Am J Orthod Dentofac Orthop 2004;126:7-15.

Sidhu MS, Kharbanda OP, Sidhu SS. Cephalometric analysis of changes produced by a modified Herbst appliance in the treatment of Class II division 1 malocclusion. Br J Orthod 1995;22:1-12.

Valant JR, Sinclair PM. Treatment effects of the Herbst appliance. Am J Orthod Dentofac Orthop 1989;95:138-147.

Wieslander L. Intensive treatment of severe Class II malocclusions with a headgear-Herbst appliance in the mixed dentition. Am J Orthod Dentofac Orthop 1984;86:1-13.

Wieslander L. Long-term effect of treatment with the headgear-Herbst appliance in the early mixed dentition. Stability or relapse? Am J Orthod Dentofac Orthop 1993;104:319-329.

Windmiller EC. The acrylic splint Herbst appliance: a cephalometric evaluation. Am J Orthod Dentofac Orthop 1993;104:73-84.

Wong GWK, So LLY, Hägg U. A comparative study of sagittal correction with the Herbst appliance in two ethical groups. Eur J Orthod 1997;19:195-204.

Chapter 8

Long-term effects on the dentoskeletal structures

Research

Immediately after Herbst treatment, overcorrected sagittal and vertical dental arch relationships with an incomplete cuspal interdigitation of the maxillary and mandibular teeth (Pancherz 1979, 1981, 1982, 1985, 1997, Obijou and Pancherz 1987, Pancherz and Ruf 2000) and a proclination of the mandibular incisors (Pancherz and Hansen 1986, Hansen et al. 1997) are common findings. As a result of recovering tooth movements especially during the first 6 months posttreatment, the occlusion settles into Class I and the mandibular incisors upright (Pancherz and Hansen 1986, Hansen et al. 1997).

On a long-term basis the stability of Class II correction seems to be more dependent on a stable cuspal interdigitation of the maxillary and mandibular teeth (Pancherz 1981, 1991, Pancherz and Hansen 1986) than on a favorable growth pattern (Pancherz and Fackel 1990, Hansen et al. 1991, Hansen and Pancherz 1992, Bock and Pancherz 2006). The long-term effects of Herbst treatment on the maxillary and mandibular dental arches (arch perimeter, arch width, available space) have been considered in one publication (Hansen et al. 1995) only.

Occlusal changes during and after Herbst treatment: a cephalometric investigation (Pancherz and Hansen 1986)

The interrelation between skeletal and dental components that contribute to sagittal changes in the occlusion during and after Herbst treatment were assessed quantitatively on lateral head films.

The subject material comprised 40 consecutively treated Class II:1 malocclusions in which no mult-

ibracket appliances were used after Herbst therapy. The mean age of the subjects at the start of treatment was 12.5 years (SD=1.1 year). Treatment time was on average 7 months (SD=1 month). The patients were re-examined 6 and 12 months posttreatment. In 16 subjects a partial anchorage system and in 24 subjects a total anchorage system of the Herbst appliance was used (see Chapter 3: Design, construction and clinical management of the Herbst appliance).

Following Herbst treatment, retention was performed in 25 subjects (an activator in 19 subjects, a maxillary plate in 1 subject and a maxillary plate together with a mandibular lingual arch wire, from first molar to first molar, or a cuspid-to-cuspid retainer in 5 subjects). No retention was performed in 15 subjects.

Lateral head films in habitual occlusion from before treatment, after treatment, 6 months and 12 months posttreatment were evaluated using the SO-Analysis (see Chapter 6: Herbst research - subjects and methods).

Treatment changes

After 7 months of Herbst treatment when the appliance was removed, a Class I dental arch relationship existed in 7 subjects and an overcorrected Class I or Class III dental arch relationship in 33 subjects. During treatment (T), overjet and sagittal molar relationship improved by an average of 6.9 mm and 6.3 mm, respectively (Fig. 8-1). This was a result of a 2.2 mm greater mandibular than maxillary growth, a 2.3 mm lingual movement of the maxillary incisors, a 2.4 mm labial movement of the mandibular incisors, a 2.0 mm distal movement of the maxillary molars and a 2.1 mm mesial movement of the mandibular molars.

Posttreatment changes

During the follow-up period of 12 months (P1 + P2) the occlusion settled into Class I in all subjects. Overjet and sagittal molar relationship recovered by an average of 2.3 mm and 1.7 mm, respectively (Fig. 8-1). About 90% of the occlusal recovery occurred during the first 6 months posttreatment (P1). In 58% of the subjects the occlusal recovery was exclusively a result of tooth movements. In 42% of the subjects an unfavorable maxillary-mandibular growth relationship did, however, contributed to a minor degree to the occlusal recovery.

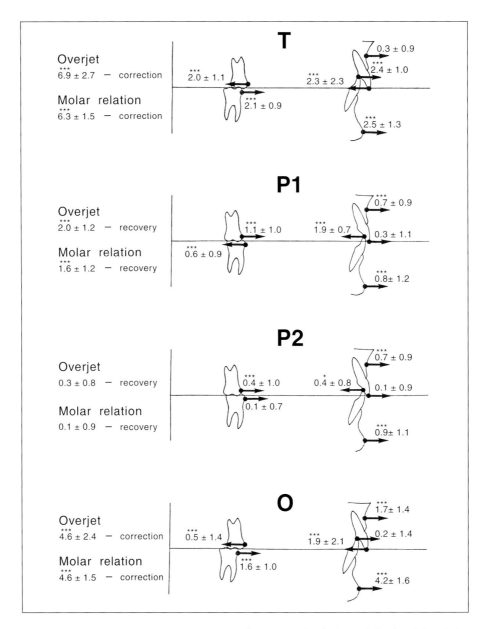

Fig. 8-1 Short-term follow-up effects of the Herbst appliance in 40 Class II:1 malocclusions: skeletal and dental changes (mm) contributing to alterations in overjet and sagittal molar relationships (SO-Analysis). Registrations (Mean and SD) during the treatment period of 7 months (T), posttreatment period 1 of 6 months (P1), posttreatment period 2 of 6 months (P2) and total observation period of 19 months (O). (*Revised from Pancherz and Hansen 1986*)

Interpretation of the results

Treatment changes

The skeletal and dental changes occurring during the active phase of Herbst treatment were previously discussed in Chapter 7.

When comparing the 16 subjects with partial anchorage with the 24 subjects with total anchorage, the maxillary molars moved posteriorly and the mandibular incisors moved anteriorly by, on average, the same amount in both anchorage forms. The results were similar to those of Franchi et al.(1999) using the acrylic splint Herbst appliance. The extension of the appliance incorporating more dental units (total anchorage), seemed thus not to reduce the strain placed on the teeth in the maxillary buccal and mandibular labial segments to a clinically significant degree. A large individual variation in treatment response existed, however (see Chapter 19: Anchorage problems).

Posttreatment changes

During the follow-up period of 12 months (P1 + P2), a 30% recovery in the sagittal dental arch relationship occurred and a stable cuspal interdigitation in Class I was established in all subjects. After settling of the teeth, the occlusion remained remarkably stable. This has also been confirmed in a long-term follow-up study by Hansen and Pancherz (1992) in which Herbst patients were re-examined at the end of growth, at least 5 years after treatment (Fig.8-2). When looking at the subjects at the end of the total observation (O) period, the mandibular incisors had, on average, returned to their original position, while the lower molars had moved forward. However, the consequent reduction in mandibular arch length did not result in anterior crowding (Hansen et al. 1997). This can be explained by the fact that a forward movement of the molars was possible in cases with a pre-treatment excess of space in the mandibular dental arch due to persisting deciduous second molars.

When comparing the 25 subjects in which retention was performed with those 15 without retention, a difference between the groups was found for the maxillary molars only. The posttreatment recovery in maxillary molar position was less in the retention than in the non-retention group. The activators used for retention in 19 of the subjects retained only the teeth in the maxillary buccal segments. In the mandible, on the other hand, the acrylic of the activator was deliberately removed from behind the anterior teeth and mesially and distally to the buccal teeth to allow for a settling of the occlusion. Thus, post-

treatment dental changes in the mandible were the same in retention and non-retention subjects (see also Chapter 25: Relapse and retention).

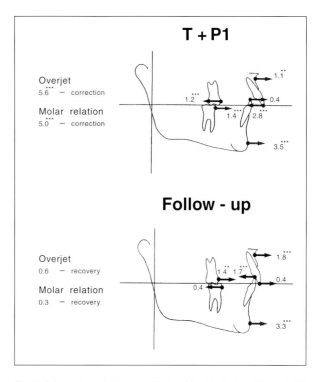

Fig. 8-2 Long-term follow-up effects of the Herbst appliance in 32 Class II:1 malocclusions: skeletal and dental changes (mm) contributing to alterations in overjet and sagittal molar relationships. Registrations (Mean) during the combined periods of 7 months of treatment (T) plus the first 6 months posttreatment (P1) (which means after the occlusion had settled) and during the follow-up period of 6.7 years. (*Revised from Hansen and Pancherz 1992*)

Long-term effects of Herbst treatment on the mandibular incisor segment: a cephalometric and biometric investigation (Hansen et al. 1997)

Mandibular incisor changes during and after Herbst treatment were analyzed with respect to tooth inclination and anterior crowding.

At the time of the examination the total sample of consecutive Class II:1 malocclusions treated with the Herbst appliance at the Department of Orthodontics, University of Lund, Sweden, comprised 152 subjects. From this sample 24 subjects (15 males and 9 females) fulfilling the following criteria were selected: (1) no permanent teeth extracted; (2) eruption of all mandibular canines before treatment; (3) total mandibular anchorage, incorporating all teeth from first molar to first molar; (4) no further treatment after Herbst therapy; (5) all subjects out of retention for at least 3 years at the final examination; (6) an observation period of at least 5 years after treatment; (7) growth completed at the end of the follow-up period (Hansen et al.1991).

The mean age of the patients before treatment was 13.0 years (SD=1.3 years) and at the follow-up 19.6 years (SD=1.2 years). The average treatment time with the Herbst appliance was 0.6 years (SD=0.1 year). The follow-up period was 6.0 years (SD=1.0 years).

Posttreatment retention (activator and mandibular cuspid-to-cuspid retainer) was performed in 17 subjects. Seven subjects were not retained.

Lateral head films and dental casts in habitual occlusion were analyzed. Registrations were performed before treatment, after treatment, 6 months posttreatment and at follow-up when growth was completed (at least 5 years after treatment).

The head film analysis comprised of angular measurement for the assessment of inclination changes of the mandibular incisors in relation to the cranial base as well as to the mandibular plane. Furthermore, linear measurements were performed to evaluate the sagittal position changes of the incisal edges of the mandibular incisors in relation to the chin (pogonion).

The biometric analysis of the dental casts comprised calculations of the available space in the mandibular anterior segment.

Treatment changes

During the 7 months of Herbst treatment the mandibular incisors were proclined (Fig. 8-3A) in relation to the cranial base by 11.3 degrees (SD=4.3 degrees) and in relation to the mandibular plane by 10.8 degrees (SD=4.3 degrees). The incisal edge moved anteriorly by 3.2 mm (SD=1.3 mm). The available space was not significantly increased and was generally unaffected by treatment (Fig. 8-4).

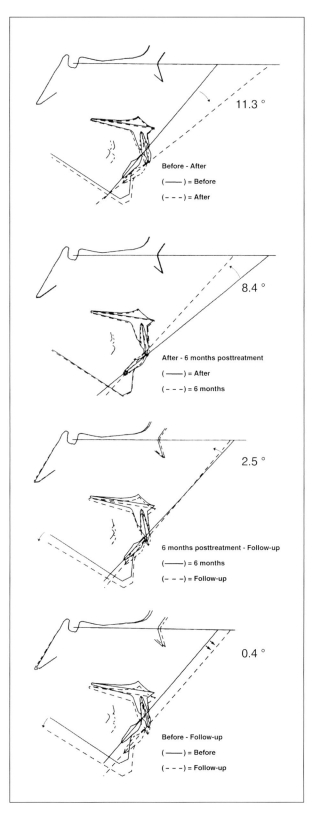

Fig. 8-3 Mean composite tracings of 24 Class II:1 malocclusions treated with the Herbst appliance. The mandibular incisor inclination changes to the cranial base are shown. (*Revised from Hansen et al. 1997*)

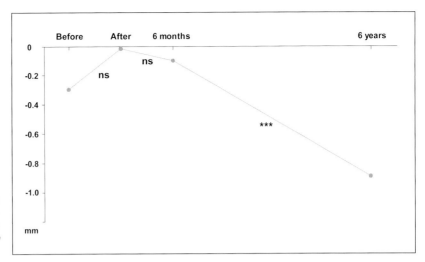

Fig. 8-4 Changes in available space (Mean) in 24 Class II:1 malocclusions treated with the Herbst appliance. A negative value indicates crowding. (*Revised from Hansen et al. 1997*)

Posttreatment changes

During the first 6 months after treatment the mandibular incisor inclination recovered (Fig. 8-3B) in relation to the cranial base by 8.4° (SD=3.6°) and in relation to the mandibular plane by 7.9° (SD=3.7°). The incisal edge moved posteriorly by 2.5 mm (SD=1.3 mm). The available space was, on average, unchanged (Fig. 8-4).

During the period from 6 months posttreatment to the end of growth the mandibular incisors recovered (retroclined) further (Fig. 8-3C) in relation to the cranial base by 2.5° (SD=4.1°), while tooth inclination remained unchanged in relation to the mandibular plane. The incisal edge moved posteriorly by 1.7 mm (SD=1.8 mm). The available space decreased by 0.8 mm (SD=0.8 mm) (Fig. 8-4).

Total observation period changes

During the period from before treatment to the end of growth, the net effect of Herbst treatment on the mandibular incisors was an almost unchanged inclination in relation to the cranial base (Fig. 8-3D) but a proclination of 2.6° (SD=4.5°) in relation to the mandibular plane. The incisal edge moved posteriorly by 0.9 mm (SD=1.8 mm). The available space decreased by 0.6 mm (SD=0.9 mm) (Fig. 8-4).

Interpretation of the results

During the treatment period the mandibular incisors proclined extensively due to difficulties in anchorage control (Pancherz and Hansen 1988). In the available space analysis, it was evident that minor spacing occurred in a few subjects. This finding was not expected, as the lower incisors were supposed to be controlled by the sectional arch wire. However, due to the incisor proclination during treatment the teeth

were placed in a larger anterior dental arch perimeter. Orthodontically moved teeth tend to return to their original position and angulation after therapy. During the first posttreatment period the lower incisors recovered, although an average net increase of 3 degrees of proclination and of 0.7 mm incisal edge advancement remained 6 months after Herbst therapy. The available arch space seemed, however, unaffected by the recovering tooth movements. During the second posttreatment period, from 6 months after treatment to the end of growth the lower incisors retroclined in relation to the cranial base but remain unchanged in relation to the mandibular plane. However, the individual variation was large. As an anterior rotation of the mandibular plane in relation to cranial base existed posttreatment (Hansen et al. 1997), the findings indicate that a change in lower incisor angulation did not compensate for the rotation of the mandible, as suggested by Björk and Skieller (1972).

During the second posttreatment period the sagittal distance of the mandibular incisor edges to the chin increased. This can also be explained by the existing anterior mandibular rotation. With the incisor inclination unchanged in relation to the mandibular plane, the incisal edge moves less forward than the chin (pogonion) during an anterior mandibular rotation.

Fudalej and Årtun (2007) found that high-angled and low-angled facial patterns were not associated with incrised risk of postretention relapse.

At the end of the follow-up period the average available space was -0.9 mm (ranging from +0.2 mm to -2.2 mm). This minor amount of crowding developing over a period of 6 years can not be considered to be the result of Herbst treatment but might rather be due to a physiologic process in connection with normal growth (Henrikson et al. 2001).

During the total observation period (treatment and posttreatment) the mandibular incisors proclined in relation to the mandibular plane, but remained unchanged in relation to the cranial base. This is in agreement with the dentoalveolar compensatory mechanism described by Björk and Skieller (1972). An average reduction of the available space of only 0.6 mm occurred during this period (Fig. 8-4). This is similar to the value seen in untreated subjects (Sinclair and Little 1983) during the same age interval.

Long-term effects of the Herbst appliance on the dental arches and arch relationships: a biometric study (Hansen et al. 1995)

The treatment and posttreatment effects of the Herbst appliance on the dental arches and arch relationships were analyzed biometrically using dental casts.

At the time of examination the total sample of consecutive Class II:1 malocclusions treated with the Herbst appliance at the Department of Orthodontics, University of Lund, Sweden, comprised 170 subjects. From this sample, 53 subjects (33 males and 20 females) fulfilling the following criteria were selected: (1) no permanent teeth extracted; (2) eruption of all permanent canines before treatment; (3) an observation period of at least 5 years after treatment; (4) growth completed at the end of the follow-up period (Hansen et al. 1991). Twenty-nine subjects received retainers (activators) for 1-2 years and 14 received fixed appliance therapy for 6-12 months after Herbst treatment.

The mean age of the subjects before treatment was 12.5 years (SD=1.2 years) and at the end of follow-up 19.3 years (SD=1.2 years). The average treatment time with the Herbst appliance was 0.6 years (SD=0.1 years). The average follow-up period was 6.1 years (SD=1.0 year).

Measurements on the dental casts were made: before treatment, after treatment, 6 months posttreatment and at follow-up, when growth was completed (at least 5 years posttreatment).

Sagittal dental arch relationships
The percentage of cases exhibiting normal, distal or mesial molar and canine relationships at each stage of examination are shown in Fig. 8-5. No gender differences existed.

During treatment the sagittal molar relationship was overcorrected in most cases, while the sagittal canine relationship was normalized. At the end of treatment, only 4% (n=2) of the cases displayed a distal molar relationship. A distal canine relationship remained in 8% (n=4) of the cases. In the long-term (an average of 6 years after treatment), Herbst therapy resulted in a a normal sagittal molar relationship as well a normal canine relationship in 68% (n=36) of the subjects.

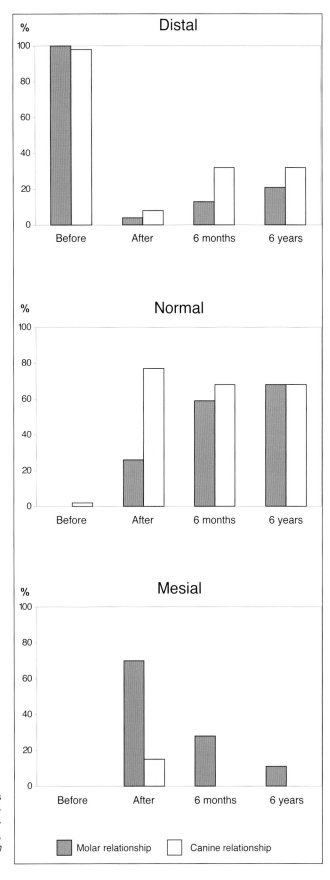

Fig. 8-5 Sagittal molar and canine relationships in 53 Class II:1 malocclusions treated with the Herbst appliance. The percentage of cases with a distal, normal and mesial relationship is given. Registrations from before and after treatment, 6 months and 6 years posttreatment. (*Revised from Hansen et al. 1995*)

Overjet

The mean values of overjet observed at each examination are shown in Fig. 8-6.

During treatment, the overjet was overcorrected in most cases. The average overjet reduction was 6.8 mm (from 8.4 mm to 1.6 mm). During the first 6 months posttreatment the overjet recovered by 1.7 mm, on average, and remained unchanged thereafter. The overjet observed at the follow-up examination was 3.7 mm which means a net reduction of 4.7 mm on average.

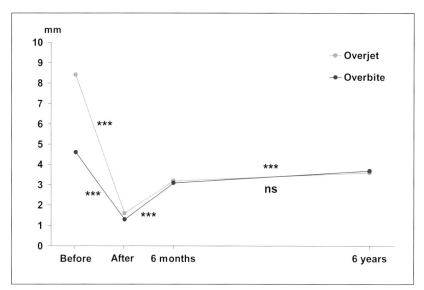

Fig. 8-6 Overjet and overbite (Mean) in 53 Class II:1 malocclusions treated with the Herbst appliance. Registrations from before and after treatment, 6 months and 6 years posttreatment. (*Revised from Hansen et al. 1995*)

Overbite

The mean values of the overbite observed at each examination are shown in Fig. 8-6.

During treatment the overbite was overcorrected in most cases. The average overbite reduction was 3.4 mm (from 4.6 mm to 1.2 mm). During the first 6 months posttreatment the overbite recovered by 1.7 mm and during the following 5.1 years by 0.6 mm on average. The overbite observed at the follow-up examination was 3.6 mm which means a net reduction of 1.0 mm on average.

Arch perimeter

The maxillary and mandibular arch perimeters were measured between the distal contact points of the second premolars (or second deciduous molars). The mean values of the arch perimeter measurements observed at each examination are shown in Fig. 8-7.

During treatment the arch perimeter increased by 2.7 mm in the maxilla and by 0.9 mm in the mandible, on average. During the first and second observation periods after treatment, the arch perimeter decreased by more than 2 mm in each period in both the maxilla and in the mandible. At the time of follow-up, the arch perimeter had decreased 2.1 mm in the maxilla and 3.3 mm in the mandible when compared to the pretreatment values.

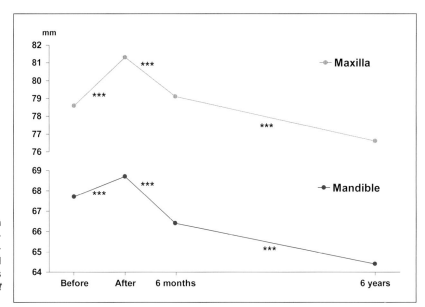

Fig. 8-7 Maxillary and mandibular arch perimeters (Mean) in 53 Class II:1 malocclusions treated with the Herbst appliance. Registrations from before and after treatment, 6 months and 6 years posttreatment. (*Revised from Hansen et al. 1995*)

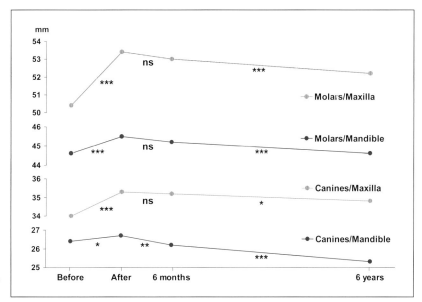

Fig. 8-8 Maxillary and mandibular intermolar and intercanine arch widths (Mean) in 53 Class II:1 malocclusions treated with the Herbst appliance. Registrations from before and after treatment, 6 months and 6 years posttreatment. (*Revised from Hansen et al. 1995*)

Arch width

The mean values of the maxillary and mandibular intermolar and intercanine arch widths observed at each examination are given in Fig. 8-8.

During treatment the maxillary and mandibular arch widths in the molar and canine areas increased. During the first and second observation period after treatment, the increase of the maxillary molar and canine dental arch widths accomplished during treatment remained virtually stable, while the mandibular molar and canine arch widths recovered.

At the time of follow-up, the maxillary intermolar arch width had increased by 1.8 mm and the maxillary intercanine arch width by 0.9 mm when compared to the pretreatment values. The mandibular intermolar arch width, on the other hand, was unchanged and the intercanine arch width had decreased by 1.0 mm in comparison to the pretreatment value.

Interpretation of the results

As 33 cases had either activators for retention or multibracket appliances after Herbst treatment, while 20 cases had no retainers, it must be acknowledged that this could have influenced the results, especially those of the first posttreatment period.

However, the effects of the retention appliances seemed to be small and the only significant difference found between the retention and non-retention groups was for the mesial movement of the maxillary molars, which was less in the retention subjects (Pancherz and Hansen 1986).

Sagittal dental arch relationships

The Herbst appliance corrected or overcorrected both molar and canine sagittal relationships in most cases. However, treatment was more effective in the molar than in the canine region (Fig. 8-5). This was most likely due to the maxillary anchorage system: the molars connected to the first premolars on each side, were pushed posteriorly by the telecope mechanism (Pancherz and Hansen 1986). The canines, on the other hand, were not directely engaged in the maxillary anchorage system.

As the occlusion was settling, some recovery was noted during the first posttreatment period both in sagittal molar and canine relationship. During the second posttreatment period, when the settling of the occlusion was over, the molar and canine relationships seemed to be rather stable.

Overjet and overbite

The overjet and overbite were reduced in all patients during treatment. Although both overjet and overbite increased posttreatment (especially during the first 6 months posttreatment) (Fig. 8-6), the amount of change was of minor clinical significance. The posttreatment changes might well be explained by the recovery of incisor tooth position (Pancherz and Hansen 1986) and the settling of the occlusion.

Arch perimeter

The arch perimeter increased during treatment both in the maxilla and in the mandible (Fig. 8-7). The increase in the maxilla was most probably due to the distal movement of the maxillary molars as shown in previous investigations (Pancherz 1982, Pancherz and Hansen 1986, Pancherz and Anehus-Pancherz 1993). In the mandible the increase in arch perimeter could be explained by the proclination of the lower incisors (Pancherz and Hansen 1986, Hansen et al. 1997). In the first posttreatment period, the shortening of the arch perimeter was probably caused by the recovery of maxillary and mandibular tooth positions (Pancherz and Hansen 1986, 1988). In the long-term perspective, changes in arch perimeters could be considered to be due to normal growth changes (Moyers et al. 1976).

Arch width

The maxillary intermolar width increased during Herbst treatment (Fig.8-8). This was most likely due to the force from the telescope mechanism directed to the upper molars in a both distal and buccal direction. Despite the subsequent reduction in intermolar width during the first and second posttreatmet periods, a net increase during the total observation period was found in the majority of the subjects. This net increase was more pronounced in the male than in the female sample. The gender dimorphism found was in accordance with normal dental development (Moyers et al. 1976, van der Linden 1983).

The maxillary intercanine width increased less during Herbst treatment than the intermolar width (Fig.8-8). In comparison to normal dental development (Moyers et al. 1976, van der Linden 1983), the expansion in the maxillary intercanine width must be considered to be a result of Herbst treatment. This may be explained by the mode of action of the appliance, as the premolars were connected to the molars by a lingual sectional arch wire and the canines to the premolars by a labial sectional arch wire. Thus, the premolars and the canines will be moved in a distal-buccal direction into a broader part of the maxillary arch when the telescope mechanism moves the maxillary molars posteriorly. Some relapse in intercanine width occurred during the first and second posttreatment periods. However, at the end of the observation period a net increase in maxillary intercanine width existed.

The mandibular intermolar width was increased to some extend during Herbst treatment (Fig.8-8). This expansion was probably not a result of the forces from the Herbst appliance but rather a compensatory expansion, secondary to the maxillary expansion. The expansion was larger when compared to normal dental development (Moyers et al. 1976, van der Linden 1983). During the first and second posttreatment periods, however, a decrease in mandibular intermolar width was found. Thus, on a long-term basis, the intermolar width remained unchanged.

The mandibular intercanine width was also increased during Herbst treatment (Fig. 8-8). As mandibular intercanine width tends to decrease after the age of 12 years (Moyers et al. 1976, van der Linden 1983), the expansion seen in the Herbst subjects may be considered to be an effect of treatment. The expansion was, however, small and of no clinical significance. Some relapse in intercanine width was found during the first and second posttreatment periods. At the end of the follow-up period the majority of the subjects displayed a constricted intercanine width, which corresponds to normal dental development (Moyers et al. 1976, van der Linden 1983).

Clinical examples

From the group of 40 Herbst subjects (Pancherz and Hansen 1986), the dental casts of the first ten subjects are presented. The casts were from before treatment, after treatment and from follow-up 12 months posttreatment (Fig. 8-9). One of the 40 cases, No. 23 (Case 8-1), is presented in detail in Fig. 8-10.

Case 8-1 (Fig. 8-10)
13-year-old male treated with the Herbst appliance for 6 months. At the end of treatment Class III dental arch relationships existed. Treatment was started with a banded Herbst appliance with partial maxillary and total mandibular anchorage. After 2 months of therapy, maxillary anchorage was increased by incorporating the front teeth into the anchorage (total anchorage). A maxillary plate and a mandibular lingual arch wire (from molar to molar) was used for retention after Herbst treatment. No other treatment was performed. The occlusion settled into Class I during the first 6 months posttreatment.

Treatment changes (T)
Overjet was reduced by 9.7 mm. This was accomplished by a 7.4 mm greater mandibular than maxillary growth, a 0.1 mm lingual movement of the maxillary incisors and a 2.2 mm labial movement of the mandibular incisors. Sagittal molar relationship was improved by 10.9 mm. Besides the difference in mandibular-maxillary growth, this was a result of a 2.4 mm posterior movement of the maxillary molars and a 1.1 mm anterior movement of the mandibular molars.

Posttreatment changes (P1+P2)
During the follow-up period of 12 months, overjet recovered by 1.6 mm and sagittal molar relationship by 3.6 mm. These recovering changes were partly a result of an unfavorable mandibular-maxillary growth relationship and partly due to tooth movements. From the group of 24 Herbst subjects (Hansen et al. 1997), four cases (Cases 8-2 to 8-5) are presented to show the large individual variation in mandibular anterior crowding developing long-term.

Case 8-2 (Fig. 8-11)
13.9-year-old female treated with the Herbst appliance for 7 months and followed for 5 years posttreatment. The available space was -0.1 mm before treatment, 0 mm after treatment, -0.8 mm 6 months posttreatment and -0.9 mm 5 years posttreatment.

Case 8-3 (Fig. 8-12)
12.6-year-old male treated with the Herbst appliance for 7 months and followed 5 years posttreatment. The available space was -0.2 mm before treatment, 0.1 mm posttreatment, -0.2 mm 6 months posttreatment and -0.8 mm 5 years posttreatment.

Case 8-4 (Fig. 8-13)
12.2-year-old male treated with the Herbst appliance for 6 months and followed 5 years posttreatment. The available space was 0 mm before treatment, 0 mm posttreatment, +0.3 mm 6 months posttreatment and -1.8 mm 5 years posttreatment.

Case 8-5 (Fig. 8-14)
13.7-year-old male treated with the Herbst appliance for 7 months and followed 5 years posttreatment. The available space was +0.3 mm before treatment, +0.3 mm after treatment, +0.2 mm 6 months posttreatment and -1.9 mm 5 years posttreatment.

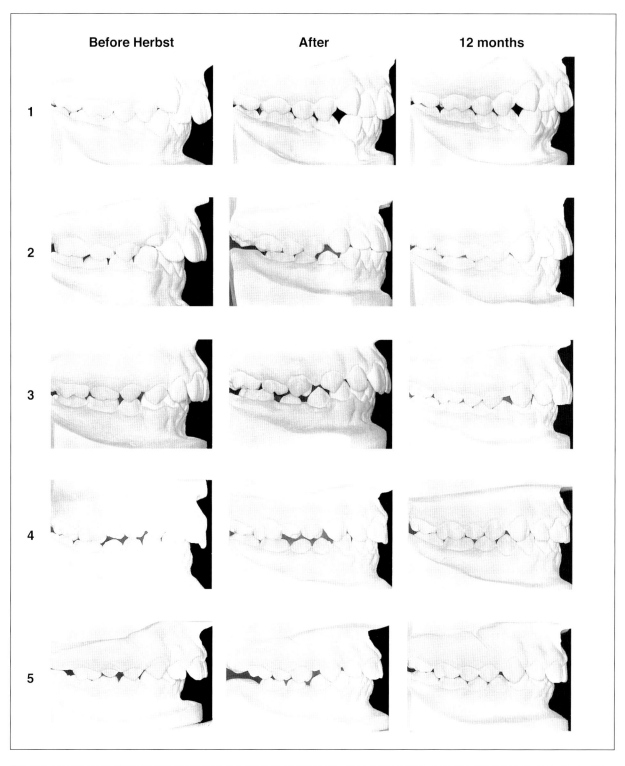

Fig. 8-9 Plaster casts of the first 10 cases from the group of 40 Class II:1 subjects treated exclusively with the Herbst appliance (Pancherz and Hansen 1986). Registrations from before treatment, after treatment and 12 months posttreatment. Postreatment stability of the occlusion was seen in all cases except for the cases 6, 7, and 8. (*Revised from Pancherz 1981*)

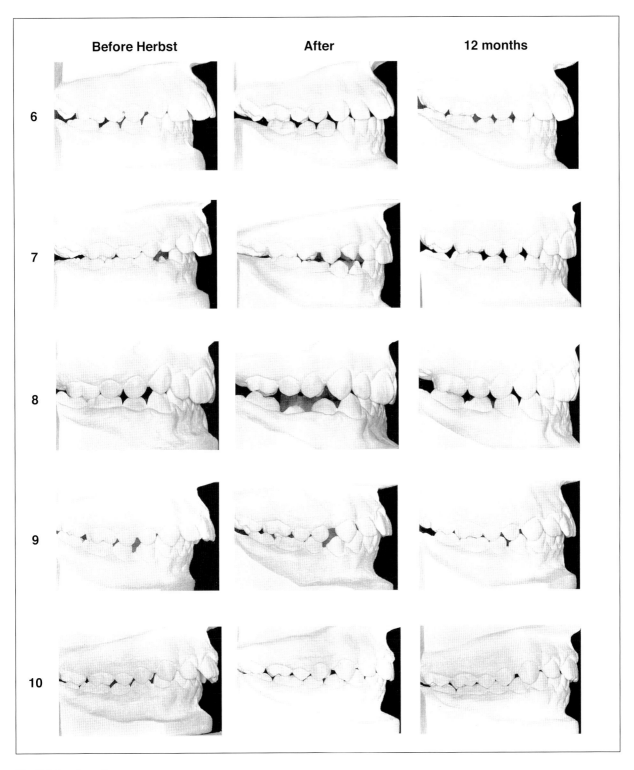

Before Herbst   **After**   **12 months**

6

7

8

9

10

Fig. 8-9 (continued)

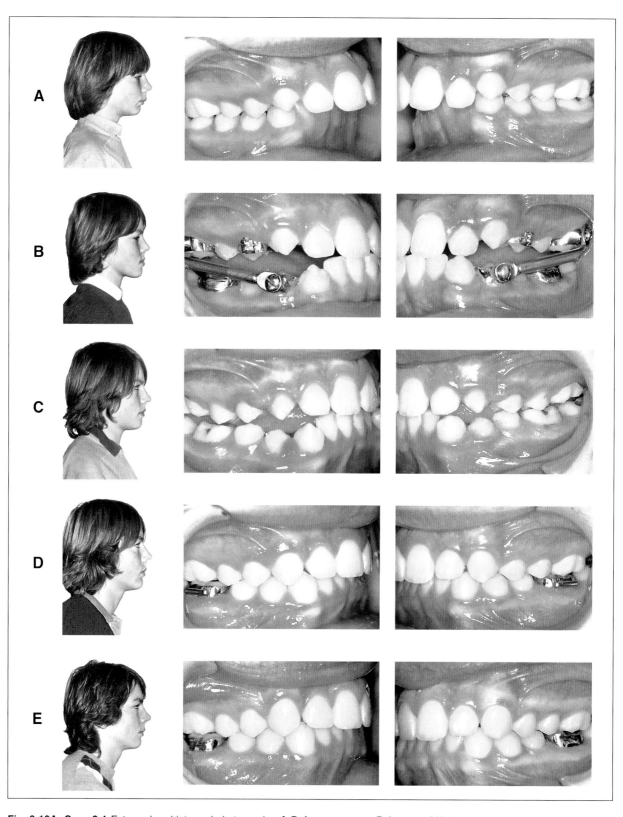

Fig. 8-10A   Case 8-1 Extraoral and intraoral photographs. **A** Before treatment. **B** At start of Herbst treatment. **C** After 6 months of treatment when the appliance was removed. **D** 6 months posttreatment. **E** 12 months posttreatment. (*Revised from Pancherz and Hansen 1986*)

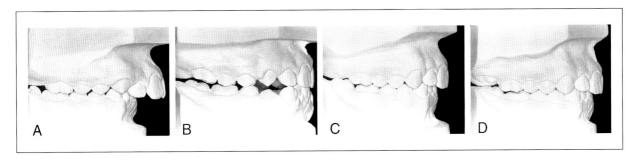

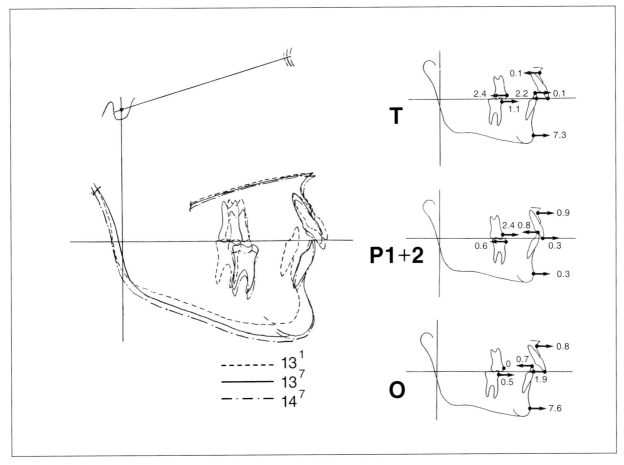

Fig. 8-10B Case 8-1 Plaster casts. **A** Before treatment. **B** After 6 months of Herbst treatment. **C** 6 months posttreatment. **D** 12 months posttreatment. Cephalometric tracings superimposed on the nasion-sella line with sella as registration point. Diagrammatic representation (SO-Analysis) of sagittal skeletal and dental changes (mm) occurring during the treatment period (T), posttreatment period of 12 months (P1+P2) and total observation period (O) of 18 months. (*Revised from Pancherz and Hansen 1986*)

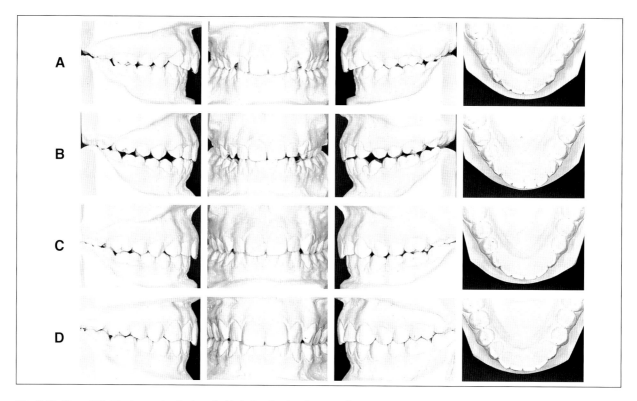

Fig. 8-11 Case 8-2 Plaster casts of a female Herbst patient at the age of 13.9 years. **A** Before treatment. **B** After 7 months of Herbst treatment. **C** 6 months posttreatment. **D** 5 years posttreatment. *(Revised from Hansen et al. 1997)*

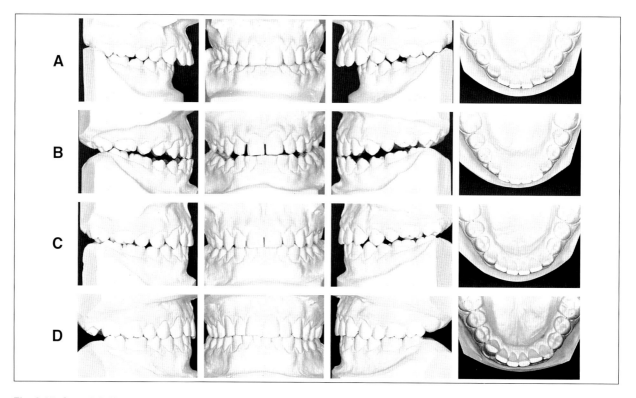

Fig. 8-12 Case 8-3 Plaster casts of a male Herbst patient at the age of 12.6 years. **A** Before treatment. **B** After 7 months of Herbst treatment. **C** 6 months posttreatment. **D** 5 years posttreatment. (*Revised from Hansen et al. 1997*)

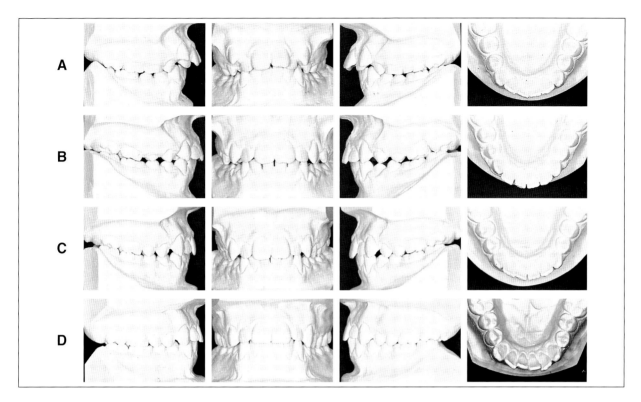

Fig. 8-13 Case 8-4 Plaster casts of a male Herbst patient at the age of 12.2 years. **A** Before treatment. **B** After 6 months of Herbst treatment. **C** 6 months posttreatment. **D** 5 years posttreatment. (*Revised from Hansen et al. 1997*)

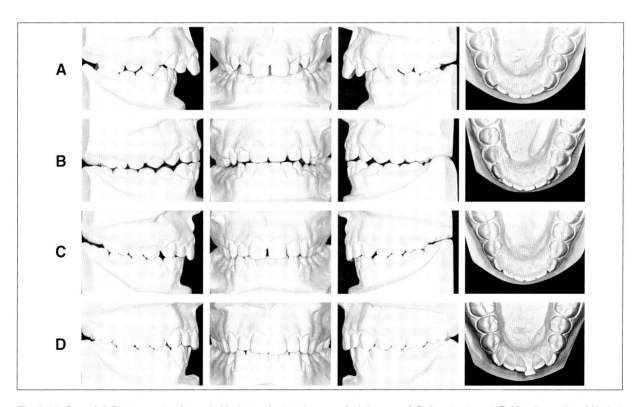

Fig. 8-14 Case 8-5 Plaster casts of a male Herbst patient at the age of 13.7 years. **A** Before treatment. **B** After 7 months of Herbst treatment. **C** 6 months posttreatment. **D** 5 years posttreatment. (*Revised from Hansen et al. 1997*)

Conclusions and clinical implications

- As Herbst treatment is performed during a relatively short period, the dentition will be in a state of instability after the appliance is removed. Posttreatment supervision of the settling of the occlusion is necessary. For retention as well as for making interocclusal adjustments possible, an activator is recommended.
- Proclination of the mandibular incisors during Herbst treatment did not result in incisor crowding after treatment.
- On a long-term basis, Herbst treatment generally resulted in normal sagittal molar and canine relationships, and in a reduction of overjet and overbite.
- Although maxillary and mandibular arch perimeters increased during treatment, in the long-term the arch perimeters followed a normal developmental pattern.
- The increase in maxillary intermolar and intercanine arch widths during treatment remained rather stable after treatment. The mandibular intermolar and intercanine widths seemed, in the long-term, to be unaffected by treatment.
- In a long-term perspective, the development of incisor crowding is probably associated with normal craniofacial growth changes. From the clinical point of view this justifies the retention of the mandibular incisors at least until the end of the growth period.

References

Björk A, Skieller V. Facial development and tooth eruption. Am J Orthod 1972;62:339-383.

Bock N, Pancherz H. Herbst treatment of Class II:1 malocclusions of the retrognathic and prognathic facial type. Angle Orthod 2006;76:930-941

Franchi L, Baccetti T, McNamara JA. Treatment and posttreatment effects of acrylic splint Herbst appliance therapy. Am J Orthod Dentofac Orthop 1999;115:429-438.

Fudalej P, Årtun J, Mandibular growth rotation effects on postretention stability of mandibular incisor alignmet. Angle Orthod 2007; 77:199-205.

Hansen K, Pancherz H, Hägg U. Long-term effects of the Herbst appliance in relation to the treatment growth period: a cephalometric study. Eur J Orthod 1991;13:471-481.

Hansen K, Pancherz H. Long-term effects of Herbst treatment in relation to normal growth development: a cephalometric study. Eur J Orthod 1992;14:285-295.

Hansen K, Iemamnueisuk P, Pancherz, H. Long-term effects of the Herbst appliance on the dental arches and arch relationships: a biometric study. Br J Orthod 1995;22:123-134.

Hansen K, Koutsonas TG, Pancherz H. Long-term effects of Herbst treatment on te mandibular incisor segment: a cephalometric and biometric investigation. Am J Orthod Dentofac Orthop 1997;112:92-103.

Henrikson J, Persson M, Thilander B. Long-term stability of dental arch form in normal occlusion from 13 to 31 years of age. Eur J Orthod 2001;23:51-61.

Moyers RE, van der Linden FPGM, Riolo, ML, McNamara JA. Standards of human occlusal development. Monograph 5, Craniofacial growth series. Ann Arbor: Center for Human Growth and Development, The University of Michigan 1976.

Obijou C, Pancherz H. Herbst appliance treatment of Class II, Division 2 malocclusions. Am J Orthod Dentofac Orthop 1997;112:287-291.

Pancherz H. Treatment of Class II malocclusions by jumping the bite with the Herbst appliance. A cephalometric investigation. Am J Orthod 1979;76:423-442.

Pancherz H. The effect of continuous bite jumping on the dentofacial complex: a follow-up study after Herbst appliance treatment of Class II malocclusions. Eur J Orthod 1981;3:49-60.

Pancherz H. The mechanism of Class II correction in Herbst appliance treatment. A cephalometric investigation. Am J Orthod 1982;82:104-113.

Pancherz H. The Herbst appliance – Its biologic effects and clinical use. Am J Orthod 1985;87:1-20.

Pancherz H. The nature of Class II relapse after Herbst appliance treatment: a cephalometric long-term investigation. Am J Orthod Dentofac Orthop 1991;100:220-233.

Pancherz H. The modern Herbst appliance. In: TM Graber, T Rakosi, AG Petrovic (eds). Dentofacial Orthopedics with Functional Appliances. St. Louise: Mosby 1997:336-366.

Pancherz H, Anehus-Pancherz M. The headgear effect of the Herbst appliance: a cephalometric long-term study. Am J Orthod Dentofac Orthop 1993;103:510-520.

Pancherz H, Fackel U. The skeletofacial growth pattern pre- and postdentofacial orthopaedics. A long-term study of Class II malocclusions treated with the Herbst appliance. Eur J Orthod 1990;12:209-218.

Pancherz H, Hansen K. Occlusal changes during and after Herbst treatment: a cephalometric investigation. Eur J Orthod 1986;8:215-228.

Pancherz H, Hansen K. Mandibular anchorage in Herbst treatment. Eur J Orthod 1988;14:285-295.

Pancherz H, Ruf S. The Herbst appliance: research based updated clinical possibilities. World J Orthod 2000;1:17-31.

Sinclair PM, Little RM. Maturation of untreated normal occlusion. Am J Orthod 1983;83:114-123.

Van der Linden FPGM. Development of the dentition. Quintessence Books, Chicago 1983.

Chapter 9

The headgear effect of the Herbst appliance

Research

In orthodontics and dentofacial orthopedics, part of the Class II correction strategy is to move the maxillary teeth, especially the molars, posteriorly. The classical way to do this is with a headgear (Kloehn 1961). As a headgear is removable, its effect is dependent on the cooperation of the patient. Therefore, fixed non-compliance appliances for maxillary molar distalization have been developed such as the Pendulum (Hilgers 1992) and the Distal Jet (Carano and Testa 1996).

The Herbst appliance, being fixed, also works independently of patient compliance and has a "headgear effect" which has been verfied in many well controlled clinical studies in both growing (Pancherz 1979, 1982, Wieslander 1984, Pancherz and Hansen 1986, Pancherz and Anehus-Pancherz 1993, Ruf and Pancherz 1997, Konik et al. 1997) and nongrowing (Ruf and Pancherz 1999) Class II subjects. In these investigations, it has been shown that the ability of the appliance to move the maxillary buccal teeth (premolars and molars) posteriorly results in 23% to 42% of the Class II molar correction seen during Herbst therapy.

The headgear effect of the Herbst appliance: a cephalometric long-term study (Pancherz and Anehus-Pancherz 1993)

The short- and long-term effects of the Herbst appliance on the maxillary complex were evaluated on lateral head films.

At the time of examination the total sample of consecutive Class II:1 malocclusions treated with the Herbst appliance at the Department of Orthodontics, University of Lund, Sweden, comprised of 118 patients. Herbst therapy resulted in Class I or overcorrected Class I dental arch relationships in all 118 cases. After Herbst treatment, 39 subjects received multibracket appliances. Of the remaining 79 subjects, those 45 subjects who were followed at least 5 years (5 to 10 years) after Herbst therapy were surveyed. All patients were treated during the adolescent growth period (Pancherz and Hägg 1985). At the end of the observation period, growth was finished in all cases but one.

The mean age of the subjects before treatment was 12.4 years (SD=1.1 years) and at follow-up 19.4 years (SD=1.4 years). The average treatment time with the Herbst appliance was 0.6 years. The follow-up period was 6.4 years. A partial anchorage system of the Herbst appliance was used in 19 subjects and a total anchorage system in 26 subjects (see Chapter 3: Design, construction and clinical management of the Herbst appliance)

Posttreatment retention (activator with and without a mandibular cuspid-to-cuspid retainer) for 1 to 2 years was performed in 29 of the subjects. 16 subjects were not retained.

At the time of follow-up, 9 subjects exhibited a Class II molar relapse (a deviation of more than half cusp width from Class I relationship) whereas 36 subjects were considered stable.

In the evaluation of the immediate treatment effects, 30 untreated Class II subjects of the same age and skeletofacial morphology as the Herbst group were used as controls. In the evaluation of the long-term effects of Herbst therapy, an ideal occlusion group, the Bolton Standards (Broadbent et al. 1975) was used for comparison.

In the Herbst patients, lateral head films with the mouth wide open (in order to identify the maxillary teeth more easily) were evaluated. The radiographs were taken before and after 0.6 years (SD=0.1 years) of Herbst treatment, 0.5 years (SD=0.0 years) after treatment when the occlusion had settled (Pancherz and Hansen 1986) and 6.4 years (SD=1.0 years) after treatment.

In the untreated Class II control group, mouth open lateral head films from before and after 0.5 years (SD=0.4 years) were evaluated.

In the Bolton Standards (comprising 16 males and 16 females) the composite head film tracings in habitual occlusion were evaluated at the ages of 11 and 18 years. For this group, adjustments were made for radiographic enlargement of 5.5% in order to adapt it to the radiographs of the Herbst and Class II control samples.

All registrations were made on tracings of the roentgenograms. The maxillary occlusal line (OL) and occlusal line perpendicular (OLP) through sella (S) were used as a reference grid for linear measurements (Pancherz 1982). The grid and the nasion-sella line (NSL) from the first tracing were transferred to the following tracings in a series after superimposition of the head films on the stable bone structures of the anterior cranial base (Björk and Skieller 1983).

Sagittal molar position changes (Fig. 9-1)

During the treatment period (T1) of 0.6 years, the maxillary permanent first molars were distalized in 96% of the Herbst subjects (maximum 4.5 mm), whereas tooth position was unchanged in 4% of the subjects. On average, the molars were distalized 2.1 mm (p<0.001). In the untreated Class II control group, the molars moved mesially by an average of 0.3 mm (p<0.001).

During the first posttreatment period (P1) of 0.5 years, the molars moved mesially (recovery in molar position) in 84% of the Herbst subjects (maximum 4.0 mm). No changes in molar position were seen in 16 subjects. On average, the molars moved mesially by 1.1 mm (p<0.001).

During the second posttreatment period (P2) of 5.9 years, the molars moved further mesially in 73% of the subjects (maximum 5.5 mm). No changes in molar position were seen in 27% of the subjects. On average, the molars moved mesially by 1.6 mm (p<0.001).

During the total observation period (O) of 7.0 years, net effect of distal molar movement during Herbst treatment was found in 27% of the subjects (maxi-

mum 3.5 mm). In 60% of the subjects the molars had moved mesially (maximum 4.0 mm). No changes in molar position were seen in 13% of the subjects. On average, the molars had moved mesially by 0.6 mm (p<0.05) and thus 0.4 mm less than in the Bolton control group.

Vertical molar position changes (Fig. 9-2)

During the treatment period (T1), the maxillary permanent first molars were intruded in 69% of the Herbst subjects (maximum 3.5 mm). In 4% of the subjects extrusive molar movements occurred (maximum 1.0 mm). No changes in vertical molar position were seen in 27% of the subjects. On average, the molars were intruded by 0.7 mm (p<0.001). In the untreated Class II control group the molars extruded an average of 0.4 mm (p<0.001).

During the first posttreatment period (P1), the molars extruded in 89% of the Herbst subjects (maximum 2.5 mm). No changes in vertical molar position were seen in 11% of the subjects. On average, the molars extruded by 1.1 mm (p<0.001).

During the second posttreatment period (P2), extrusive molar movements were seen in all Herbst subjects (maximum 7.5 mm). On average, the molars extruded by 3.5 mm (p<0.001).

During the total observation period (O), extrusive molar movements were seen in all Herbst subjects (maximum 7.5 mm). On average, the molars extruded by 3.9 mm (p<0.001), which was comparable to the changes in the Bolton control group.

Interpretation of the results

The 9 subjects with Class II molar relapse and the 36 subjects without relapse had a comparable dentoskeletal morphology before treatment, responded equally during therapy and were comparable with respect to the early posttreatment changes (P1). During the second posttreatment period (P2), however, adverse molar changes were more pronounced in the relapse than in the stable cases. Two relapse promoting factors (Pancherz 1994) could explain the difference in the adverse molar tooth movements seen in the two groups: (1) a lip-tongue dysfunction habit e.g. atypical swallowing pattern at the end of the total observation period was noted in all relapse cases but in none of the stable cases, and (2) an unstable cuspal interdigitation existed in 8 (89%) of the relapse but in only 2 (6%) of the stable cases.

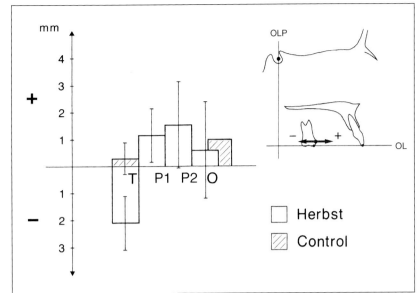

Fig. 9-1 Sagittal maxillary molar position changes (Mean, SD) in 45 Class II:1 malocclusions treated with the Herbst appliance. Registrations during four observation periods: treatment period of 0.6 years (T), posttreatment period 1 of 0.5 years (P1), posttreatment period 2 of 5.9 years (P2) and total observation period of 7.0 years (O). The untreated Class II control group (T) and the Bolton Standards control group (O) are shown. *(Revised from Pancherz and Anehus-Pancherz 1993)*

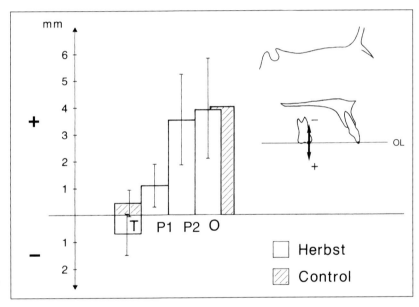

Fig. 9-2 Vertical maxillary molar position changes (Mean, SD) in 45 Class II:1 malocclusions treated with the Herbst appliance. Registrations during four observation periods: treatment period of 0.6 years (T), posttreatment period 1 of 0.5 years (P1), posttreatment period 2 of 5.9 years (P2) and total observation period of 7.0 years (O). The untreated Class II control group (T) and the Bolton Standards control group (O) are shown. *(Revised from Pancherz and Anehus-Pancherz 1993)*

Treatment changes

The telescope mechanism of the Herbst appliance produces a posterior-upward directed force on the maxillary molars. The force system can be compared to that of a high-pull headgear. During treatment the teeth were distalized and intruded. No differences in the amount of sagittal and vertical molar movements were found when comparing the two anchorage systems (partial and total) used (Pancherz and Hansen 1986).

Posttreatment changes

During the first 0.5 years after the Herbst appliance was removed the treatment changes reverted to a great extent and the molars moved anteriorly and extruded. Similar findings were found for headgear treatment (Wieslander and Buck 1974, Melsen 1978). During the following 5.9 years after treatment, the molar changes were mainly a result of normal growth development (Riolo et al. 1974, Broadbent et al. 1975). A difference between the retention and non-retention cases was found for the sagittal molar position only. During the first posttreatment period (P1) the recovery in sagittal molar position was less in the retention than in the non-retention subjects (Pancherz and Hansen 1986). On a long-term basis, however, no group differences were found.

Obviously, the retention period was too short for stabilizing sagittal tooth position changes. Concerning vertical molar position, the activators used for retention after Herbst treatment were not meant to retain vertical tooth position. On the contrary, the acrylic covering the occlusal surfaces was removed to enhance vertical eruption of the molars for further improvement of the overbite.

Neither erupted or unerupted second molars, nor the presence or absence of third molars were found to influence the short- and long-term effects of the Herbst appliance on the sagittal and vertical position of the maxillary first molars.

Clinical examples

Five Class II:1 patients are presented in Figs. 9-3 and 9-4 to illustrate the headgear effect of the Herbst appliance on the maxillary dentition.

Case 9-1 (Fig. 9-3)
12-year-old female with maxillary incisor crowding treated with the Herbst appliance (7 months) for correcting the Class II malocclusion and to create space for the incisors by distalizing the teeth in the lateral segments (headgear effect). Final tooth alignment was accomplished with a multibracket appliance.

Case 9-2 (Fig. 9-3)
12-year-old male with maxillary incisor crowding treated with the Herbst appliance (8 months) for correcting the Class II malocclusion and to create space for the incisors by distalizing the teeth in the lateral segments (headgear effect). Final tooth alignment was accomplished with a multibracket appliance. Note that incisor tooth alignment started already at the end of the Herbst-phase by the use of a sectional arch wire.

Case 9-3 (Fig. 9-3)
18-year-old female with maxillary incisor crowding treated with the Herbst appliance (8 months) for correcting the Class II malocclusion and to create space for the incisors by distalizing the teeth in the lateral segments (headgear effect) Final tooth alignment was accomplished with a multibracket appliance. Note that incisor tooth alignment started already at the end of the Herbst-phase by the use of a sectional arch wire.

Case 9-4 (Fig. 9-3)
24-year-old female with deficient space for the impacted permanent canines. The deciduous canines are persisting. Herbst treatment (12 months) was performed for correcting the Class II malocclusion and to create space for the permanent canines by distalizing the teeth in the lateral segments (headgear effect). Final tooth alignment was accomplished with a multibracket appliance. Note that incisor tooth alignment started already at the end of the Herbst-phase by the use of a sectional arch wire.

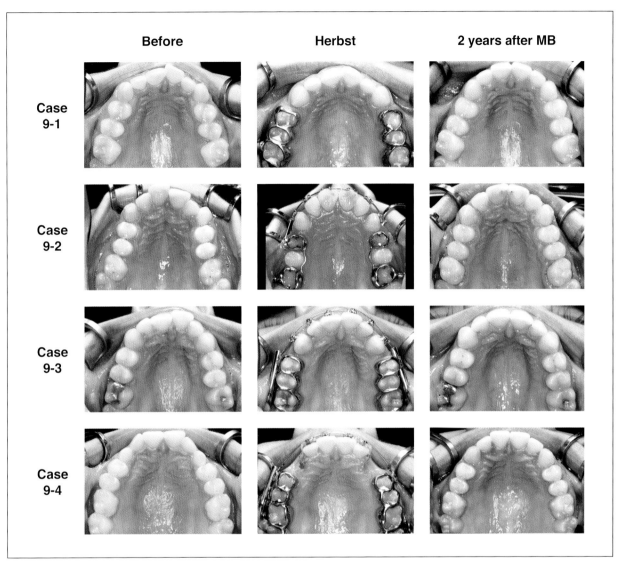

	Before	Herbst	2 years after MB

Case 9-1

Case 9-2

Case 9-3

Case 9-4

Fig. 9-3 Cases 9-1 to 9-4 Headgear effect of the Herbst appliance on the maxillary dentition in four treated Class II:1 malocclusions (Cases 9-1 and 9-2: 12 years of age, Case 9-3: 18 years of age and Case 9-4: 24 years of age). Note the gain of space for the incisors and canines as a result of distal movement of the teeth in the lateral segments (molars and premolars). Registrations at before treatment, during Herbst treatment and 2 years after mulibracket (MB) appliance treatment.

Case 9-5 (Fig. 9-4)

28-year-old female. Herbst treatment (11 months) was performed for correcting the Class II malocclusion. The case demonstrates an extremely intrusive effect of the appliance on the maxillary lateral teeth (high-pull headgear effect). Final tooth alignment was accomplished with a multibracket appliance.

Before

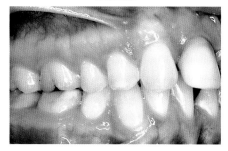

Herbst

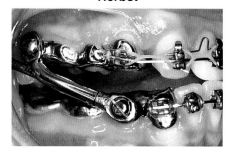

End Herbst

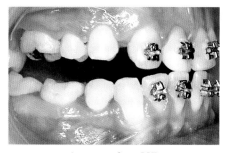

1 year after MB

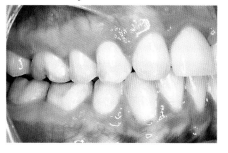

Conclusions and clinical implications

The Herbst appliance has a pronounced high-pull headgear effect on the maxillary molars.

- During treatment, the molars in the study presented were distalized on a general (96% of the subjects) and intruded on a frequent (69% of the subjects) basis.
- In case of inadequate retention, the treatment changes were prone to recover, especially during the first 0.5 years posttreatment (the molars moved anteriorly and extruded.
- In order to avoid recovering molar position changes posttreatment, a maxillary plate with first molar clasps or a circumferential palatal arch wire attached to the molars are recommended as retention devices. An activator is unreliable for retaining tooth position.
- The clinician should take advantage of the headgear effect of the Herbst appliance in order to create space for crowded maxillary incisors and / or canines and thus possibly avoid extractions of permanent teeth.

Fig. 9-4 Case 9-5 Headgear effect of the Herbst appliance on the maxillary dentition in a 28-year-old female with a Class II:1 malocclusion. Note the pronounced intrusive effect of the appliance on the first molar and first and second premolars. Registrations at before treatment, during Herbst treatment, at the end of Herbst treatment and 1 year after multibracket (MB) appliance treatment.

References

Björk A, Skieller V. Normal and abnormal growth of the mandible. A synthesis of longitudinal cephalometric implant studies over a period of 25 years. Eur J Orthod 1983;5:1-46.

Broadbent BHSr, Broadbent BHJr, Golden W. Bolton Standards of dentofacial development growth. St Louis: C.V. Mosby Company, 1975.

Carano A, Testa M. The distal jet for upper molar distalization. J Clin Orthod 1996;30:374-380.

Hilgers JJ. The Pendulum appliance for Class II non-compliance therapy. J Clin Orthod 1992;26:706-714.

Kloehn SJ. Evaluation of cervical anchorage force in treatment. Angle Orthod 1961;31:91-104.

Konik M, Pancherz H, Hansen K. The mechanism of Class II correction in late Herbst treatment. Am J Orthod Dentofac Orthop 1997;112:87-91.

Melsen B. Effects of cervical anchorage during and after treatment: an implant study. Am J Orthod 1978;73:526-540.

Pancherz H. Treatment of Class II malocclusions by jumping the bite with the Herbst appliance. A cephalometric investigation. Am J Orthod 1979;76:423-442.

Pancherz H. The mechanism of Class II correction in Herbst appliance treatment. A cephalometric investigation. Am J Orthod 1982;82:104-113.

Pancherz H. Früh- oder Spätbehandlung mit der Herbst-Apparatur – Stabilität oder Rezidiv? Inf Orthod Kieferorthop 1994;26:437-445.

Pancherz H, Anehus-Pancherz M. The headgear effect of the Herbst appliance: A cephalometric long-term study. Am J Orthod Dentofac Orthop 1993;103:510-520.

Pancherz H, Hansen K. Occlusal changes during and after Herbst treatment: a cephalometric investigation. Eur J Orthod 1986;8:215-228.

Pancherz H, Hägg U. Dentofacial orthopedics in relation to somatic maturation. An analysis of 70 consecutive cases treated with the Herbst appliance. Am J Orthod 1985;88:273-287.

Riolo ML, Moyers RE, McNamara JA, Hunter WS. An atlas of craniofacial growth. Monograsph 2. Craniofacial Growth Series. Ann Arbor: Center of Human Growth and Development, University of Michigan, 1974.

Ruf S, Pancherz H. The mechanism of Class II correction during Herbst therapy in relation to the vertical jaw base relationship: a cephalometric roentgenographic study. Angle Orthod 1997;67:271-276.

Ruf S, Pancherz H. Dentoskeletal effects and facial profile changes in young adults treated with the Herbst appliance. Angle Orthod 1999;69:239-246.

Wieslander L. Intensive treatment of severe Class II malocclusions with a headgear Herbst appliance in the early mixed dentition. Am J Orthod 1984;86:1-13.

Wieslander L, Buck DL. Physiologic recovery after cervical traction therapy. Am J Orthod 1974;66:294-301.

Chapter 10

Effects on TMJ growth

Research

Three possible adaptive processes in the temporo-mandibular joint (TMJ) are thought to contribute to the increase in mandibular prognathism seen during Herbst treatment: (1) condylar modeling, (2) glenoid fossa modeling and (3) condylar position changes within the fossa. In animal experiments (monkeys, rats) it has been clearly demonstrated that mandibular protrusion procedures (splints, Herbst appliance) result in modeling processes at the condyle and the glenoid fossa (see Chapter 5: Experimental studies on bite jumping).

In clinical Herbst studies using TMJ roentgenograms, orthopantomograms, computerized tomograms and bone scintigrams, modeling processes of the mandibular condyle or the glenoid fossa were shown occasionally in single patients (Pancherz 1979, Wieslander 1984, Decrue and Wieslander 1990; Paulsen 1997; Paulsen et al. 1995, 1998, Kitai et al. 2002).

In several magnetic resonance imaging (MRI) Herbst studies on consecutively treated adolescent and adult subjects, condylar and glenoid fossa modeling were verified on a regular basis (Ruf and Pancherz 1998a,b, 1999a). Furthermore, using lateral head films the different TMJ adaptive processes have been assessed metrically (Ruf and Pancherz 1998a,b, 1999a; Pancherz et al. 1998, Pancherz and Fischer 2003). The scientific evidence on the effect of the Herbst appliance on TMJ growth will be presented by reviewing four publications.

1. Temporomandibular joint growth adaptation in Herbst treatment. A prospective magneticresonance imaging and cephalometric roentgenographic study (Ruf and Pancherz 1998a)

2. Temporomandibular joint growth adaptation in young adults during Herbst appliance treatment. A prospective magnetic resonance imaging and cephalometric roentgenographic study (Ruf and Pancherz 1998b) [Article in German]

3. Temporomandibular joint remodeling in adolescents and young adults during Herbst treatment: a prospective longitudinal magnetic resonance imaging and cephalometric radiographic investigation (Ruf and Pancherz 1999a)

In the above three publications the possible adaptive TMJ growth processes which contribute to the increase in mandibular prognathism accomplished by Herbst appliance therapy (condylar modeling, glenoid fossa modeling and condyle-fossa relationship changes) were analyzed using magnetic resonance imaging.

The total subject material comprised 25 adolescent and 14 young adult Class II patients treated with the Herbst appliance. In the first publication (Ruf and Pancherz 1998a) 15 adolescent subjects with a mean age of 13.5 years, and in the second publication (Ruf and Pancherz 1998b) 10 young adults with a mean age of 16.7 years were analyzed. In the third publication (Ruf and Pancherz 1999a) 25 adolescents with a mean age of 12.8 years were compared with 14 young adults with a mean age of 16.5 years. The treatment time with the Herbst appliance was on average 7 months for the adolescents and 8.5 months for the young adults.

Adolescence was defined by the hand-wrist radiographic stages MP3-E to MP3-G and young adulthood by the hand-wrist radiographic stages R-IJ or R-J according to Hägg and Taranger (1980) (see Chapter 6: Herbst research - subjects and methods). Parasagittal MRIs in closed mouth (proton density weighted MRI sequences) and mouth open (T2-weighted MRI sequences) positions were screened: before treatment (T0), at start of treatment with the Herbst appliance in place (T1), after 6-12 weeks of Herbst treatment (T2) and after removal of the Herbst appliance (T3).

The MRIs were analyzed visually for possible signs of TMJ modeling as well as metrically to document possible condylar position changes within the fossa. The metric MRI analysis was performed according to the method described by Kamelchuk et al (1996) (Fig. 10-1).

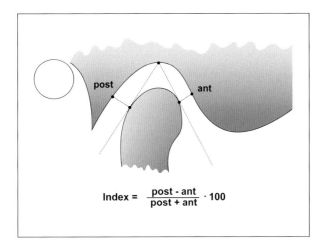

Fig. 10-1 Method for assessment of anterior (ant) and posterior (post) joint spaces (mm) on the magnetic resonance images (Kamelchuk et al. 1996). To eliminate problems with differences in joint size when comparing the individuals, a *Joint Space Index* was calculated.

Condylar modeling (Figs. 10-2 and 10-3)
At start of Herbst treatment (T1), the mandible in all subjects was advanced to an incisal edge-to-edge position. Thereby the condyles became positioned on top of the articular eminence. After 6 to 12 weeks of Herbst treatment (T2), the condyles were partially relocated in the fossa. At T2, signs of modeling in the posterior-superior area of the condyle in form of a distinct area of increased signal intensity (=bright area) located immediately below a signal-poor zone (=dark area) surrounding the condyle were seen in 48 of the 50 TMJs of the adolescents (Fig. 10-2) and

in 26 of the 28 TMJs of the young adults (Fig. 10-3). In the young adults this area of increased signal intensity was situated between two signal-poor zones: one surrounding the condyle and the other one situated above of the bone marrow (=gray area). This "bone marrow" demarcation line was missing in the adolescent subjects.

In the young adults the bright area at the condyle could still be seen at the time of removal of the appliance (T3) and occasionally the area even increased in brightness when compared to T2. On the other hand, for all adolescent subjects a decrease in signal intensity between T2 and T3 was characteristic. Thus, in most adolescents a normal condylar MRI appearance without signs of modeling was seen at the time of appliance removal (T3).

Glenoid fossa modeling
At T2 and/or T3, signs of glenoid fossa modeling could be seen in 36 of the 50 TMJs of the adolescents and in 22 of the 28 TMJs of the young adults. In all subjects the adaptive processes were located at the anterior surface of the postglenoid spine. In most subjects the amount of glenoid fossa modeling was less than the amount of condylar modeling. Furthermore, fossa modeling seemed to be more pronounced in young adults then in adolescents.

Condyle-fossa relationship (Figs. 10-4 and 10-5)
In most adolescent and young adult Herbst subjects the analysis of the condyle-fossa relationship (Ruf and Pancherz 1998a,b) revealed a tendency for an anterior positioning of the condyle (positive Index value) both pre- and posttreatment. The average change of the Index during treatment indicated a slightly anterior positioning of the condyle, which was larger in the young adults (+2.4) than in the adolescents (+1.6). However, none of these condyle-fossa relationship changes were statistically significant. Furthermore, a large individual variation existed.

Right   Left

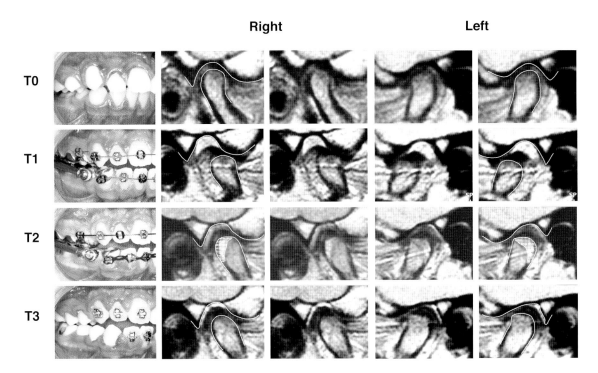

Fig. 10-2 Case 10-1 Intraoral photographs and magnetic resonance images of the left and right temporomandibular joint of a boy aged 12 years. **T0**: Before Herbst treatment. **T1**: At start of Herbst treatment. **T2**: After 12 weeks of Herbst treatment. **T3**: After removal of the Herbst appliance. Note the increased signal intensity (=bright area) in the posterior superior aspect of the condyle at T2. The streak artefacts seen on the images at T1, T2 and T3 are caused by the metal of the Herbst splints and the brackets. *(Revised from Ruf and Pancherz 1998a)*

Right   Left

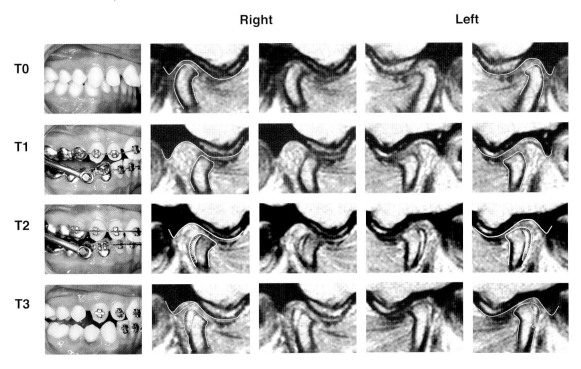

Fig. 10-3 Case 10-2 Intraoral photographs and magnetic resonance images of the left and right temporomandibular joint of a young man aged 20 years. **T0**: Before Herbst treatment. **T1**: At start of Herbst treatment. **T2**: After 12 weeks of Herbst treatment. **T3**: After removal of the Herbst appliance. Note the increased signal intensity (=bright area) in the posterior superior aspect of the condyle at T2 and T3 as well as the dark bone marrow demarcation line. A disc displacement without reduction was present before treatment and could not be reduced. *(Revised from Ruf and Pancherz 1999a)*

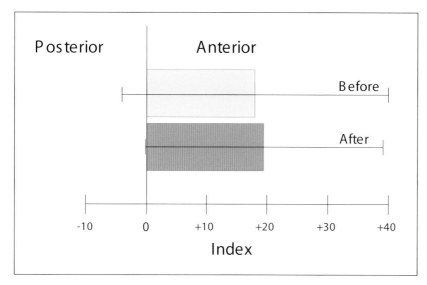

Fig. 10-4 Average left and right *Joint Space Index* in 15 adolescent Herbst patients (Ruf and Pancherz 1998a) before and after treatment (Mean, SD). A positive index value implies an anterior condylar position in the glenoid fossa, while a negative value indicates a posterior condylar position.

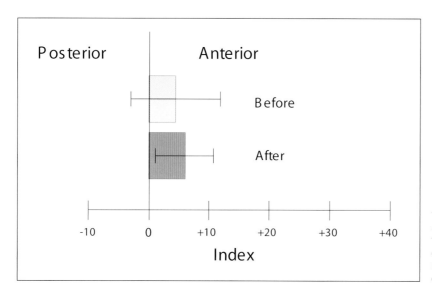

Fig. 10-5 Average left and right *Joint Space Index* in 10 young adult Herbst patients (Ruf and Pancherz 1998b) before and after treatment (Mean, SD). A positive index value implies an anterior condylar position in the glenoid fossa, while a negative value indicates a posterior condylar position.

Interpretation of the results

Both the adolescents and the young adults were successfully treated to a Class I or overcorrected Class I dental arch relationship. This was a result of a combination of dental and skeletal changes (Ruf and Pancherz 1999b).

Condylar modeling

In interpreting the MR images the following has to be taken into account. During condylar growth a significant increase in cartilage matrix, which consists of 80-90% of water, takes place (Bosshardt-Luehrs and Luder 1991). The hydrogen proton of the water molecule is highly susceptible to the effects of the magnetic fields due to the high electronegativity of

oxygen. In the proton-density-weighted MRIs used in the presented studies, the contrast of the image reflects the differences in proton density (relative number of hydrogen protons per unit volume) between the tissues. Tissues with a high proton density have a high signal and therefore appear bright, while tissues with a low proton density have a low signal and appear dark on the MRI. An increase in the relative number of hydrogen protons per unit volume is thus reflected as an area of high signal (*bright area*).

Therefore, the increase in MR signal intensity (bright area) on the posterior-superior aspect of the condyle found in the MRIs of adolescent and young adult

Herbst subjects most probably corresponds to the histologically proven hyperplasia of the prechondro-blastic-chondroblastic area demonstrated in animal Herbst studies (Peterson and McNamara 2003, McNamara et al. 2003). While in adolescent Herbst patients this would be the result of a stimulation of the active cells in the prechondroblastic zone, in the young adult Herbst patients it would be a reactivation of the inactive ("sleeping") cells in this zone. The stimulation or reactivation of cartilage growth results in bony apposition at the posterior surface of the condyle and lengthening of the mandible. For further details on condylar growth stimulation in animal studies see Chapter 5: Experimental studies on bite jumping.

In adult Herbst patients, in contrast to adolescent subjects, the bright MR signal in the posterior area of the condyle seen at T2 still persisted at T3. Also, in the aforementioned histological animal studies (Peterson and McNamara 2003, McNamara et al. 2003), the quantitative analysis of the thickness of the condylar cartilage revealed that in adult monkeys condylar cartilage thickness only changed slightly between treatment week 12 and 24, while in adolescent monkeys the thickness decreased. Furthermore, as mentioned earlier, in the young adult Herbst patients the area of condylar modeling was located between two signal-poor (dark) zones. The inner dark zone most probably corresponded to the continuous bony plate at the cartilage-bone interface which is characteristic of the adult condylar morphology (McNamara et al. 1982, Luder and Schroeder 1992, McNamara et al. 2003). This cartilage-bone interface becomes invaded by blood vessels in young adult monkeys, responding to protrusive function with cartilage hypertrophy (McNamara et al. 1982). As this bony plate at the cartilage-bone interface is missing in growing animals (McNamara et al. 1982, Luder and Schroeder 1992, Peterson and McNamara 2003), no inner dark zone was detectable in the MRIs of adolescent Herbst patients.

Glenoid fossa modeling
Histological animal studies have shown that the temporal bone of the glenoid fossa adapts to Herbst treatment both in juvenile and adult monkeys (Peterson and McNamara 2003, McNamara et al. 2003) with bone formation along the anterior border and bone resorption on the posterior border of the post-glenoid spine. Thereby, the normal posterior directed fossa displacement is reverted in an anterior direc

tion. The change in glenoid fossa growth direction has also been verified cephalometrically by Pancherz and Fischer (2003).
Fossa modeling as visualized by MRI in 36 of the 50 investigated TMJs of the adolescents and in 22 of the 28 TMJs of the young adult Herbst subjects, occurred at a later treatment stage than condylar modeling. A similar delay in temporal bone response was shown histologically in young adult (McNamara et al. 2003) but not in juvenile (Peterson and McNamara 2003) Herbst treated monkeys.
An explanation for the delayed MRI visualization of glenoid fossa modeling in comparison with the histological findings in adolescent animals might be the difference between the adaptive processes of the temporal bone (periosteal ossification) and the condyle (endochondral ossification). The periosteal ossification is not associated with large increases in water content of the tissue and does not seem to result in a marked change in MR signal intensity. Thus, the bone apposition along the postglenoid spine is visualized later in the MRI, at the time when the newly formed bone consolidates. Furthermore, fossa adaptation in the Herbst patients was less extensive than in the animals, which may be due to the fact that the size of the postglenoid spine in humans is reduced compared to that of monkeys (Hinton and McNamara 1984).

Condyle-fossa relationship
Theoretically, the increase in mandibular prognathism during Herbst treatment could be the result of anterior mandibular posturing. However, the results of the MRI joint space analysis clearly demonstrate that no significant change in condylar position within the glenoid fossa occurred during treatment either in adolescent or in young adult Herbst patients.

4. Amount and direction of temporomandibular joint growth changes in Herbst treatment: a cephalometric long-term investigation (Pancherz and Fischer 2003)

Temporomandibular joint growth changes (condyle and glenoid fossa) were assessed quantitatively on lateral head films. From the original patient material of 118 consecutive Class II, division 1 malocclusions treated with the Herbst appliance at the Department of Orthodontics, University of Lund, Sweden, 35 subjects (23 boys and 12 girls) with available head films (in habitual occlusion and mouth open) were examined: before treatment (T0), after 7.5 months of treatment (T3), 7.5 months posttreatment, when the occlusion had settled (T4) and 3 years posttreatment (T5). For simplicity only the male group of 35 subjects will be presented. The mean pretreatment age of these males was 13.2 years.

A sample of 12 untreated male Class II division 1 malocclusions was used as controls. All control subjects had lateral head films (in habitual occlusion and mouth open) corresponding to the examination times T0 and T3. The average age of the control group was 11.8 years. The average observation period amounted to 7.5 months.

The habitual occlusion head films in a series (T0, T3, T4, T5) were superimposed on the T0 film using the stable bone structures of the anterior cranial base and the mandible (Björk and Skieller 1983).

Condylar growth (Fig. 10-6) was assessed as a positional change of the anatomic condylar point (Co) using a mandibular superimposition of the head films. The Co point was identified on the mouth-open radiographs and transferred to the mouth-closed radiographs. Measurements were performed relative to the RL/RLp reference grid (see Chapter 6: Herbst research – subjects and methods).

Glenoid fossa displacement was assessed as a positional change of the Co point using a cranial base superimposition of the head films. The method is described in Chapter 6: Herbst research – subjects and methods.

Condylar growth (Fig. 10-7)

During the treatment period (T0-T3) condylar growth in the Herbst subjects was directed significantly posteriorly (mean=2.2 mm) and superiorly (mean=3.1 mm) and proved also to be larger than in the untreated control subjects. The group differences were more pronounced for sagittal (mean=2.1 mm) than for vertical (mean=1.5 mm) condylar growth. During the posttreatment periods (T3-T4, T4-T5), condylar growth was more vertically oriented than during the treatment period (T0-T3). Furthermore, the amount of posttreatment growth was reduced in comparison to that during the treatment period.

Glenoid fossa displacement (Fig. 10-8)

During the treatment period (T0-T3) the glenoid fossa in the Herbst subjects was displaced significantly anteriorly (mean=0.4 mm) and inferio (mean=1.3 mm). In the untreated control subjects the amount of fossa displacement was small and the direction was opposite to that found in the Herbst subjects. During the posttreatment periods (T3-T4, T4-T5) fossa displacement reverted to a posterior direction.

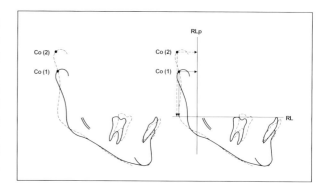

Fig. 10-6 Method for the assessment of condylar growth (Co). **A**: Mandibular base superimposition. **B**: Measurement of condylar growth (Co point changes) in relation to the RL/RLp reference grid. *(Revised from Pancherz and Fischer 2003)*

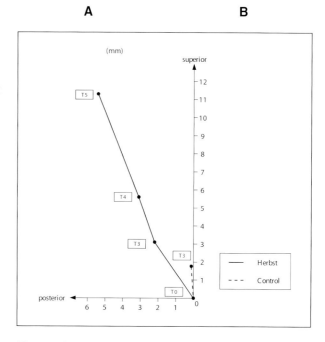

Fig. 10-7 Average condylar growth (Co point changes assessed after mandibular superimposition of head films) in 23 male Herbst subjects and 12 male control subjects. **T0**: Before treatment. **T3**: After 7.5 months of Herbst treatment. **T4**: 7.5 months posttreatment when the occlusion had settled. **T5**: 3 years posttreatment. *(Revised from Pancherz and Fischer 2003)*

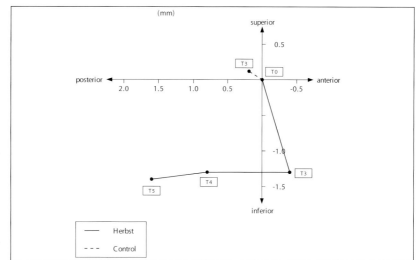

Fig. 10-8 Average glenoid fossa displacement (Co point changes assessed after cranial base superimposition of head films) in 23 male Herbst subjects and 12 male control subjects. **T0**: Before treatment. **T3**: After 7.5 months of Herbst treatment. **T4**: 7.5 months posttreatment when the occlusion had settled. **T5**: 3 years posttreatment. *(Revised from Pancherz and Fischer 2003)*

Interpretation of the results

In interpreting the presented findings it must be remembered that anteriorly directed fossa displacement and posteriorly directed condylar growth are advantageous for Class II correction as these changes result in an anterior positioning of the mandible.

In the treatment period (T0-T3), condylar growth in the Herbst subjects was not only larger than in the untreated controls but also more posteriorly-superiorly directed. This was the result of the modeling processes induced on the posterior-superior aspect of the condyle (Ruf and Pancherz 1998a,b, Ruf and Pancherz 1999a). A similar redirection of growth was described metrically in prepubertal Herbst patients (Pancherz and Littmann 1989) and histologically in growing Herbst monkeys (Peterson and McNamara 2003). Woodside et al. (1983), on the other hand, found that Herbst treatment stimulated condylar growth in the vertical direction only.

In the first posttreatment period (T3-T4) of 7.5 months, the amount of condylar growth was reduced in relation to that in the treatment period and the direction of growth became more vertically upward. This is in agreement with the clinical findings of Johnston (1999). Subnormal condylar growth, immediately following appliance removal, has also been reported in rat experiments (Chayanupatkul et al. 2003) and was attributed to an insufficient maturation of the newly formed bone, which predisposes its resorption.

In the second posttreatment period (T4-T5) of 2.4 years, the more vertically upward-directed condylar growth seen in the period T3-T4 was maintained.

The amount and direction of growth seemed to correspond to that of normal growth (Buschang and Santos-Pinto 1998).

Physiologically, the fossa is displaced in a posterior and inferior direction during growth development (Buschang and Santos-Pinto 1998, Björk and Skieller 1983). During Herbst treatment (T0-T3), however, the fossa was displaced anteriorly and inferiorly. As mentioned before, this reversal in growth direction is due to the bone apposition along the anterior border of the postglenoid spine seen in the MRIs of the Herbst patients (Ruf and Pancherz 1998a,b; Ruf and Pancherz 1999a) as well as in the histological sections of the Herbst monkeys (Peterson and McNamara 2003; McNamara et al. 2003).

During the posttreatment periods (T3-T4, T4-T5), the glenoid fossa displacement reverted back to a posterior direction. When looking at the total observation period (T0-T5), the glenoid fossa was displaced in a posterior and inferior direction, corresponding to normal growth (Buschang and Santos-Pinto 1998, Björk and Skieller 1983).

Conclusion and clinical implications

In both adolescent and young adult Herbst subjects, the growth of the condyle can be stimulated and the glenoid fossa displaced anteriorly. These TMJ adaptive processes will result in mandibular advancement, which will contribute to treatment of skeletal Class II malocclusions.

References

Björk A, Skieller V. Normal and abnormal growth of the mandible. A synthesis of the longitudinal cephalometric implant studies over a period of 25 years. Eur J Orthod 1983;5:1-46.

Bosshardt-Luehrs CPB, Luder HU. Cartilage matrix production and chondrocyte enlargement as contributors to mandibular condylar growth in monkeys *(Macaca fascicularis)*. Am J Orthod Dentofac Orthop 1991;100:362-369.

Buschang PH, Santos-Pinto A. Condylar growth and glenoid fossa displacement during childhood and adolescence. Am J Orthod Dentofac Orthop 1998;113:437-442.

Chayanupatkul A, Rabie ABM, Hägg U. Temporomandibular response to early and late removal of bite-jumping devices. Eur J Orthod 2003;25:465-470.

Decrue A, Wieslander L. Veränderungen der Fossa articularis nach Vorverlagerung der Mandibula mittels Herbstapparatur. Zahnärztl Prax 1990;41:360-365.

Hägg U, Taranger J. Skeletal stages of the hand and wrist as indicators of the pubertal growth spurt. Acta Odontol Scand 1980;38:187-200.

Hinton RJ, McNamara JA Jr. Temporal bone adaptations in response to protrusive function in juvenile and young adult rhesus monkeys *(Macaca mulatta)*. Eur J Orthod 1984;6:155-174.

Johnston LE. Growing jaws for fun and profit: a modest proposal. In: McNamara JA (ed). Growth modification: what works, what doesn't, and why. Monograph No. 35, Craniofacial Growth Series, Center for Human growth and development, University of Michigan, Ann Arbor 1999:63-86.

Kamelchuk LS, Grace MGA, Major PW. Post-imaging temporomandibular joint space analysis. J Craniomand Pract 1996;14:23-29.

Kitai N, Kreiborg S, Bakke M, Paulsen HU, Moller E, Darvan TA, Pedersen H, Takada K. Three-dimensional magnetic resonance imaging of the mandible and masticatory muscles in a case of juvenile chronic arthritis treated with the Herbst appliance. Angle Orthod. 2002;72:81-87.

Luder HU, Schroeder HE. Light and electron microscopic morphology of the temporomandibular joint in growing and mature crab-eating monkeys *(Macaca fascicularis)*: the condylar calcified cartilage. Anat Embryol 1992;185:189-199.

McNamara JA Jr, Hinton RJ, Hoffman DL. Histological analysis of temporomandibular joint adaptation to protrusive function in young adult rhesus monkeys *(Macaca mulatta)*. Am J Orthod 1982;82:288-298.

McNamara JA, Peterson JE, Pancherz H. Histologic changes associated with the Herbst appliance in adult rhesus monkeys *(Macaca mulatta)*. Sem Orthod 2003;9:26-40.

Pancherz H. Treatment of Class II malocclusions by jumping the-bite with the Herbst appliance. Am J Orthod 1979;76:423-442.

Pancherz H, Fischer S. Amount and direction of temporomandibular joint growth changes in Herbst treatment: a cephalometric long-term investigation. Angle Orthod 2003;73:493-501.

Pancherz H, Littmann C. Morphologie und Lage des Unterkiefers bei der Herbst-Behandlung. Eine kephalometrische Analyse der Veränderungen bis zum Wachstumsabschluss. Inf Orthod Kieferorthop 1989;21:493-513.

Pancherz H, Ruf S, Kohlhas P. "Effective condylar growth" and chin position changes in Herbst treatment: a cephalometric roentgenographic long-term study. Am J Orthod Dentofac Orthop 1998;114:437-446. Paulsen HU. Changes of the condyles of 100 patients treated with the Herbst appliance from puberty to adulthood: a long-term radiographic study. Eur J Orthod 1997;19:657-668.

Paulsen HU, Karle A, Bakke M, Herskind A. CT-scanning and radiographic analysis of temporomandibular joints and cephalometric analysis in a case of Herbst treatment in late puberty. Eur J Orthod 1995;17:165-175.

Paulsen HU, Rabol A, Sorensen S. Bone scintigraphy of human temporomandibular joints during Herbst treatment: a case report. Eur J Orthod 1998;20:369-374.

Peterson JE, McNamara JA. Temporomandibular joint adaptatons associated with Herbst appliance treatment in juvenile rhesus monkeys *(Macaca mulatta)*. Sem Orthod 2003;9:12-25.

Ruf S, Pancherz H. Temporomandibular joint growth adaptation in Herbst treatment. A prospective magnetic resonance imaging and cephalometric roentgenographic study. Eur J Orthod 1998a;20:375-388.

Ruf S, Pancherz H. Kiefergelenkwachstumsadaptation bei jungen Erwachsenen während Behandlung mit der Herbst-Apparatur. Eine prospektive magnetresonanztomographische und kephalometrische Studie. Inf Orthod Kieferorthop 1998b;30:735-750.

Ruf S, Pancherz H. Temporomandibular joint remodeling in adolescents and young adults during Herbst treatment: a prospective longitudinal magnetic resonance imaging and cephalometric radiographic investigation. Am J Orthod Dentofac Orthop 1999a;115:607-618.

Ruf S, Pancherz H. Dentoskeletal effects and facial profile changes in young adults treated with the Herbst appliance. Angle Orthod 1999b;69:239-246.

Wieslander L. Intensive treatment of severe Class II malocclusions with a headgear-Herbst appliance in the early mixed dentition. Am J Orthod 1984;86:1-13.

Woodside DG, Altuna G, Harvold E, Herbert M, Metaxas A. Primate experiments in malocclusion and bone induction. Am J Orthod 1983;83:460-468.

Chapter 11

Effects on mandibular growth and morphology

Research

As early as 1895 Roux described the ability of bones to react to alterations in mechanical load by morphological changes. In numerous animal studies (monkeys and rats) using different kinds of mandibular protrusion appliances it has been shown that temporomandibular (TMJ) adaptations occur in response to altered mandibular function (see Chapter 5: Experimental studies on bite jumping).

In dentofacial orthopedics of Class II malocclusions using removable functional appliances such as the Activator, Bionator, Fränkel or the Twin-block there is, however, disagreement about the ability of these appliances to affect mandibular condyle growth (Gianelli et al. 1983, Creekmore and Radney 1983, McNamara et al. 1985, Vargervik and Harvold 1985, Pancherz 1984, Heij et al. 1989, Mamandras and Allen 1990, Jakobsson and Paulin 1990, De-Vincenzo 1991, Hashim 1991, Mills 1991, Nelson et al. 1993, Woodside 1998, Toth and McNamara 1999, Mills and McCulloch 2000, Ruf et al. 2001, O´Brian et al. 2003, Araujo et al. 2004, Cozza et al. 2004, Gill and Lee 2005, Türkkahraman and Sayin 2006).

With respect to the Herbst appliance, on the other hand, there is ample proof that TMJ adaptation to protrusive mandibular function is possible and that mandibular morphologic changes occur (Pancherz 1979, 1982, Wieslander 1984, Pancherz and Littmann 1988, 1989, Paulsen 1997, Paulsen et al. 1988, 1995, Pancherz et al. 1998, Ruf and Pancherz 1998, 1999). Furthermore, it has been shown that these changes are dependent on the maturity level of the patient (Pancherz and Littmann 1988). The scientific evidence of TMJ growth adaptation and mandibular morphologic changes during and after Herbst treatment will be presented by reviewing two publications.

1. Somatic maturity and mandibular morphologic changes during Herbst treatment. (Pancherz and Littmann 1988) [Article in German]

Mandibular growth and morphologic changes occurring during Herbst treatment of Class II:1 malocclusions were analyzed with respect to the patients` level of somatic maturation.

At the time of examination the total male sample of Class II:1 malocclusions treated with the Herbst appliance at the Department of Orthodontics, University of Lund, Sweden, comprised 71 subjects. Of these, 65 were assigned to the group of "Herbst subjects". Herbst treatment was performed during an average period of 6 months. In the remaining 6 individuals and in an additional 14 male Class II:1 subjects with the same dentoskeletal morphology as the Herbst subjects, pretreatment growth records and lateral head films existed, covering an average period of 6 months. These 20 subjects were assigned as the "Control subjects" group.

Longitudinal growth records of standing height over a period of 5 to 10 years were used for the assessment of somatic maturation of both the Herbst and Control subjects (Pancherz and Hägg 1985). From the growth records, individual velocity curves were constructed and three growth periods were established (see Chapter 22: Treatment timing) to which the patients were assigned:

Prepeak – 30 Herbst subjects and all 20 Control
          subjects
Peak   – 26 Herbst subjects
Postpeak – 9 Herbst subjects

Mouth-open lateral head films from before and after Herbst treatment as well as before and after the control period were analyzed using mandibular tracings. The reference points for the head film analysis are shown in Fig 11-1. The angular and linear measurements used for the assessment of mandibular growth and morphologic changes are presented in Figs. 11-2 and 11-3. For the assessment of growth changes at the condyle and at the inferior and posterior borders of the mandible (bone apposition and resorption) the tracings from "before" and "after" were superimposed, using the stable reference structures of the mandible (Björk and Skieller 1983) for orientation. The lines ML, CLs and CLp from the first tracing were transferred to the second tracing and used as reference lines for the measurements (Fig. 11-4).

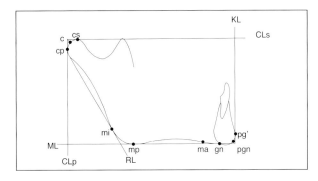

Fig. 11-1 Reference points and lines used for the assessment of mandibular growth and morphologic changes. (*Revised from Pancherz and Littmann 1988*)

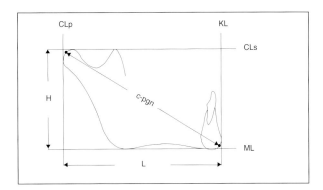

Fig. 11-2 Linear measurements for the assessment of mandibular growth and morphologic changes. (*Revised from Pancherz and Littmann 1988*)

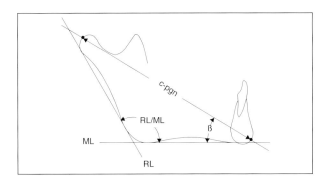

Fig. 11-3 Angular measurements for the assessment of mandibular growth and morphologic changes. (*Revised from Pancherz and Littmann 1988*)

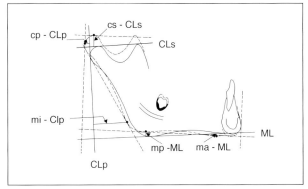

Fig. 11-4 Linear measurements for the assessment of mandibular growth changes (bone modeling) at the condyle and at the lower and posterior borders of the mandible. Superimposition of mandibular tracings using the stable mandibular reference structures (Björk and Skieller 1983) for orientation. (*Revised from Pancherz and Littmann 1988*)

Comparison of Herbst and Control subjects

In order to assess the therapeutic influence of Herbst treatment on mandibular growth and morphology, the prepeak Herbst and Control subjects were compared. The following changes were seen. The increase in mandibular base length (c-pgn) (Fig. 11-5A) and mandibular horizontal length (L) (Fig. 11-5B) was larger in the Herbst than in the Control subjects. The increase in the gonion angle (RL/ML) and the reduction of the ß-angle (Fig. 11-5A) was a result of Herbst therapy. The posterior directed condylar growth (cp-CLp) and the bone resorption at the posterior part of the lower mandibular border (mp-ML) was larger in the Herbst than in the Control subjects (Fig. 11-5C).

Comparison of prepeak and peak Herbst subjects

The following mandibular growth and morphologic changes were larger in the peak than in the prepeak

Herbst subjects: the increase in mandibular base length (c-pgn) (Fig. 11-5A) and mandibular height (H) (Fig 11-5B), the posterior directed (cp-CLp) as well as the superior directed (cs-CLs) condylar growth (Fig.11-5C), and bone resorption at the posterior part of the mandibular lower border (mp-ML) (Fig. 11-5C).

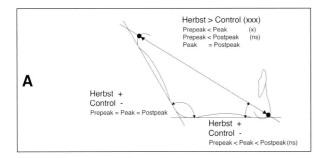

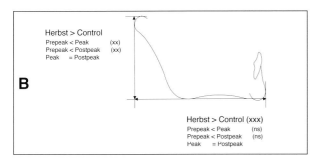

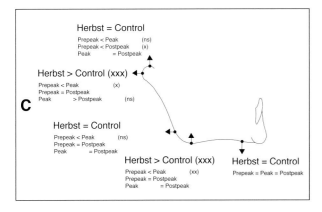

Fig. 11-5 Mandibular growth and morphologic changes during 6 months (of treatment) in 65 males treated with the Herbst appliance and in 20 male Control subjects, all with a Class II:1 malocclusion. Treatment of the Herbst subjects in three somatic maturation periods: Prepeak (n=30), Peak (n=26) and Postpeak (n=9). All Controls were in the Prepeak priod. **A**: Mandibular base length, gonion angle and ß-angle. **B**: Mandibular horizontal length and mandibular height. **C**: Bone modeling processes at the condyle and at the mandibular inferior and posterior borders. xxx indicates significance at 0.1 % level, xx at 1 % level, x at 5 % level and ns indicates no significance.

Comparison of prepeak and postpeak Herbst subjects

Mandibular growth and morphologic group differences were found for only two variables: the increase in mandibular height (H) (Fig. 11-5B) and in vertically directed condylar growth (cs-CLs) was larger in the postpeak than in the prepeak Herbst subjects.

Comparison of peak and postpeak Herbst subjects

Similar changes in mandibular growth and morphology were registered in the two groups of Herbst subjects.

Interpretation of the results

When interpreting the findings it must be remembered that untreated Control subjects were available for only the prepeak period but not for the peak and postpeak periods.

The most obvious finding was that Herbst treatment stimulated condylar growth in a posterior direction (cp-CLp). As a result of this, mandibular base length (c-pgn) and mandibular horizontal length (L) were increased. Due to the change in condylar growth direction together with the bone resorption at the posterior part of the lower mandibular border (mp-ML), the gonion angle (RL/ML) was increased and the ß-angle was reduced.

The possibility of condylar growth stimulation, especially in a posterior direction, by anterior displacement of the mandible has been verified histologically in several animal experiments (see Chapter 5: Experimental studies on bite jumping) and with the aid of magnetic resonance imaging in Herbst subjects (Ruf and Pancherz 1998, 1999) (see Chapter 10: Effects on TMJ growth). The resorption at the lower border of the mandible at point mp is thought to result from an altered muscle function pattern during therapy as found electromyographically by Pancherz and Anehus-Pancherz (1980) (see Chapter 15: Effects on muscular activity).

When comparing Herbst subjects treated at different growth periods it became obvious that the somatic developmental stage of the patients had an influence on mandibular growth and morphological changes occurring during therapy. Thus, the increase in the amount of posterior directed condylar growth (cp-CLp) and mandibular base length (c-pgn) was largest in the peak and smallest in the prepeak subjects. Bone resorption at the posterior part of the mandibular lower border (mp-ML), on the other hand, was larger in the prepeak than in the peak subjects. Consequently, these changes affected the increase in mandibular height (H), which was less in the prepeak than in the peak subjects.

The group difference in the amount of posterior directed condylar growth was most probably because of the differences in basic growth rate, which, of course, was largest in the subjects treated during the peak period. On top of the basic growth, an equal amount of stimulated growth was added, irrespective of the maturation of the subjects (Hägg et al. 1987).

The larger increase in mandibular height (H) in the postpeak subjects when compared to the prepeak subjects was certainly due to the larger amount of superior directed condylar growth (cs-CLs) and the smaller amount of bone resorption at point mp found in the postpeak subjects.

2. Mandibular morphology and position in Herbst treatment. A cephalometric analysis of changes to the end of growth. (Pancherz and Littmann 1989) [Article in German]

This publication is concerned with the long-term effects of Herbst treatment on mandibular growth and morphology.

The sample examined was based on the same 71 male Class II:1 subjects presented previously (Pancherz and Littmann 1988). The first 12 of these 71 Herbst subjects were followed to the end of their growth, on average 7 years after treatment. From the previous group of 20 untreated male Class II:1 Control subjects (Pancherz and Littmann 1988), 10 were re-examined at the end of growth. The total observation period of these 10 individuals was, on average, 7 years.

Mouth-open lateral head films from before and after Herbst treatment as well as at the end of growth were evaluated. The head films of the Control subjects were evaluated at comparable time intervals as those of the Herbst subjects. The analyzing method was the same as that used previously (Pancherz and Littmann 1988).

Treatment period (T) changes

Although the number of subjects in the Herbst and Control groups was smaller than that in the previous study (Pancherz and Littmann 1988), the results were comparable (Fig. 11-6A to C).

Posttreatment period (P) changes

Most treatment changes reverted posttreatment according to the following results. In comparison to the Controls the increase in mandibular base length (c-pgn) (Fig. 11-6A) and mandibular horizontal length (L) (Fig. 11-6B) was less in the Herbst subjects. The gonion angle (RL/ML) was reduced more and the ß-angle was increased more in the Herbst than in the Control subjects (Fig. 11-6A). The amount of posterior directed condylar growth (cp-CLp) was less in the Herbst treated cases than in the Control cases (Fig. 11-6C). Finally, bone apposition at the posterior part of the mandibular lower border (mp-ML) took place in the Herbst subject while continuing resorption occurred in the Controls (Fig. 11-6C). The group difference in mandibular bone modeling affected the mandibular height (H), which was increased more in the Herbst than in the Control subjects (Fig. 11-6B).

Total observation period (O) changes

A comparison between the Herbst and Control subjects revealed differences for only three variables: The ß-angle (Fig. 11-6A) as well as the mandibular height (H) (Fig. 11-6B) were increased more in the Herbst than in the Controls (Fig. 11-6B) and bone apposition at point mp (mp-ML) (Fig. 11-6C) occurred in the Herbst subjects while bone resorption was seen in the Controls.

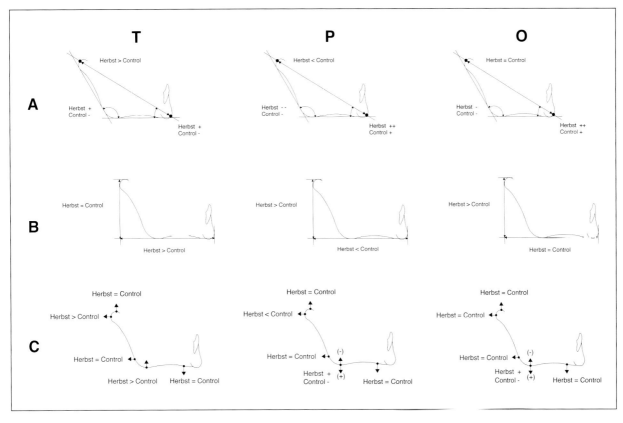

Fig. 11-6 Long-term mandibular growth and morphologic changes in 12 males treated with the Herbst appliance and in 10 male Control subjects, all with a Class II:1 malocclusion. **T**: Treatment period of 6 months. **P**: Posttreatment period of 7 years (to the end of growth). **O**: Total observation period of 7.5 years. **A**: Mandibular base length, gonion angle and ß-angle. **B**: Mandibular horizontal length and mandibular height. **C**: Bone modeling processes at the condyle and at the mandibular inferior and posterior borders.

Interpretation of the results

The results of this investigation revealed that most of the changes accomplished during Herbst treatment reverted after treatment. Thus, with the exception of the bone modeling at the posterior part of the mandibular lower border (mp-ML) with its impact on mandibular height (H), Herbst treatment seemed to have only a temporary influence on mandibular growth and morphology.

The reversible growth changes at point mp, when comparing the treatment and posttreatment periods, were thought to result from an alteration in the masseter muscle activity pattern (see Chapter 15: Effects on muscular activity). During treatment, the bone resorption, which was larger than normally occur during growth (Björk and Skieller 1972), resulted from a reduced masseter activity (Pancherz and Anehus-Pancherz 1980). The posttreatment bone apposition (instead of normally occurring resorption) was then due to increased masseter activity, beyond the pretreatment level (Pancherz 1995).

Conclusions and clinical implications

- Herbst treatment stimulates condylar growth in a posterior direction. As a consequence, the mandibular length and the gonion angle are increased while the ß-angle is reduced.
- The increase in condylar growth and mandibular length is larger in subjects treated during the peak period of pubertal growth than in subjects treated during the prepeak and postpeak periods.
- Mandibular treatment changes tend to revert posttreatment.
- Even if Herbst treatment seems not to have any decisive long-term influence on mandibular growth and morphology, the increase in mandibular length at the time of treatment is most important for the correction of the existing Class II malocclusion during that period. Posttreatment, a solid Class I cuspal interdigitation of the teeth will help to maintain the result, in spite of recovering mandibular growth changes.

105

References

Araujo AM, Buschang PH, Melo ACM. Adaptive condylar growth and mandibular remodelling changes with bionator therapy – an implant study. Eur J Orthod 2004;26:515-522.

Björk A, Skieller V. Facial development and tooth eruption. An implant study at the age of puberty. Am J Orthod 1972;62:339-383.

Björk A, Skieller V. Normal and abnormal growth of the mandible. A synthesis of longitudinal cephalometric implant studies over a period of 25 years. Eur J Orthod 1983;5:1-46.

Creekmore TD, Radney LJ. Fränkel appliance therapy: orthopedic or orthodontic? Am J Orthod 1983;83:89-108.

Cozza P, De Toffol L, Iacopini L. An analysis of the corrective contribution in activator treatment. Angle Orthod 2004;74:741-748.

DeVincenzo JP. Changes in mandibular length during and after successful correction of Class II malocclusions, using a functional appliance. Am J Orthod Dentofac Orthop 1991;99:241-257.

Gianelli AA, Brosnan P, Martingnoni M, Berstein L. Mandibular growth, condyle position and Fränkel appliance therapy. Angle Orthod 1983;53:131-142.

Gill DS, Lee RT. Prospective clinical trial comparing the effects of conventional Twin-block and mini-block appliances: Part 1. Hard tissue changes. Am J Orthod Dentofac Orthop 2005;127:465-472.

Hashim H. Analysis of activator treatment changes. Aus Orthod J 1991;12:100-104.

Hägg U, Pancherz H, Taranger J. Pubertal growth and orthodontic treatment. In: Carlson DS, Ribbens KA (eds). Craniofacial growth during adolescence. Monograph 20, Craniofacial Growth Series. Ann Arbor: Center for Human Growth and Development. The University of Michigan 1987:87-115.

Heij DG, Callaert H, Opdebeek HM. The effect of amount of protrusion built into the Bionator on condylar growth and displacement: a clinical study. Am J Orthod Dentofac Orthop 1989;95:401-409.

Jakobsson SO, Paulin G. The influence of activator treatment on skeletal growth in Angle Class II:1 cases: a roentgenocephalometric study. Eur J Orthod 1990;12:174-184.

McNamara JA, Bookstein FL, Shaugnessy TG. Skeletal and dental changes following functional regulator therapy on Class II patients. Am J Orthod 1985;88:91-110.

Mamandras AH, Allen LP. Mandibular response to orthodontic treatment with the Bionator appliance. Am J Orthod Dentofac Orthop 1990;97:113-120.

Mills JR. The effect of functional appliances on the skeletal pattern. Br J Orthod 1991;18:267-275.

Mills CM, McCulloch KJ. Posttreatment changes after successful correction of Class II malocclusions with the twin block appliance. Am J Orthod Dentofac Orthop 2000;118:24-33.

Nelson C, Harkness M, Herbison P. Mandibular changes due to functional appliance treatment. Am J Orthod Dentofac Orthop 1993;104:153-161.

O`Brian K, Wright J, Conboy F, Sanjie YW, Mandall N, Chadwick S, Conolly I, Cook P, Birnie D, Hammond M, Harradine N, Lewis D, McDade C, Mitchell L, Murray A, O´Neill J, Read M, Robinson S, Roberts-Harry D, Sandler J, Shaw I. Effectiveness of early orthodontic treatment with the Twin-block appliance: A multicenter, randomized controlled trial. Part 1: Dental and skeletal effects. Am J Orthod Dentofac Orthop 2003;124:234-243.

Paulsen HU. Changes of the condyles of 100 patients treated with the Herbst appliance from puberty to adulthood. Eur J Orthod 1997;19:657-668.

Paulsen HU, Rabol, A, Sorensen S. Bone scintograpy of human mandibular joints during Herbst treatment: a case report. Eur J Orthod 1988;20:369-374.

Paulsen HU, Karle A, Bakke M, Herskind A. A CT-scanning and radiographic analysis of temporomandibular joints and cephalometric analysis in a case of Herbst treatment in late puberty. Eur J Orthod 1995;17:657-668.

Pancherz H. Treatment of Class II malocclusions by jumping the bite with the Herbst appliance. A cephalometric investigation. Am J Orthod 1979;76:423-442.

Pancherz H. The mechanism of Class II correction in Herbst appliance treatment. A cephalometric investigation. Am J Orthod 1982;82:104-113.

Pancherz H. A cephalometric analysis of skeletal and dental changes contributing to Class II correction in activator treatment. Am J Orthod 1984;85:125-134.

Pancherz H. The Herbst appliance. Sevilla: Editorial Aguiram 1995:1-74.

Pancherz H, Anehus-Pancherz M. Muscle activity in Class II, Division 1 malocclusions treated by bite jumping with the Herbst appliance. Am J Orthod 1980;78:321-329.

Pancherz H, Hägg U. Dentofacial orthopedics in relation to somatic maturation. An analysis of 70 consecutive cases treated with the Herbst appliance. Am J Orthod 1985;88:273-287.

Pancherz H, Littmann C. Somatisch Reife und morphologische Veränderungen des Unterkiefers bei der Herbst-Behandlung. Inf Orthod Kieferorthop 1988;20:455-470.

Pancherz H, Littmann C. Morphologie und Lage des Unterkiefers bei der Herbst-Behandlung. Eine kephalometrische Analyse der Veränderungen bis zum Wachstumsabschluss. Inf Orthod Kieferorthop 1989;21:493-513.

Pancherz H, Ruf, S, Kohlhas P. "Effective condylar growth" and chin position changes in Herbst treatment: a cephalometric roentgenographic long-term study. Am J Orthod Dentofac Orthop 1998;114:437-446.

Ruf S, Pancherz H. Temporomandibular joint adaptation in Herbst treatment:a prospectivemagneticresonanceimaging and cephalometric roentgenographic study. Eur J Orthod 1998;20:375-388.

Ruf S, Pancherz H. Temporomandibular joint remodeling in adolescents and young adults during Herbst treatment: a prospective longitudinal magnetic resonance imaging and cephalometric radiographic investigation. Am J Orthod Dentofac Orthop 1999;115:607-618.

Ruf S, Baltromejus S, Pancherz H. Effective condylar growth and chin position changes in activator treatment: a cephalometric roentgenographic study. Angle Orthod 2001;71:4-11.

Toth RL, McNamara JA. Treatment effects produced by the Twin-block appliance and the FR-2 appliance of Fränkel compared with an untreated Class II sample. Am J Orthod Dentofac Orthop 1999;116:597-609.

Türkkahraman H, Sayin MÖ. Effects of activator and headgear treatment: comparison with untreated Class II subjects. Eur J Orthod 2006;28:27-34.

Vargervik K, Harvold EP. Response to activator treatment in Class II malocclusion. Am J Orthod 1985;88:242-251.

Wieslander L. Intensive treatment of severe Class II malocclusions with a headgear-Herbst appliance in the mixed dentition. Am J Orthod Dentofac Orthop 1984;86:1-13.

Woodside DG. Do functional appliances have an orthopedic effect? Am J Orthod Dentofac Orthop 1998;113:11-14.

Chapter 12

"Effective TMJ growth"

Research

The main goal in dentofacial orthopedics of skeletal Class II malocclusions is to develop the mandible in an anterior direction. In Herbst therapy, the increase of mandibular prognathism can be explained by three adaptive processes in the temporomandibular joint (TMJ): (1) increased condylar growth due to condylar modeling, (2) anterior glenoid fossa displacement due to fossa modeling and (3) anterior positioning of the condyle within the fossa due to condylar displacement. However, mandibular rota-tion during treatment also affects the position of the chin: an anterior rotation will result in an increase and a posterior rotation in a decrease of mandibular prognathism. In previous Herbst studies, the three TMJ adaptive mechanisms have been analyzed as single factors by the use of lateral head films (Pancherz 1979, 1981, Wieslander 1984, Pancherz and Hägg 1985, Pancherz and Littmann 1989, Pancherz and Fischer 2003), orthopantomograms (Paulsen 1997), computerized tomography scans (Paulsen et al. 1995), bone scintigraphs (Paulsen et al. 1988) and magnetic resonance imaging (MRI) (Ruf and Pancherz 1998, 1999).

Although measurements of condylar and fossa changes are difficult to perform with any degree of accuracy, the method of Creekmore (1967) makes it possible to overcome this problem by using an arbitrary condylar reference point. With the Creekmore approach the "effective TMJ growth" is assessed. This is a summation of the above mentioned three adaptive processes in the TMJ (condylar modeling, glenoid fossa modeling and condylar-fossa relationship changes). The "effective TMJ growth" is measured on lateral head films.

In three long-term Herbst studies, the "effective TMJ growth" was assessed (Pancherz et al. 1998, Pancherz and Fischer 2003, Pancherz and Michaelidou 2004). In one of the studies (Pancherz and Michaelidou 2004), the "effective TMJ growth" was related to the facial type of the patients (see Chapter 18: Treatment of hyper- and hypodivergent Class II:1 malocclusions).

The scientific evidence on "effective TMJ growth" in Herbst treatment will be surveyed by presenting one publication.

"Effective condylar growth" and chin position changes in Herbst treatment: a cephalometric roentgenographic long-term study (Pancherz et al.1998)

In this long-term investigation of patients treated with the Herbst appliance, an analysis was performed of the "effective TMJ growth" and its effect on the chin, considering mandibular rotation in the evaluation.

The sample investigated comprised 98 subjects (59 males and 39 females) with complete records, selected from 118 consecutive Class II:1 malocclusions treated successfully with the Herbst appliance at the Department of Orthodontics, University of Lund, Sweden. Following Herbst treatment, no active treatment was performed in 79 of the subjects. For the final tooth alignment, in 19 subjects further treatment with multibracket appliances was carried out for an additional year. Posttreatment retention (activator, upper plate, mandibular cuspid-to-cuspid retainer) for 1 to 2 years was performed in 65 subjects while, 33 subjects had no retainers.

Lateral head films in habitual occlusion were analyzed at the following times: before treatment (T1), after 7 months (6 to 13 months) of treatment when the appliance was removed (T2), 7 months (6 to 13 months) posttreatment when the occlusion had settled (T3) (Pancherz and Hansen 1986) and at follow-up 3 years (2 to 5 years) posttreatment (T4). The mean age of the subjects at T1 was 12.6 years (SD=1.2 years) and at T4 16.3 years (SD=1.3 years) In order to visualize the different steps of examination, the intraoral photos of a typical Herbst subject (Case 12-1) are shown in Fig. 12-1.

The Bolton Standards (Broadbent et al. 1975) were used as control sample. In the comparison of the Herbst and Bolton groups, the Bolton data were interpolated to suit the age and examination intervals of the Herbst patients.

The lateral head films of the Herbst patients and the tracings of the Bolton Standards were evaluated. The linear roentgenographic enlargement of 7% in the Herbst group was not compensated for. The enlargement of the Bolton tracings varied between 5.5% and 5.8% and was adapted to that of the Herbst patients.

The methods for the assessment of "effective TMJ growth" (a summation of condylar modeling, glenoid fossa modeling and condylar position changes in the fossa), chin position change and mandibular rotation are presented in Chapter 6: Herbst research-subjects and methods. The point Co (arbitrary condylar point) was used as reference for "effective TMJ growth", the point Pg (pogonion) as reference for chin position changes and the line RL as reference for mandibular rotation.

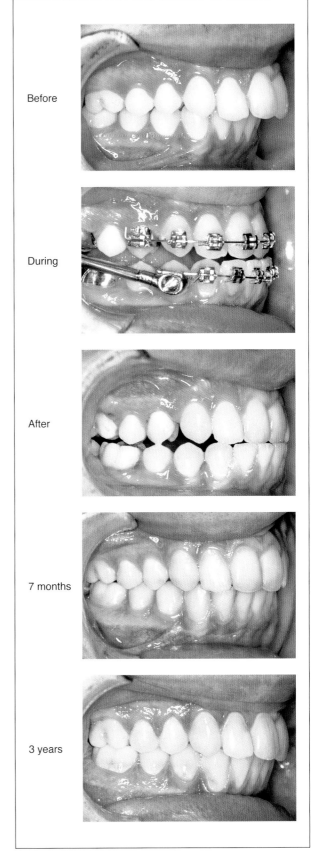

Before

During

After

7 months

3 years

Fig. 12-1 Case 12-1 Herbst treatment of a 14-year-old male. Registrations at before treatment, during treatment, after 7 months of treatment when the appliance was removed (note overcorrected sagittal and vertical dental arch relationships), 7 months posttreatment (note the settling of the occlusion) and 3 years posttreatment. No retention was used in this patient.

"Effective TMJ growth" (Figs. 12-2 and 12-3)

During the treatment period (T1 to T2) of 7 months, the Co point in the Herbst group changed its position in an almost equal upward (mean=3.1 mm) and backward (mean=2.8 mm) direction (Fig. 12-2). Compared to the Bolton group, the Co change in the Herbst group was about three times as large in the horizontal and twice as large in the vertical direction.

When comparing the male and the female subjects of the Herbst group (Fig. 12-3), no gender differences with respect to the direction of Co changes during the different examination periods were found. However, the amount of changes were more extensive in the male subjects, especially in the T3 to T4 period.

During the first posttreatment period of 7 months (T2 to T3), the direction of Co change in the Herbst group was, on average, almost completely vertically upward and the amount (mean=1.0 mm) was reduced to one third of that seen in the T1 to T2 period (Fig. 12-2). Compared to the Bolton group, the amount of vertical Co change was, on average, approximately only one half.

During the second posttreatment period (T3 to T4) of 2.5 years, the Co point in the Herbst group changed its position more in an upward (mean=4.4 mm) than in a backward (mean=1.4 mm) direction (Fig. 12-2). In the Bolton group, the amount of the Co change was, on average, larger than in the Herbst group, and the direction of change was predominantly vertically upward. At T4 the Co point was, on average, positioned 2.8 mm more posteriorly in the Herbst group than in the Bolton group.

Chin position change (Figs. 12-2 and 12-3)

During the treatment period (T1 to T2) of 7 months, the Pg point in the Herbst group changed its position in a more downward (mean=3.9 mm) than forward (mean=2.2 mm) direction (Fig. 12-2). In comparison to the Bolton group, the Pg change in the Herbst group was approximately five times as large in the vertical and twice as large in the horizontal direction. During the first posttreatment period (T2 to T3) of 7 months, the amount of Pg change in the Herbst group was dramatically reduced in comparison to that seen in the T1 to T2 period and the direction was equally (0.5 mm) forward and downward (Fig. 12-2).

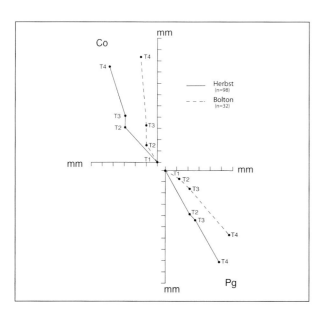

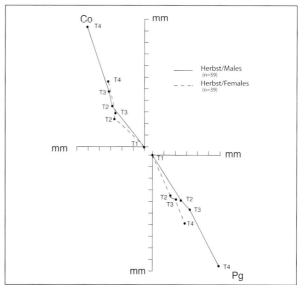

Fig. 12-2 "Effective TMJ growth" (Co) and chin position changes (Pg) in 98 Herbst patients. Registrations at before treatment (T1), after 7 months of treatment when the appliance was removed (T2), 7 months posttreatment (T3) and 3 years posttreatment (T4). The corresponding changes in the Bolton Standards are shown. (*Revised from Pancherz et al. 1998*)

Fig. 12-3 "Effective TMJ growth" (Co) and chin position changes (Pg) in 59 male and 39 female Herbst patients. Registrations at before treatment (T1), after 7 months of treatment when the appliance was removed (T2), 7 months posttreatment (T3) and 3 years posttreatment (T4). (*Revised from Pancherz et al. 1998*)

Compared with the Bolton group, the amount of Pg change in the Herbst group was, on average, only half. The direction was, however, the same in both groups.

During the second posttreatment period (T3 to T4) of 2.5 years, the Pg point in the Herbst group changed its position less forward (mean=2.1 mm) than downward (mean=3.7 mm) (Fig.12-2). In the Bolton group, the amount of Pg change was, on average, somewhat larger than in the Herbst group, and the direction of change was more horizontally forward. At T4 the Pg point was, on average, positioned 2.4 mm more downward and 0.9 mm more backward in the Herbst than in the Bolton group.

When the males and the females of the Herbst group were compared (Fig. 12-3), a tendency for relatively more horizontally directed Pg changes were noted in the males during the different examination periods. Furthermore, the amount of change was larger in the male than in the female subjects, especially during the T3 to T4 period.

Mandibular rotation

During the treatment period (T1 to T2) of 7 months, the mandible (line RL) in the Herbst group rotated posteriorly (mean=0.4°). This was twice as much as in the Bolton group (mean=0.2°).

During the first posttreatment period (T2 to T3) of 7 months, the RL in the Herbst group rotated anteriorly by, an average of 0.3°. In the Bolton group, no RL rotation was, on average, noted during this period.

During the second posttreatment period (T3 to T4) of 2.5 years, the RL in the Herbst group rotated further anteriorly by an average of, 0.3°. In the Bolton group, the RL rotated anteriorly by an average of, 1.3°, which was four times larger than in the Herbst group.

When considering the total examination period (T1 to T4), an anterior RL rotation was found in both examination groups. This, however, was five times larger in the Bolton (mean=1.1°) than in the Herbst (mean=0.2°) group.

When comparing the male and female subjects of the Herbst group during the T1 to T2 period, posterior RL rotation was, on average, more than three times larger in the females (mean=0.7°) than in the males (mean=0.2°). During the T2 to T3 period, anterior RL rotation was comparable in the two gender groups (mean=0.3°). During the T3 to T4 period, anterior RL rotation was twice as large in the male (mean=0.4°) than in the female (mean=0.2°) subjects.

Interpretation of the results

In interpreting the findings it must be emphasized that a large individual variation existed for all variables at all times of examination.

The results of this study clearly showed the large influence of mandibular rotation on the direction of chin position changes. Without jaw rotation, the changes in chin position are a mirror image of the "effective TMJ growth" (Fig. 12-4). In cases with anterior mandibular rotation, the chin moves relatively more forward (Fig. 12-5) and in cases with posterior rotation the chin moves relatively more downward (Fig. 12-6). Several processes are involved in mandibular rotation (Solow 1980), such as "effective TMJ growth", vertical maxillary jaw growth, vertical maxillary and mandibular dentoalveolar growth and steepness of the incisal guidance during mandibular advancement. With the use of the mandibular superimposition technique of Björk and Skieller (1983) the RL line (defined on the T1 head film) could be compared with an implant line (Björk and Skieller, 1983). Its change during the different examination periods shows the true jaw bone rotation not masked by remodeling processes at the lower border of the mandibular corpus (Björk and Skieller 1972, 1983, Kruse 1999).

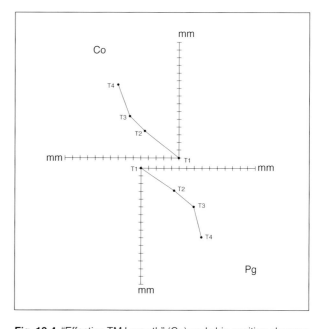

Fig. 12-4 "Effective TMJ growth" (Co) and chin position changes (Pg) in a 14-year-old boy treated with the Herbst appliance for 6 months. Registrations at before treatment (T1), after treatment when the appliance was removed (T2), 6 months posttreatment (T3) and 4 years posttreatment (T4). No mandibular rotation occurred during the examination period. (*Revised from Pancherz et al. 1998*)

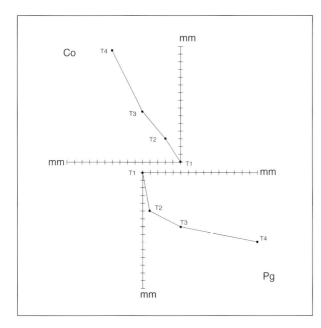

Fig. 12-5 "Effective TMJ growth" (Co) and chin position changes (Pg) in a 12-year-old boy treated with the Herbst appliance for 8 months. Registrations at before treatment (T1), after treatment when the appliance was removed (T2), 1 year posttreatment (T3) and 3 years posttreatment (T4). An anterior mandibular rotation of 4.0° occurred during the posttreatment period T2 to T4. (*Revised from Pancherz et al. 1998*)

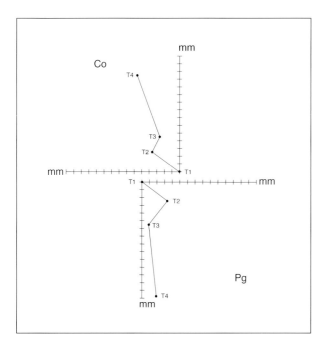

Fig. 12-6 "Effective TMJ growth" (Co) and chin position changes (Pg) in a 11-year-old boy treated with the Herbst appliance for 7 months. Registrations at before treatment (T1), after treatment when the appliance was removed (T2), 6 months posttreatment (T3) and 3 years posttreatment (T4). A posterior mandibular rotation of 2.5° occurred during the posttreatment period T3 to T4. (*Revised from Pancherz et al. 1998*)

Treatment changes

During 7 months of treatment (T1 to T2), "effective TMJ growth" in the Herbst group was directed horizontally backward and about three times larger than that of the Bolton group (Fig. 12-3). This could primarily be explained by the stimulating effect of the Herbst appliance on sagittal condylar growth (Pancherz 1979, Pancherz and Hägg 1985, Pancherz and Littmann 1989, Ruf and Pancherz 1998). However, glenoid fossa modeling (Pancherz 1979, Woodside et al. 1987, Decrue and Wieslander 1990, Ruf and Pancherz 1998, Pancherz and Fischer 2003) would certainly also contribute to the changes of "effective TMJ growth" seen during treatment. Repositioning of the condyle within the fossa (Hansen et al. 1990, Ruf and Pancherz 1998), on the other hand, was thought to be of minor importance for the "effective TMJ growth" during Herbst treatment.

As a result of the "effective TMJ growth", the chin moved forward and downward (Fig. 12-2). The amount of the downward-directed chin changes was about five times larger in the Herbst than in the Bolton group. The increased vertical component of the chin position changes was certainly the result of posterior mandibular rotation when the jaw was advanced to an incisal edge-to-edge position during treatment (Fig. 12-1).

Posttreatment changes

During the first posttreatment period (T2 to T3) of 7 months, "effective TMJ growth" recovered in the Herbst group (Pancherz 1981, Pancherz and Littmann 1989). At the same time, the chin moved relatively more horizontally forward (Fig. 12-3). This was because of an anterior mandibular rotation when the occlusion was settling (Fig. 12-1).

During the second posttreatment period (T3 to T4) of 2.5 years, "effective TMJ growth" and chin position changes in the Herbst group can be considered to result from normal growth development. In comparison to the Bolton Standards, the "effective TMJ growth" of the Herbst sample was directed more horizontally backward whereas the direction of chin movement was more vertically downward (Fig. 12-2). This was owing to the fact that anterior mandibular rotation in the Herbst group was only one fourth of that seen in the Bolton group.

Differences between gender

During the treatment period (T1 to T2) and first posttreatment period (T2-T3), the amount and direction of "effective TMJ growth" and chin position changes were comparable in the male and female subjects.

During the second posttreatment period (T3 to T4), however, the males exhibited changes twice as large as the females (Fig. 12-3). This can be explained by gender differences in growth potential during the age period of 14 to 16 years, in which the males still grew actively whereas the females had almost finished their growth (Taranger and Hägg 1980).

Conclusions and clinical implications

- In Herbst treatment, "effective TMJ growth" (a summation of condylar modeling, glenoid fossa modeling and condylar position changes in the fossa) in combination with mandibular rotation decides the position of the chin.
- During the treatment period, "effective TMJ growth" is relatively more backward directed and larger than that in untreated subjects with normal occlusion. During the first posttreatment period of 0.6 years, "effective TMJ growth" recovers with respect to both the direction and the amount of changes. Thereafter "effective TMJ growth", (direction and amount) tends to be "normal".
- Chin position changes during and after Herbst therapy are a mirror image of "effective TMJ growth" provided no mandibular rotation occurs.
- In subjects with anterior mandibular rotation, relatively more forward, and in subjects with posterior mandibular rotation, relatively more backward directed chin position changes result.

References

Björk A, Skieller V. Facial development and tooth eruption. An implant study at the age of puberty. Am J Orthod 1972;62:339-383.

Björk A, Skieller V. Normal and abnormal growth of the mandible. A synthesis of longitudinal cephalometric implant studies over a period of 25 years. Eur J Orthod 1983;5:1-46.

Broadbent BH, Broadbent BH Jr, Golden WH. Bolton Standards of dentofacial development. St. Louis: CV Mosby 1975.

Creekmore TD. Inhibition or stimulation of vertical growth of the facial complex: its significance to treatment. Angle Orthod 1967;37:285-297.

Decrue A, Wieslander L. Verlagerung der Fossa articularis nach Vorverlagerung der Mandibula mittels Herbstapparatur. Zahnärztl Praxis 1990;41:360-365.

Hansen K, Pancherz H, Petersson A. Long-term effects of the Herbst appliance on the craniomandibular system with special reference to the TMJ. Eur J Orthod 1990;12:244-253

Kruse J. Rotationsformen des Unterkiefers bei der Herbst-Behandlung. Eine röntgenkephalometrische Untersuchung der Langzeitveränderungen der Total-, Matrix- und Intramatrix-Rotation. Diss. med. dent. (Thesis), Giessen 1999.

Paulsen HU. Changes of the condyles of 100 patients treated with the Herbst appliance from puberty to adulthood. Eur J Orthod 1997;19:657-668.

Paulsen HU, Karle A, Bakke M, Herskind A. A CT-scanning and radiographic analysis of temporomandibular joints and cephalometric analysis in a case of Herbst treatment in late puberty. Eur J Orthod 1995;17:657-668.

Paulsen HU, Rabol, A, Sorensen S. Bone scintograpy of human mandibular joints during Herbst treatment: a case report. Eur J Orthod 1988;20:369-374.

Pancherz H. Treatment of Class II malocclusions by jumping the bite with the Herbst appliance. A cephalometric investigation. Am J Orthod 1979;76:423-442.

Pancherz H. The effect of continuous bite jumping on the dentofacial complex: a follow-up study after Herbst appliance treatment of Class II malocclusions. Eur J Orthod 1981;3:49-60.

Pancherz H, Fischer S. Amount and direction of temporomandibular joint growth changes in Herbst treatment: a cephalometric long-term investigation. Angle Orthod 2003;73:493-501.

Pancherz H, Hägg U. Dentofacial orthopedics in relation to somatic maturation, An analysis of 70 consecutive cases treated with the Herbst appliance. Am J Orthod 1985;88:273-287.

Pancherz H, Hansen K. Occlusal changes during and after Herbst treatment: a cephalmetric investigation. Eur J Orthod 1986;8:215-228.

Pancherz H, Littmann C. Morphologie und Lage des Unterkiefers bei der Herbst-Behandlung. Eine kephalometrische Analyse der Veränderungen bis zum Wachstumsabschluss. Inf Orthod Kieferorthop 1989;21:493-513.

Pancherz H, Michaelidou C. Temporomandibular joint changes in hyperdivergent and hypodivergent Herbst subjects. A long-term roentgenographic study. Am J Orthod Dentofac Orthop 2004;126:153-161.

Pancherz H, Ruf S, Kohlhas P. "Effective condylar growth" and chin position changes in Herbst treatment: a cephalometric roentgenographic long-term study. Am J Orthod Dentofac Orthop 1998;114:437-446.

Ruf S, Pancherz H. Temporomandibular joint adaptation in Herbst treatment: a prospective magnetic resonance imaging and cephalometric roentgenographic study. Eur J Orthod 1998;20:375-388.

Ruf S, Pancherz H. Temporomandibular joint remodeling in adolescents and young adults during Herbst treatment: a prospective longitudinal magnetic resonance imaging and cephalometric radiographic investigation. Am J Orthod Dentofac Orthop 1999;115:607-618.

Solow B. The dentoalveolar compensatory mechanism: background and clinical implications. Br J Orthod 1980;7:145-161.

Taranger J, Hägg U. The timing and duration of adolescent growth. Acta Odont Scand 1980;38:57-67.

Wieslander L. Intensive treatment of severe Class II malocclusions with a headgear-Herbst appliance in the mixed dentition. Am J Orthod Dentofac Orthop 1984;86:1-13.

Woodside DG, Metaxas A, Altuna G. The influence of functional appliance therapy on glenoid fossa remodeling. Am J Orthod 1987;92:181-198.

Chapter 13

Effects on the skeletofacial growth pattern

Research

In dentofacial orthopedics of Class II malocclusions it has been claimed that normalization of the skeletal- and soft-tissue morphology at an early age would provide a basis for continuing normal development of these structures (Angle 1907, Fränkel 1967, Bass 1983, Wieslander 1984). This has, however, never been proven. On the contrary, there are several clinical (Melsen 1978, Hooymaayer et al. 1989, Pancherz and Littmann 1989, Pancherz and Fackel 1990, Hägg 1992) and experimental (Petrovic et al. 1981, McNamara and Bryan 1987) studies indicating that the original skeletofacial growth pattern can be altered only temporarily by dentofacial orthopedic means.

The skeletofacial growth pattern pre- and post-dentofacial orthopaedics. A long-term study of Class II malocclusions treated with the Herbst appliance (Pancherz and Fackel 1990)

Using lateral head films in habitual occlusion, the skeletofacial growth changes before and after a 7-month period of Herbst treatment were assessed in 17 male Class II:1 subjects. The pre- and posttreatment periods in each subject were of equal lengths and amounted to an average of 2.5 years. No treatment was performed during the two control periods.

The mean ages of the subjects at the different times of examination were 10.3 years at the beginning of the pretreatment period, 12.9 years at the start of Herbst treatment, 13.6 years at the end of Herbst treatment and 16.1 years at the end of the posttreatment period. Herbst treatment in all subjects was performed before or at the pubertal peak of growth. Posttreatment retention was performed in 8 of the 17 subjects using an upper Hawley plate and a lower cuspid to cuspid retainer. During the pretreatment period of 2.5 years, the Class II:1 malocclusion remained unchanged. Following that period, Herbst treatment resulted in Class I or overcorrected Class I dental arch relationships in all 17 subjects. During the posttreatment period of 2.5 years, the occlusion settled into Class I in 14 subjects while a partial dental relapse, due to a persisting tongue dysfunction habit, was seen in 3 subjects.

The results of the investigation are visualized by superimposed facial polygons (see Chapter 17: Treatment of the retrognathic and prognathic facial type, Fig. 17-1). The average growth changes occurring during the three examination periods are given in Fig. 13-1.

When comparing the average growth changes occurring during the treatment period of 7 months with those of the pretreatment control period of 2.5 years it was found that during Herbst treatment maxillary growth was inhibited and redirected, mandibular growth increased, anterior mandibular growth rotation arrested, intermaxillary jaw relationship improved, the skeletal profile straightened and the gonion angle increased.

During the posttreatment period of 2.5 years a rebound occurred for several of the treatment changes: maxillary position, mandibular inclination and gonion angle.

Maxillary and mandibular growth directions were comparable in both control periods: the inclination of the maxilla in relation to the cranial base remained unchanged, the mandible rotated anteriorly and the gonion angle was reduced in both periods. When looking at individual cases, however, large variations in the growth were seen (see Clinical examples).

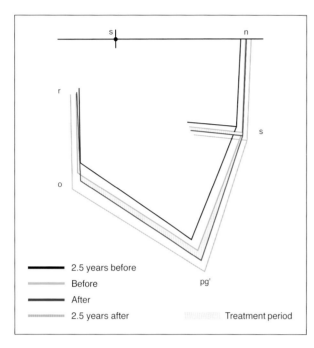

—— 2.5 years before	
—— Before	pg'
—— After	
⸱⸱⸱⸱⸱ 2.5 years after	▓▓▓ Treatment period

Fig. 13-1 Superimposed facial polygons based upon the mean values from 17 male subjects treated with the Herbst appliance. *(Revised from Pancherz and Fackel 1990)*

Interpretations of the results

The skeletofacial growth pattern existing before treatment seemed to prevail, on average, after treatment. Thus, after the orthopedic interventive period, maxillary and mandibular growth seemed to strive to catch up with their earlier patterns. The increase in the gonion and mandibular plane angles during Herbst treatment can be explained by the fact that condylar growth was redirected posteriorly and bone was resorbed at the posterior part of the mandibular lower border (Pancherz and Littmann 1989). The subsequent decrease in the two angles posttreatment resulted from a change in condylar growth in a more vertical direction in combination with bone apposition at the posterior part of the mandibular lower border (Pancherz and Littmann 1989). Similar changes in the gonion angle were reported to occur in mandibular protrusion experiments in monkeys (McNamara and Bryan 1987).

Long-term effects of Herbst treatment in relation to normal growth development: a cephalometric study (Hansen and Pancherz 1992).

Using lateral head films, the short- and long-term effects of Herbst treatment in relation to "normal" growth records of subjects exhibiting excellent occlusion (Bolton Standards) were assessed.

At the time of the examination, the total sample of consecutive Class II:1 malocclusions treated with the Herbst appliance at the Department of Orthodontics, University of Lund, Sweden, comprised of 170 subjects. From this sample 32 subjects (16 males and 16 females) fulfilling the following criteria were selected: (1) the subjects had to match the control group (see below); (2) no permanent teeth extracted; (3) an observation period of at least 5 years after treatment; (4) growth completed at the time of follow-up (Hansen et al. 1991). The control group comprised the Bolton Standards (Broadbent et al. 1975). The Standards consist of composite lateral head film tracings of 32 subjects (16 males and 16 females) with excellent occlusion, followed annually from 1 year to 18 years of age. The 12 years standard was used to match the age of the Herbst sample at start of treatment. The mean age of the Herbst subjects before treatment was 12.5 years (SD=1.0 years) and at the end of the follow-up period 19.3 years (SD=1.4 years). The average treatment time with the Herbst appliance was 0.6 years (SD=0.1 year). The total observation period was, on average, 6.8 years (SD=1.1 years). Lateral head films in habitual occlusion were analyzed according to the SO-Analysis (see Chapter 6: Herbst research-subjects and methods) at three occasions:

- *Herbst sample*: before treatment, 6 months posttreatment when the occlusion had settled (Pancherz and Hansen 1986) and at follow up (Mean=6.2 years, SD=1.1 years, posttreatment). The head films from 6 months posttreatment and follow-up were superimposed on the before treatment film using the stable bone structures in the anterior cranial base for orientation (Björk and Skieller 1983). A composite tracing of the 32 Herbst subjects for each of the three examination stages was constructed.
- *Bolton sample*: at the ages 12, 13 and 18 years. The anterior cranial base structures on the composite tracings were used for superimposition of the 13 and 18 year tracings on the 12 year

tracing. In the head film analysis correction was made for the difference in linear radiographic enlargement in the Herbst (7%) and Bolton (5.9%) samples. The superimposed composite tracings of the Herbst sample and the corresponding tracings of the Bolton sample from the three times of examination are shown in Fig. 13-4.

The comparison of the Herbst and Bolton samples revealed that a retrognathic mandible existed in the Herbst sample at all three times of examination.

During the first observation period from before treatment to 6 months posttreatment (covering the treatment and occlusal settling period), the Herbst sample revealed larger mandibular growth and less maxillary growth than the Bolton sample. Sagittal mandibular growth exceeded sagittal maxillary growth by 2.4 mm in the Herbst sample and by 1.6 mm in the Bolton sample. The overjet and the sagittal molar relationship were normalized (Class I) in the Herbst group, while these parameters remained unchanged (Class I) in the Bolton group.

During the second observation period from 6 months posttreatment to the end of growth (6.2 years after treatment) mandibular and maxillary growth were larger in the Bolton sample than in the Herbst sample. Sagittal mandibular growth exceeded sagittal maxillary growth by 1.5 mm in the Herbst and 3.1 mm in the Bolton samples. With respect to changes in sagittal occlusion there was a clinical insignificant rebound in overjet and molar relationship in the Herbst group. The occlusion, however, stayed Class I. In the Bolton group the overjet and molar relationship remained unchanged (Class I).

During the total observation period from before treatment to the end of growth mandibular and maxillary growth were larger in the Bolton than in the Herbst sample. Sagittal mandibular growth exceeded sagittal maxillary growth with 3.9 mm in the Herbst sample and with 4.1 mm in the Bolton sample. The overjet and the sagittal molar relationship were normalized (Class I) in the Herbst group and remained unchanged (Class I) in the Bolton group.

Interpretation of the results
Jaw relationship
During the first observation period a favorable growth pattern was registered for the Herbst sample. This was certainly an effect of the Herbst appliance (Pancherz 1982). As mentioned above, mandibular growth exceeded maxillary growth by 2.4 mm. In the Bolton sample the corresponding figure was 1.6 mm. The changes in the growth pattern improved the jaw base relationship in all Herbst individuals except one (Hansen and Pancherz 1992). However, only a few subjects reached a value that was comparable with a "normal" jaw base relationship (Bolton Standards). During the second observation period the jaw base relationship continued to improve (sagittal mandibular growth exceeding sagittal maxillary growth) in both samples. The improvement was, however, larger in the Bolton group. The findings at the end of the examination period revealed that the mean difference in jaw base relationship was about the same before treatment and at the time of follow up (before: Herbst/Bolton= -6.1 mm; follow-up: Herbst/Bolton= -6.3 mm). Thus, in spite of the favorable changes occurring during Herbst treatment (Pancherz 1982), jaw growth was not normalized on a long-term basis (Pancherz and Fackel 1990).

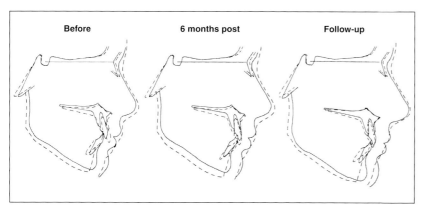

| Before | 6 months post | Follow-up |

Fig. 13-4 Computer calculated composite tracings of 32 Class II:1 malocclusions treated with the Herbst appliance (- - - - -) and composite tracings of 32 subjects exhibiting excellent occlusion (Bolton Standards) (———). Registrations before treatment (12-year-Bolton Standard), 6 months posttreatment (13-year-Bolton Standard) and at follow-up 6.2 years posttreatment (18-year-Bolton Standard).
(Revised from Hansen and Pancherz 1992)

Dental arch relationship
During the first observation period both overjet and sagittal molar relationship were significantly improved in the Herbst sample. In addition to the mandibular skeletal changes mentioned above, this was accomplished by maxillary and mandibular dental changes: the maxillary teeth were moved posteriorly and the mandibular teeth were moved anteriorly (Pancherz 1982, Pancherz and Hansen 1986). Although a minor rebound in overjet and sagittal molar relationship occurred during the second observation period, the dental arch relationship was normalized on a long-term basis in the Herbst sample.

Clinical examples

Two boys with a Class II:1 malocclusion (Cases 13-1 and 13-2) illustrating differences in growth pattern during the three examination periods are presented.

Case 13-1 (Fig. 13-2a,b)
A 12-year-old male was treated with the Herbst appliance for 7 months. The pre- and posttreatment examination periods were 2 years each. The boy originally had a small mandibular plane angle (ML/NSL=26°), which was unchanged during the examination period of 4.6 years. Sagittal maxillary growth was restrained during Herbst treatment but recovered posttreatment. The mandible was positioned forward during treatment and dropped back posttreatment. The gonion angle was opened by 4° during therapy, but recovered completely thereafter.

Case 13-2 (Fig. 13-3a,b)
A 14-year-old male was treated with the Herbst appliance for 6 months. The pre- and posttreatment examination periods were 3 years each. The boy originally had an increased mandibular plane angle (ML/NSL=37°), which was reduced during the examination period of 6.5 years. Sagittal maxillary growth was restrained during Herbst treatment but recovered posttreatment. The mandible was positioned forward during treatment and continued to grow forward posttreatment. The gonion angle was opened by 3° during therapy, but recovered completely thereafter.

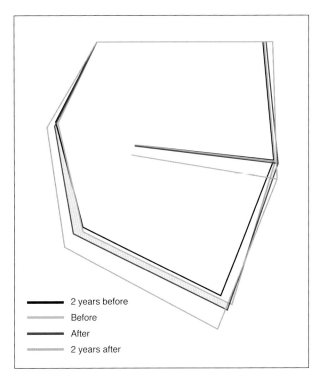

— 2 years before
Before
After
2 years after

Fig. 13-2a Case 13-1 12-year-old male with a Class II:1 malocclusion treated with the Herbst appliance for 7 months. Superimposed facial polygons. *(Revised from Pancherz and Fackel 1990)*

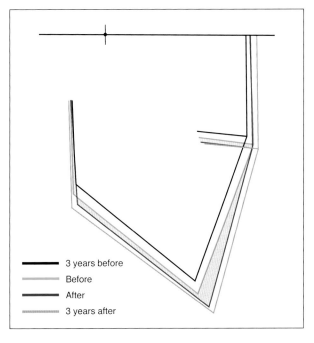

— 3 years before
Before
After
3 years after

Fig. 13-3a Case 13-2 14-year-old male with a Class II:1 malocclusion treated with the Herbst appliance for 6 months. Superimposed facial polygons. *(Revised from Pancherz and Fackel 1990)*

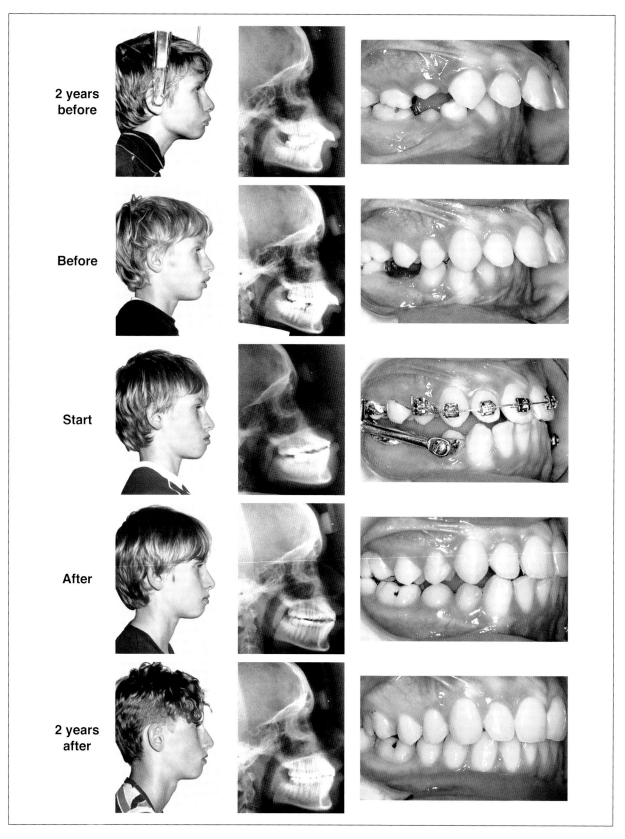

Fig. 13-2b Case 13-1 12-year-old male with a Class II:1 malocclusion treated with the Herbst appliance for 7 months. Profile photos, lateral head films and intraoral photos. *(Revised from Pancherz and Fackel 1990)*

117

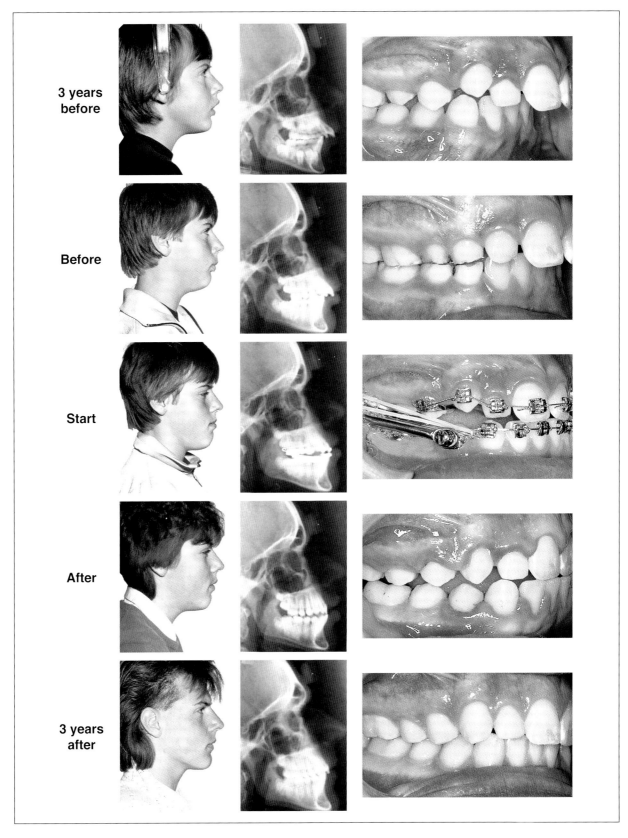

Fig. 13-3b Case 13-2 14-year-old male with a Class II:1 malocclusion treated with the Herbst appliance for 6 months. Profile photos, lateral head films and intraoral photos. *(Revised from Pancherz and Fackel 1990)*

Conclusions and clinical implications

- Dentofacial orthopedics using the Herbst appliance in early adolescent Class II:1 subjects seems to have only a temporary impact on the existing skeletofacial growth pattern. In spite of the recovering growth changes after Herbst treatment a stable occlusion will counteract an occlusal relapse (as seen in 14 of the 17 subjects investigated). Thus, a solid Class I interdigitation of the teeth after Herbst therapy or any dentofacial orthopedic measure will be of utmost importance for a stable long-term treatment result (Pancherz, 1991).
- In comparison to normal growth development (Bolton Standards), Herbst treatment can, on a long-term basis, improve the basal jaw base relationship but not normalize it. The dental effects of the Herbst appliance as part of the treatment outcome can compensate for an unfavorable jaw base relationship.

References

Angle E. Malocclusions of the teeth. 7th edn. Philadelphia: SS White Dental MFG Co, 1907.

Bass, N. Orthopedic coordination of dentofacial development in skeletal Class II malocclusions in the conjunction with edgewise therapy Part I and II. Am J Orthod 1983;84:361-383, 466-499.

Björk A, Skieller V. Normal and abnormal growth of the mandible. A synthesis of longitudinal cephalometric implant studies over a period of 25 years. Eur J Orthod 1983;5:1-46.

Broadbent BHSr, Broadbent BHJr, Golden W. Bolton Standards of dentofacial development growth. St Louis: C.V. Mosby Company, 1975.

Fränkel R. Funktionskieferorthopädie und der Mundvorhof als apparative Basis. Berlin: V.E.B. Verlag Volk & Gesundheit, 1967.

Hägg U. Change of mandibular growth direction by means of a Herbst appliance? A case report. Am J Orthod Dentofac Orthop 1992;102:456-463.

Hansen K, Pancherz H. Long-term effects of Herbst treatment in relation to normal growth development: a cephalometric study. Eur J Orthod 1992;14:285-295.

Hansen K, Pancherz H, Hägg U. Long-term effects of Herbst treatment in relation to the treatment growth period: a cephalometric study. Eur J Orthod 1991;13:471-481.

Hooymaayer J, van der Linden FPGM, Boersma, H. Post treatment facial development in corrected class II division 1 anomalies. J Dent Res 1989;68:632.

McNamara JA, Bryan FA. Long-term mandibular adaptations to protrusive function: an experimental study in Macaca mulatta. Am J Orthod 1987;92:98-108.

Melsen B. Effects of cervical anchorage during and after treatment: an implant study. Am J Orthod 1978;73:526-540.

Pancherz H. The mechanism of Class II correction in Herbst appliance treatment. Am J Orthod 1982;82:104-113.

Pancherz H. The nature of Class II relapse after Herbst appliance treatment: a cephalometric long-term investigation. Am J Orthod Dentofac Orthop 1991;100:220-233.

Pancherz H, Fackel U. The skeletofacial growth pattern pre- and postdentofacial orthopeadics. A long-term study of Class II malloclusions treated with the Herbst appliance. Eur J Orthod 1990;12:209-218.

Pancherz H, Hansen K. Occlusal changes during and after Herbst treatment. Eur J Orthod 1986;8:215-228.

Pancherz H, Littmann C. Morphologie und Lage des Unterkiefers bei der Herbst-Behandlung. Eine kephalometrische Analyse der Veränderungen bis zum Wachstumsabschluss. Inf Orthod Kieferorthop 1989;21:493-513.

Petrovic A, Stutzmann, Gasson N. The final length of the mandible: is it genetically determined? In Carson DS, ed. Craniofacial Biology, Monograph 10, Craniofacial growth series. Ann Arbor: Center of Human Growth and Development, The University of Michigan, 1981:105-126.

Wieslander, L. Intensive treatment of severe Class II malocclusions with a headgear-Herbst appliance in the early mixed dentition. Am J Orthod 1984;86:1-13.

Chapter 14

Effects on the facial profile

Research

In accordance with the Caucasian beauty ideal we undoubtedly prefer a fairly straight facial profile. As a convex profile is the prominent feature in many Class II malocclusions one of the objectives in orthodontic therapy is to improve facial esthetics by reducing facial profile convexity.

In growing Class II:1 subjects, the short-term effects of Herbst therapy on the facial profile have been analyzed by Pancherz (1979) and Eicke and Wieslander (1990), and the long-term effects by Pancherz and Anehus-Pancherz (1994). In adult Herbst subjects the facial profile changes were considered in three investigations (Ruf and Pancherz 1999, 2004, 2006). A systematic review on soft tissue facial profile changes with fixed functional appliances (Herbst, Jasper Jumper, MARA, Forsus spring) has been performed by Flores-Mir et al. (2006).

The scientific evidence on the topic of facial profile changes in Herbst treatment will be presented by scrutinizing two publications.

1. Facial profile changes during and after Herbst appliance treatment (Pancherz and Anehus-Pancherz 1994)

In this retrospective study the short- and long-term effects of Herbst therapy on the hard and soft tissue facial profile were evaluated using lateral head films. The subject material comprised of 49 Class II:1 cases (32 males and 17 females) treated successfully with the banded type of Herbst appliance (see Chapter 3: Design, construction and clinical management

of the Herbst appliance) at the Department of Orthodontics, Univesity of Lund, Sweden. The mean age of the subjects at start of therapy was 12.7 years (SD=1.2 years). Treatment was performed during a period of 6-8 months (Mean=7 months) and the patients were followed for 5-10 years (Mean=6.2 years) posttreatment. Before treatment all subjects had a full Class II molar relationship, an overjet of at least 6 mm and a minimum ANB angle of 5°. The Herbst therapy resulted in Class I or overcorrected Class I dental arch relationships with a normal overjet in all cases. At the time of follow-up the overjet was unchanged and the molar relationship in Class I. Following Herbst treatment no further active treatment was carried out. Retention (upper plate, activator, mandibular cuspid to cuspid retainer) for 1- 2 years was performed in 35 subjects. At the time of follow-up the subjects were out of retention for a minimum of 4 years. No retention was performed in 14 subjects. Lateral head films in habitual occlusion and the lips in relaxed position were examined. The radiographs were taken before treatment (prior to the placement of the appliance, after 7 months of treatment (when the appliance was removed), 6 months posttreatment (when the occlusion had settled and at follow-up (6.2 years posttreatment). The short- and long-term changes of the hard and soft tissue profile convexity and the lip position were assessed. As a gender difference existed only for the hard tissue profile convexity angle (the males had straighter profiles than the females at all times of examination) the male and female samples were pooled in the presentation of the results.

Treatment changes

After 7 months of treatment the hard tissue and soft tissue (including and excluding the nose) profile convexities (Fig. 14-1) were reduced and the distances of the upper and lower lips to the Esthetic line (E-line) (Fig. 14-2) had increased (the lips had become more retrusive).

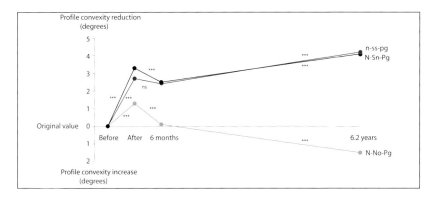

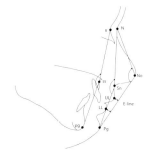

Fig. 14-1 Facial profile convexity changes in 49 adolescent Class II:1 malocclusions treated with the Herbst appliance. Mean changes in hard tissue profile convexity (n-ss-pg), soft tissue profile convexity excluding the nose (N-Sn-Pg) and soft tissue profile convexity including the nose (N-No-Pg).

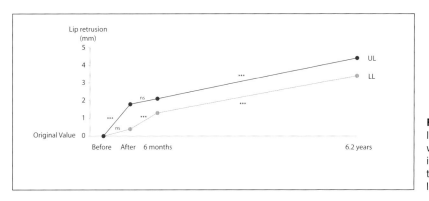

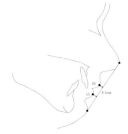

Fig. 14-2 Lip position changes in 49 adolescent Class II:1 malocclusions treated with the Herbst appliance. Mean changes in the position of the upper lip (UL) and the lower lip (LL) in relation to the Esthetic line (E-line).

Posttreatment changes

During the first posttreatment period of 6 months a minor rebound in the hard tissue and soft tissue (excluding the nose) profile convexities had occurred while a complete rebound had taken place for the soft tissue profile convexity including the nose (Fig. 14-1). The distances of the upper and lower lips to the E-line had increased further (lip retrusion was enhanced) (Fig. 14-2).

During the following posttreatment period of 5.7 years the hard tissue and soft tissue (excluding the nose) profile convexities were reduced again while the soft tissue profile convexity including the nose had increased further (Fig. 14-1). The distances of the upper and lower lips to the E-line had also increased further (lip retrusion was enhanced) (Fig. 14-2).

Total observation period changes

During the total observation period of 6.8 years the hard tissue and soft tissue (excluding the nose) profile convexities were reduced while the soft tissue profile convexity incuding the nose had increased) (Fig. 14-1). The distances of the upper and lower lips to the E-line had increased (lip retrusion was enhanced) (Fig. 14-2).

Interpretations of the results

In interpreting the findings it must be pointed out that a large individual variation in facial profile convexity changes existed both in the treatment and posttreatment periods.

Treatment changes

As has been shown previously (Chapter 7: Short-term effects on the dentoskeletal structures), the Herbst appliance increases mandibular prognathism, moves the upper dentition posteriorly and the mandibular dentition anteriorly. This will result in a straightening of the hard and soft tissue profiles. Due to the forward movement of the chin, the upper lip will consequently be placed in a retrusive position relative to the E-line. The lower lip, on the other hand, follows the movement of the mandible and chin and its relation to the E-line will be affected only to a minor degree. Thus the upper to lower lip relationship will be improved.

Early posttreatment changes

Immediately after Herbst treatment, overcorrected sagittal dental arch relationships in combination with an incomplete cuspal interdigitation existed in all subjects. Due to relapsing tooth movements and settling of the occlusion (Pancherz and Hansen 1986) as well as recovering jaw growth (Pancherz and Fackel 1990) during the first 6 months posttreatment, the hard and soft tissue profile convexities increase. However, part of the soft tissue profile changes including the nose may be attributed to an increase in nasal growth as well (Subtelny 1959, Meng et al. 1988). Furthermore, nasal growth will also result in a retrusion of the lips in relation to the E-line.

As the posture of the lips is closely related to the teeth (Subtelny 1959) and the lower incisors are more prone to relapse (lingual tipping), than the upper (labial tipping) the lower lip may become retrusive in relation to the upper lip.

Late posttreatment changes

In the period from 6 months posttreatment to 5.7 years posttreatment the largest part of the facial profile changes seen were most certainly a result of the normal posttreatment growth development. As a consequence of mandibular growth with forward movement of the chin the hard tissue and soft tissue (excluding the nose) profile convexity will be reduced, while due to continuing nasal growth the soft tissue profile convexity including the nose will increase. Furthermore, due to both chin and nose growth the distances of the upper and lower lips to the E-line will increase as well.

2. Herbst/Multibracket appliance treatment of Class II, division 1 malocclusions in early and late adulthood (Ruf and Pancherz 2006)

In this prospective study of consecutive adult Class II:1 malocclusions treated with the Herbst/Multibracket appliance, the effects of therapy on the hard and soft tissue profile were evaluated using lateral head films. The subject material comprised 23 adult Class II:1 cases (4 males and 19 females) treated non-extraction with a cast splint Herbst appliance (see Chapter 3: Design, construction and clinical management of the Herbst appliance) in a first phase and a multibracket appliance (MB) in a second phase. All patients were treated at the Department of Orthodontics, University of Giessen, Germany. The mean pretreatment age was 21.9 years (15.7 – 44.4 years). Using the method of Hägg and Taranger (1980), adulthood was defined by the pretreatment hand radiographic stages R-IJ (4 subjects) and R-J (19 subjects). At the end of treatment all subjects had reached the stage R-J. The average treatment time was 22 months (Herbst = 9 months, MB = 13 months). Before treatment the average overjet was 8.9 mm (SD=2.7 mm). All subjects were treated successfully to a Class I occlusion with a normal overjet.

Lateral head films in habitual occlusion from before treatment, after the Herbst phase and after the MB phase were analyzed. The treatment changes of the hard and soft tissue profile convexity and the lip position were assessed.

Due to the small number of male subjects (n=4), gender differences were not considered and the male and female samples were pooled.

Changes during the Herbst phase

During 9 months of Herbst treatment the hard tissue and soft tissue profile (including and excluding the nose) convexities were reduced (Fig. 14-3). The largest reduction was seen for the soft tissue profile convexity excluding the nose. The upper lip became more retrusive and the lower lip more protrusive in relation to the E-line (Fig. 14-4).

Changes during the MB phase

During 13 months of MB treatment after the Herbst treatment phase, a partial rebound in the hard and soft tissue profile convexity measures occurred. This was especially the case for the soft tissue profile convexity including the nose (Fig. 14-3). Upper lip position did not change significantly while lower lip position rebounded (Fig. 14-4).

Total treatment changes

During 22 months of Herbst/MB appliance treatment, the profile convexity (all three variables) was significantly reduced. The largest reduction was seen for the soft tissue profile convexity excluding the nose (Fig. 14-3). The upper lip became significantly more retrusive while the lower lip rebounded to its original position (Fig. 14-4).

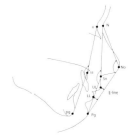

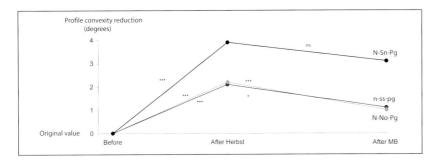

Fig. 14-3 Facial profile convexity changes in 23 adult Class II:1 malocclusions treated with the Herbst/Multibracket appliance. Mean changes in hard tissue profile convexity (n-ss-pg), soft tissue profile convexity excluding the nose (N-Sn-Pg) and soft tissue profile convexity including the nose (N-No-Pg).

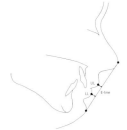

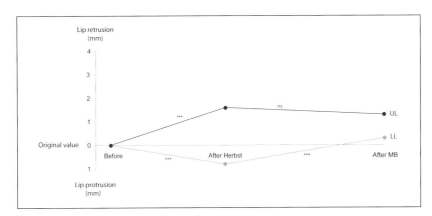

Fig. 14-4 Lip position changes in 23 adult Class II:1 malocclusions treated with the Herbst/Multibracket appliance. Mean changes in the position of the upper lip (UL) and the lower lip (LL) in relation to the Esthetic line (E-line).

Interpretations of the results

Herbst treatment of adult Class II:1 malocclusions has been shown to be very successful (Ruf and Pancherz 1999, 2004, 2006). Basically the overjet correction mechanism is similar to that seen in adolescent subjects (Pancherz and Hansen 1986), altough the skeletal contribution is less. Therefore, it is not surprising that the facial profile changes were comparable in the adolescent (Fig. 14-1) and adult (Fig. 14-3) subjects. The only difference seen was for the lower lip position during the Herbst phase: in the adolescent subjects the lower lip to E-line relationship was hardly changed (Fig. 14-2) while in the adult subjects the lower lip became more protrusive (Fig. 14-4). An explanation could be that in adult subjects nose growth is less pronounced than in adolescent subjects. Thus, the E-line would be less affected in the older than in the younger subjects.

Clinical examples

Three adolescent (Case 14-1 to Case 14-3) and three adult (Case 14-4 to Case 14-6) Class II:1 subjects treated with the Herbst appliance are presented. The facial profile photos and lateral head films are shown. The adolescent subjects were exclusively treated with a banded Herbst appliance for 6 months and followed to adulthood 6-8 years after therapy. The adult subjects were treated with a cast splint Herbst appliance for 8 -12 months followed by a MB appliance for 14 - 22 months. The treatment was successful and stable in all subjects.

Case 14-1 (Fig. 14-5)

A 12-year-old female was treated with the Herbst appliance for 6 months. No retention was performed after therapy. The patient was re-examined at the age of 19 years, 6 years posttreatment. A continuous facial profile convexity reduction occurred during and after treatment. The upper to lower lip relationship was improved. Nose growth was minimal.

Case 14-2 (Fig. 14-5)

A 13-year-old male was treated with the Herbst appliance for 6 months. No retention was performed after therapy. The patient was re-examined at the age of 22 years, 8 years posttreatment. The facial profile convexity was reduced during treatment and remained almost unchanged during the follow-up period. The nose growth was minimal.

Case 14-3 (Fig. 14-5)

A 11-year-old female was treated with the Herbst appliance for 6 months. No retention was performed after therapy. The patient was re-examined at the age 20 years, 8 years posttreatment. The facial profile convexity was reduced during treatment. The upper to lower lip relationship was improved. Due to a large nose growth posttreatment the face had a bimaxillary retrognathic look at the time of follow-up.

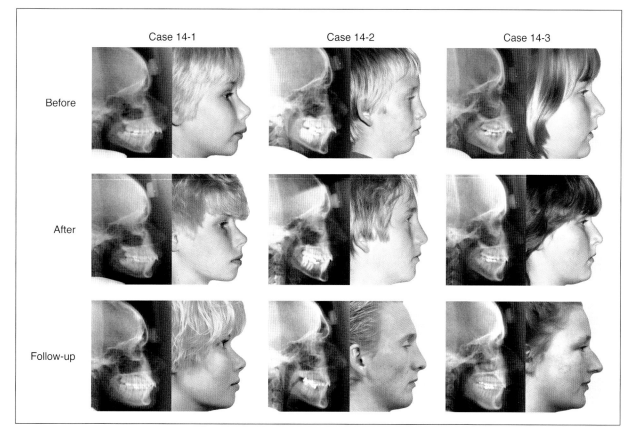

Fig. 14-5 Facial profile changes in three adolescent (Cases 14-1 to 14-3) Class II:1 maloccusions treated successfully with the Herbst appliance. Registrations at before treatment, after treatment and at follow-up (in adulthood, 6-8 years after therapy).

Case 14-4 (Fig. 14-6)

A 22-year-old female was treated with the Herbst appliance for 12 months followed by an MB appliance for 14 months. The patient had previously been treated unsuccessfully at the age of 12 years with a MB appliance and extractions of 4 premolars. The facial profile convexity was reduced by therapy and the upper to lower lip relationship was improved.

Case 14-5 (Fig. 14-6)

A 27-year-old female was treated with the Herbst appliance for 8 months followed by an MB appliance for 15 months. Due to severe crowding one mandibular incisor was extracted during treatment. The facial profile convexity was reduced by therapy and the upper to lower lip relationship was improved.

Case 14-6 (Fig. 14-6)

A 24-year-old male was treated with the Herbst appliance for 10 months followed by an MB appliance for 22 months. The facial profile convexity was reduced by therapy and the upper to lower lip relationship was improved.

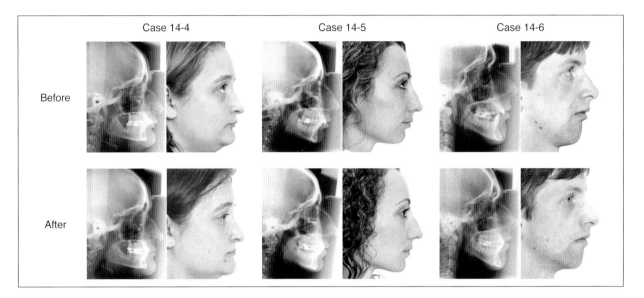

Fig. 14-6 Facial profile changes in three adult (Cases 14-4 to 14-6) Class II:1 maloccusions treated successfully with the Herbst / MB appliance. Registrations at before treatment and after treatment.

Conclusions and clinical implications

In both adolescent and adult Class II:1 subjects the Herbst appliance has an advantageous effect on the facial profile.
- The facial hard and soft tissue profiles are straightened consistently.
- The soft tissue profile excluding the nose is affected more than the hard tissue profile and the soft tissue profile including the nose.
- The upper lip becomes retrusive in relation to the E-line while the lower lip is relatively unaffected by therapy.

- The most favorable facial profile changes during treatment are seen in subjects with a retrognathic mandible (chin), a retrusive lower lip and a protrusive upper lip.
- Due to posttreatment growth changes the long-term effects of Herbst therapy on the facial profile are variable and unpredictable.

References

Eicke C, Wieslander L. Weichteilprofilveränderungen durch Therapie mit dem Herbst-Scharnier. Schweiz Monatsschr Zahnmed 1990;100:149-153.

Flores-Mir C, Major MP, Major PW. Soft tissue changes with fixed functional appliances in Class II division 1. A systematic review. Angle Orthod 2006; 76: 712-720

Hägg U, Taranger J. Skeletal stages of the hand and wrist as indicators of the pubertal growth spurt. Acta Odont Scand 1980;38:187-200.

Meng HP, Goorhuis J, Kapila S, Nanda RS.Growth changes in the nasal profile from 7 to 18 years of age. Am J Orthod Dentofac Orthop 1988;94:317-326.

Pancherz H. Treatment of Class II malocclusions by jumping the bite with the Herbst appliance. A cephalometric investigation. Am J Orthod 1979;76:423-442.

Pancherz H, Anehus-Pancherz M. Facial profile changes during and after Herbst appliance treatment. Eur J Orthod 1994;16:275-286.

Pancherz H, Fackel U. The skeletofacial growth pattern pre- and postdentofacial orthopeadics. A long-term study of Class II maloclusions treated with the Herbst appliance. Eur J Orthod 1990;12:209-218.

Pancherz H, Hansen K. Occlusal changes during and after Herbst treatment: a cephalmetric investigation. Eur J Orthod 1986;8:215-228.

Ruf S, Pancherz H. Dentoskeletal effects and facial profile changes in young adults treated with the Herbst appliance. Angle Orthod 1999;69:239-246.

Ruf S, Pancherz H. Orthognathic surgery and dentofacial orthopedics in adult Class II Division 1 treatment: Mandibular sagittal split osteotomy versus Herbst appliance. Am J Orthod Dentofac Orthop 2004;126:140-152.

Ruf S, Pancherz H. Herbst/Multibracket appliance treatment of Class II, division 1 malocclusions in early and late adulthood. A prospective cephalometric study of consecutively treated subjects. Eur J Orthod 2006; 28: 352-360.

Subtelny JD. A longitudinal study of soft tissue facial structures and their profile characteristics, defined in relation to underlying skeletal structures. Am J Orthod 1959;45:481-507.

Chapter 15

Effects on muscular activity

In the field of orthodontics and dental research electromyography (EMG) of the masticatory muscles has been used since 1949 (Moyers 1949). The masseter and temporal muscles have mainly been in the focus of attention.

It has been shown that the EMG activity is related to malocclusion and craniofacial morphology (Ahlgren 1966, Möller 1966, Ahlgren et al. 1973, Ingervall and Thilander 1974). In comparison to individuals with normal (Class I) occlusion (Ahlgren 1966, Möller 1966, Pancherz 1980a), an abnormal muscle contraction pattern has been ascertained in Class II:1 malocclusions (Moyers 1949, Grosfeld 1965, Ahlgren et al. 1973, Moss 1975, Pancherz 1980b). Thus, it can be expected that changes in occlusion and craniofacial morphology accomplished by dentofacial orthopedics will affect muscle function.It was found that treatment with removable functional appliances normalizes the muscle pattern (Grosfeld 1965, Moss 1975). With respect to the Herbst appliance this topic has been addressed in 6 publications (Pancherz and Anehus-Pancherz 1980, 1982, Sessle et al 1990, Pancherz 1995, Leung and Hägg 2001, Du and Hägg 2003).

Reviewing three publications (Pancherz 1980a, 1980b, Pancherz and Anehus-Pancherz 1980), the scientific evidence concerning the short- and long-term effects of Herbst treatment on the EMG activity of the masticatory muscles will be presented. In all three investigations the same electromyograph (Mingograph 800 from Elema-Schönander, Stockholm), electrode technique and functional parameters were used.

Direct and integrated EMG recordings were obtained from the masseter and temporal muscles bila-terally using bipolar hook electrodes (Ahlgren 1967) placed in a standardized way (see Chapter 6: Herbst research - subjects and methods, Fig. 6-8).

The EMG activity was registered during the following functions:

- *Maximal biting in intercuspal position* (mean value of five consecutive biting cycles).
- *Chewing of five peanuts* (mean value of 10 consecutive chewing cycles).

1. Temporal and masseter muscle activity in children and adults with normal occlusion. An electromyographic analysis (Pancherz 1980a)

Integrated EMG recordings were analyzed in male subjects with normal (Class I) occlusion, 12 years (n=23) and 25 years (n=21) of age. The results of the investigation revealed the following for both maximal biting and chewing (Figs. 15-1 and 15-2):

- Masseter muscle activity was greater in older than in younger subjects.
- Temporal activity was the same in both age groups.
- Masseter muscle activity was increased in relation to temporal muscle activity in the older subjects. In the younger subjects the same activity was found in the two muscles.

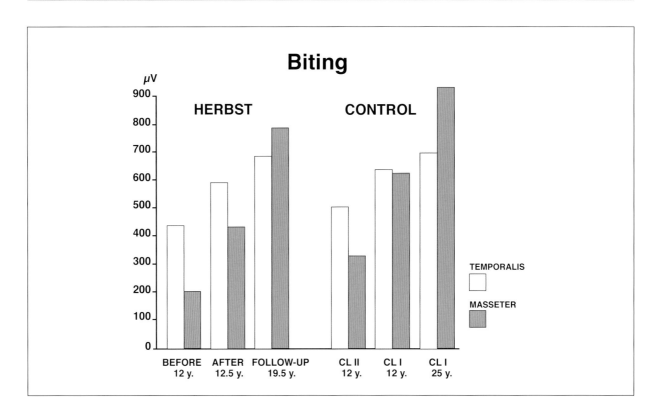

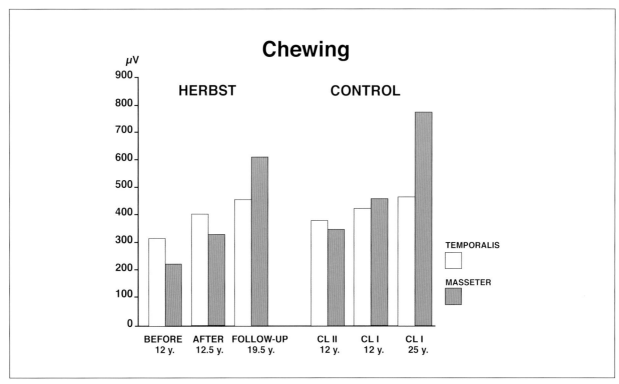

Fig. 15-1 Maximal integrated EMG activity from the temporal and masseter muscles during maximal biting in intercuspal position and during chewing of peanuts. Registrations (mean values) in 10 consecutive boys with Class II:1 maloccusion treated with the Herbst appliance and in three groups of control subjects: 23 untreated boys with Class II:1 (Cl II) malocclusion, 23 boys with normal (Cl I) occlusion and 21 male adults with normal (Cl I) occlusion. *(Revised from Pancherz 1995)*

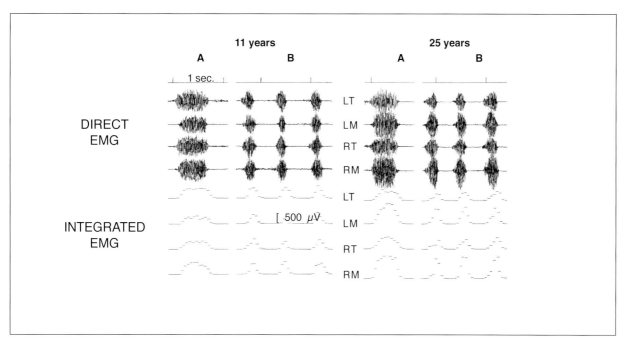

Fig. 15-2 Electromyograms during maximal biting in intercuspal position from two subjects with normal (Class I) occlusion, 11 years and 25 years of age. **A**: Maximal biting in intercuspal position. **B**: Chewing of peanuts. LT: left temporalis. LM: left masseter. RT: right temporalis. RM: right masseter. *(Revised from Pancherz 1980)*

2. Activity of the temporal and masseter muscles in Class II, Division 1 malocclusions. An electromyographic investigation (Pancherz 1980b)

Integrated EMG recordings were analyzed in 23 male Class II:1 subjects, 12 years of age, and compared to the 23 male Class I subjects, 12 years of age, from the previous publication (Pancherz 1980a). The results revealed the following (Fig. 15-1):

- During maximal biting the Class II subjects exhibited less EMG activity in the masseter and temporal muscles than the Class I subjects.
- During chewing the Class II subjects exhibited less EMG activity in the masseter than the Class I subjects. For the temporal muscle, no differences were found between the two groups.

3. Muscle activity in Class II, Division 1 malocclusions treated by bite jumping with the Herbst appliance (Pancherz and Anehus-Pancherz 1980)

Integrated EMG recordings were analyzed in 10 consecutive Class II:1 male subjects, 12 years of age, treated with the Herbst appliance (Pancherz 1979). After 6 months of treatment, normal (Class I) dental arch relationships were established in all subjects. EMG recordings were made at six occasions: (1) before treatment, (2) at the start of treatment when the appliance was placed, (3) during treatment (after 3 months), and (4) after treatment when the appliance was removed. Follow-up registrations were performed (5) 1 year and (6) 7 years posttreatment (Pancherz 1995). The results revealed the following (Figs. 15-3 and 15-4):

- Before treatment the EMG activity from the temporal and masseter muscles was less (maximal biting) than from the temporal muscle (Pancherz 1980b).
- At the start of treatment the EMG activity from the two muscles was markedly reduced during maximal biting and chewing.
- After 3 months of treatment the EMG activity of the two muscles had almost reached pretreatment values.
- After treatment the EMG activity of the two muscles exceeded pretreatment values. The increase in EMG activity was larger in the masseter than in the temporal muscle.
- During the follow-up periods of 1 year and 7 years the EMG activity had increased continuously, especially in the masseter muscle.

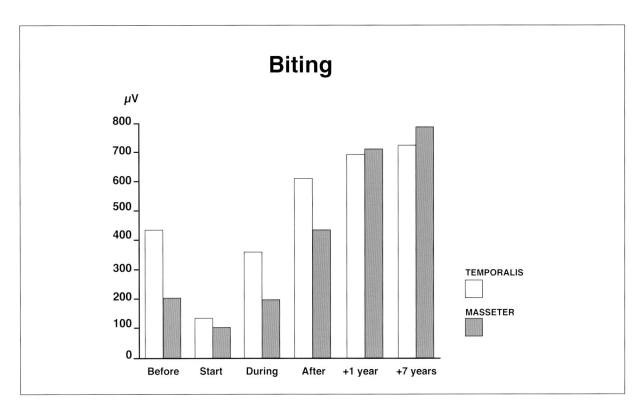

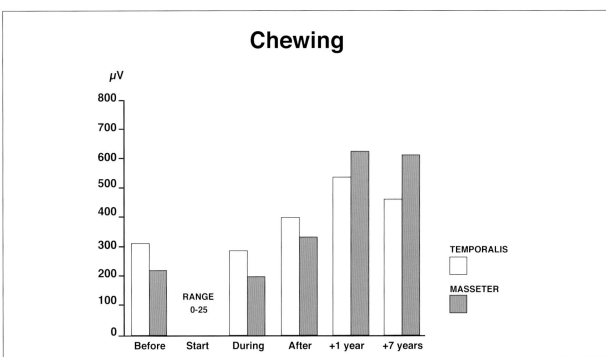

Fig. 15-3 Maximal integrated EMG activity from the temporal and masseter muscles during maximal **Biting** in intercuspal position and during **Chewing** of peanuts. Registrations (mean values) in 10 consecutive boys with Class II:1 maloccusion treated with the Herbst appliance. *Before*: Before treatment. *Start*: At start of treatment when the appliance was placed. *During*: After 3 months of treatment. *After*: After 6 months of treatment when the appliance was removed. *+1 year*: 1 year posttreatment. *+7 years*: 7 years posttreatment. *(Revised from Pancherz 1995)*

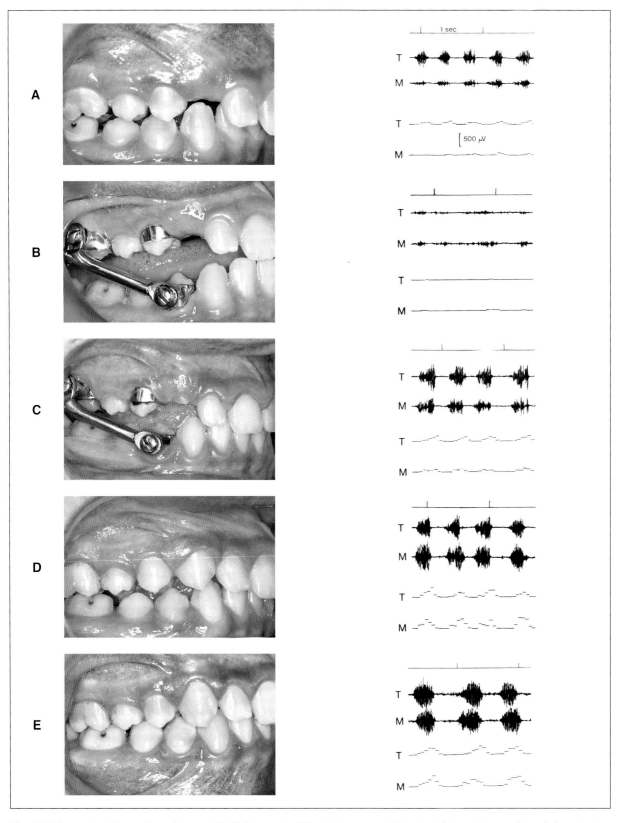

Fig. 15-4 Intraoral photographs and temporalis (T) / masseter (M) electromygrams (direct and integrated recordings during chewing of peanuts) from an 11-year-old boy treated with the Herbst appliance. **A**: Before treatment. **B**: At start of treatment when the appliance was placed. **C**: After 3 months of treatment. **D**: After 6 months of treatment when the appliance was removed. **E**: 1 year posttreatment.

Interpretation of the results

1. The increased EMG activity found in adults when compared to children with Class I occlusion may be attributed to age differences and/or an exercising effect of the muscles during normal jaw function. This would be specially true for the masseter as it is the "force muscle" while the temporalis is the "positioning muscle".

2. The impaired muscle activity found in Class II:1 malocclusions, in comparison to Class I cases, may be attributed to a diverging dentofacial morphology and unstable occlusal contact condition (incomplete Class II cuspal interdigitation) in the Class II subjects.

3. The increase in muscle activity seen in the Herbst treated Class II:1 malocclusions was probably due to an altered sagittal jaw base or dental arch relationship and a training effect of muscle function, especially of the masseter, during the appliance period. The posttreatment increase in muscle activity was most likely due to normal age changes (Pancherz 1980a). At the end of follow-up the muscle contraction pattern resembled that of untreated adult Class I occlusion subjects (Pancherz 1980a) (Fig 15-1).

Conclusions and clinical implications

In Class II:1 malocclusions Herbst treatment normalizes the muscle contraction pattern. A normal function of the masticatory muscles is certainly of utmost importance for normal development of the dentofacial structures and for posttreatment stability. Further studies in this area are, however, necessary.

References

Ahlgren J. Mechanism of mastification. Acta Odont Scand 1966;24 (Suppl 44):1-109.

Ahlgren J. An intracutaneous needle electrode for kinesidogic EMG studies. Acta Odont Scand 1967;25:15-19

Ahlgren J, Ingervall B, Thilander B. Muscle activity in normal and postnormal occlusion. Am J Orthod 1973;64:445-456.

Du X, Hägg U. Muscular adaption to gradual advancement of the mandible. Angle Orthod 2003;73:525-53.

Grosfeld O. Changes of muscle contraction patterns as a result of orthodontic treatment. Trans Eur Orthod Soc 1965;41:203-214.

Ingervall B, Thilander B. Relation between facial morphology and activity of the masticatory muscles. J Oral Rehab 1974;1:131-147.

Leung DK, Hägg U. An electromyographic investigation of the first six months of progressive mandibular advancement of the Herbst appliance in adolescents. Angle Orthod 2001;71:177-184.

Moss JP. Function – Facts or fiction? Am J Orthod 1975;67:625-646.

Moyers RE. Temporomandibular muscle contraction patterns in Angle Class II, Division 1 malocclusions: an electromyographic analysis. Am J Orthod 1949;35:837-857.

Möller E. The chewing apparatus. Acta Phys Scand 1966;69 (Suppl) 280:1-229.

Pancherz H. Treatment of Class II malocclusions by jumping the bite with the Herbst appliance. A cephalometric investigation. Am J Orthod 1979;76:423-442

Pancherz H. Temporal and masseter muscle activity in children and adults with normal occlusion. An electromyographic investigation. Acta Odont Scand 1980a;38:343-348.

Pancherz H. Activity of the temporal and masseter muscles in Class II, Division 1 malocclusions. An electromyographic investigation. Am J Orthod 1980b;77:679-688.

Pancherz H. The Herbst appliance. Editorial Aguiram, Barcelona 1995.

Pancherz H, Anehus-Pancherz M. Muscle activity in Class II, Division 1 malocclusions treated by bite jumping with the Herbst appliance. Am J Orthod 1980;78:321-329.

Pancherz H, Anehus-Pancherz M. The effect of continuous bite jumping with the Herbst appliance on the masticatory system: a functional analysis of treated Class II malocclusions. Eur J Orthod 1982;4:37-44.

Sessle BJ, Woodside P, Borque P, Gurza S, Powell J, Voudouris J, Metaxas A, Altuna G. Effect of functional appliances on jaw muscle activity. Am J Orthod Dentofac Orthop 1990;98:220-230.

Chapter 16

Effects on TMJ function

Research

There is considerable controversy in the literature with respect to the effect of the Herbst appliance (Popowich et al. 2003) and of orthodontic treatment in general (Luther 2007) on TMJ function.

Using clinical TMD screening, TMJ tomograms and magnetic resonance imaging (MRI), the effects of the Herbst appliance on TMJ and masticatory muscle function have been investigated in eight studies (Pancherz and Anehus-Pancherz 1982, Hansen et al. 1990, Foucart et al. 1998, Ruf and Pancherz 1998a, 2000, Croft et al. 1999, Pancherz et al. 1999, Arruda Aidar et al. 2006). The scientific evidence of these studies will be presented by reviewing them in chronological order.

1. The effect of continuous bite jumping with the Herbst appliance on the masticatory system: a functional analysis of treated Class II malocclusions (Pancherz and Anehus-Pancherz 1982)

The sample consisted of 20 consecutive male Class II:1 patients (11-14 years of age) treated with the Herbst appliance for an average period of 6 months. Temporomandibular function was analyzed using an anamnestic questionnaire and a clinical examination (Ingervall 1970, Carlsson and Helkimo 1972) before treatment, after 3 months of treatment, after removal of the appliance as well as 12 months posttreatment. All clinical recordings during treatment were carried out after removal of the telescope mechanism.

During Herbst treatment the lateral movement capacity of the mandible was reduced by an average of 1.9 mm, but returned to pretreatment values 12 months posttreatment. The frequency of joint tenderness increased from 20% to 45% during the first three months of treatment. However, after treatment and 12 months posttreatment, reduced prevalences of joint tenderness (15% and 10%, respectively), compared to pretreatment values, were seen. Muscle tenderness showed a corresponding development.

2. Long-term effects of the Herbst appliance on the craniomandibular system with special reference to the TMJ (Hansen et al. 1990)

The sample comprised 19 male Class II:1 patients (mean age 20.4 years) that had been treated with the Herbst appliance an average of 7.5 years earlier. Temporomandibular function was analyzed using an anamnestic questionnaire and a clinical examination (Ingervall 1970, Carlsson and Helkimo 1972). Furthermore, tomograms of both TMJs were taken. TMJ sounds could be detected in 26% and muscle tenderness in 32% of the subjects. None of the individuals exhibited joint tenderness. Structural bony changes in the TMJ were found in one condyle (Fig. 16-1). In the 19 subjects, the average condylar position corresponded to a physiologic condyle-fossa relationship.

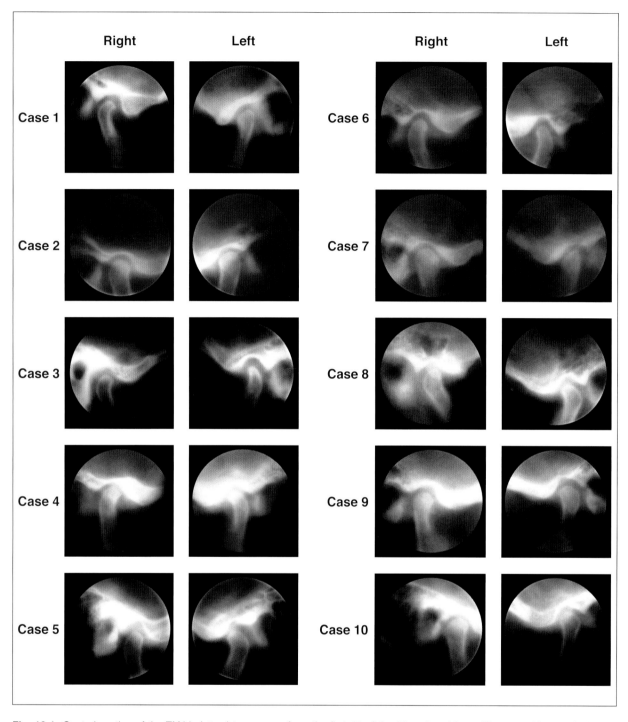

Fig. 16-1   Central section of the TMJ in lateral tomograms from the first 10 of the 19 male subjects (Cases 1-10) treated with the Herbst appliance 7.5 years previously. Note the left TMJ of Case 7, exhibiting a flattened condyle with signs of an osteophyte. *(From Hansen et al. 1990)*

3. Magnetic resonance analysis of the TMJ disc compartment in children wearing hyperpropulsors (Foucart et al. 1998) [Article in French]

The subject material comprised 10 Class II:1 patients (mean age 11.5 years) treated with a removable Herbst appliance for an average period of 8.7 months full-time plus 6.5 months night-time. Temporomandibular function was analyzed using MRI and a clinical examination (range of motion, TMJ sounds, TMJ and muscle tenderness, isometric muscle contraction). Recordings were made before treatment, once during treatment and after Herbst treatment.
Prior to treatment, none of the subjects exhibited any muscle or joint tenderness or disk displacement. During treatment, muscle and joint tenderness was noted in one subject. After treatment, a reduced condylar translation in one individual was the only clinical sign of TMD seen in the subject material. The MRIs after treatment showed varying minor degrees of disk displacement in three subjects.

4. Long-term TMJ effects of Herbst treatment: a clinical and MRI study (Ruf and Pancherz 1998a)

The sample consisted of 20 Class II patients (mean age 17.4 years) that had been treated with the Herbst appliance an average of 4 years earlier. Temporomandibular function was analyzed by means of MRIs, an anamnestic questionnaire and a clinical examination (Bumann and Lotzmann 2002).
The prevalence of anamnestic and clinical signs or symptoms of TMD was within the normal range, as reported in the literature. Partial or total disk displacement or deviation in condylar form were seen in 5 subjects (25%). The frequency of disc displacement in MRIs was not higher than in asymptomatic populations. Three subjects (15%) showed mild symptoms of TMD with either small condylar displacements or subclinical soft tissue lesions.

5. A cephalometric and tomographic evaluation of Herbst treatment in the mixed dentition (Croft et al. 1999)

The sample comprised of 37 Class II patients (mean age 9.4 years) treated with the Herbst appliance for an average period of 11 months. Condylar position was analyzed using TMJ tomograms. Recordings were made one year before Herbst treatment, immediately before removal of the Herbst appliance and an average of 2.7 years posttreatment.

The joint space analysis demonstrated only small changes in condylar position throughout the observation period. There was a tendency for the condyles to be positioned slightly forward (0.2 mm) at the end of treatment and then to fall back during the posttreatment period.

6. Mandibular articular disk position changes during Herbst treatment: a prospective longitudinal MRI study (Pancherz et al. 1999)

7. Does bite-jumping damage the TMJ? A prospective longitudinal clinical and MRI study of Herbst patients (Ruf and Pancherz 2000)

The total subject material comprised of 62 Class II patients (mean age 14.4 years) treated with the Herbst appliance for an average period of 7.2 months. In the first publication (Pancherz et al. 1999), 15 out of the 62 subjects were analyzed by means of MRI taken before treatment, during treatment (after 1, 6 and 12 weeks) as well as after treatment (after removal of the Herbst appliance). In the second publication (Ruf and Pancherz 2000), temporomandibular function was analyzed by means of MRIs taken before treatment, after treatment and one year posttreatment. Furthermore, an anamnestic questionnaire was administered and a clinical examination (Bumann and Lotzmann 2002) was performed before treatment, during treatment (after 1, 6 and 12 weeks), after treatment (after removal of the Herbst appliance) as well as 1 year posttreatment. All clinical recordings during treatment were carried out after removing the telescope mechanism.
Before Herbst treatment, the articular disk was on average, in a slightly protrusive position relative to the condyle (Fig. 16-2). At the start of treatment, the mandible was advanced to an incisal edge-to-edge position. Due to the physiologic relative movements of the disk and condyle upon mandibular protrusion, the disk attained a pronounced retrusive position. At the end of treatment, the condyle was still slightly anteriorly positioned and a retrusive disk position prevailed (Fig. 16-2). Although the condyle had returned to its original position one year posttreatment, a slight retrusive disk position could still be noted (Fig. 16-3).

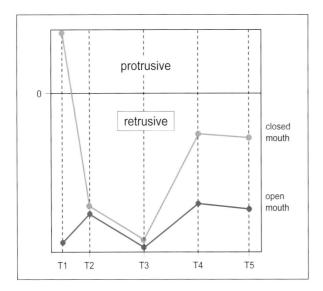

Fig. 16-2 Mean disk position in 15 Class II subjects treated with the Herbst appliance. Analysis of MRIs (central slice) from the right TMJ in closed and open mouth position. T1: Before Herbst treatment. T2: At start of Herbst treatment when the appliance was placed. T3: After 6 weeks of Herbst treatment. T4: After 13 weeks of Herbst treatment. T5: After removal of the Herbst appliance. *(Revised from Pancherz et al. 1999)*

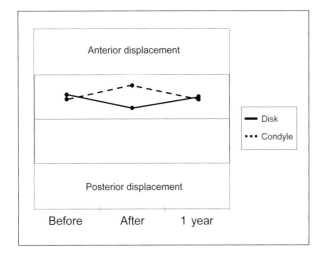

Fig. 16-3 Average changes in articular disk and condylar position from before to one year after treatment in 62 consecutive Herbst patients. The gray shaded area represents the physiologic range. *(Revised from Ruf and Pancherz 2000)*

A temporary capsulitis of the inferior stratum of the posterior attachment was induced during treatment (Fig. 16-4). The lateral part of the inferior stratum reacted more than the central part. During Herbst treatment the prevalence of a capsulitis of the lateral part of the inferior stratum of the posterior attachment changed from 24% pretreatment to 100% after 6 weeks of Herbst treatment and to 88% immediately after removal of the Herbst appliance. During the posttreatment period the capsulitis prevalence decreased to 32% six months and to 7% one year posttreatment.

Before treatment nearly 14% of the joints exhibited condylar bony changes, while this was the case for only 3% one year posttreatment.

In summary, it was found that over the entire observation period from before treatment to one year posttreatment, bite jumping with the Herbst appliance: (1) did not result in any muscular TMD; (2) reduced the prevalence of capsulitis; (3) reduced the prevalence of structural condylar bony changes; (4) did not induce any disk displacement in subjects with a physiologic pretreatment disc position; (5) resulted in a stable repositioning of the disk in subjects with a pretreatment partial disk displacement with reduction; and (6) could not recapture the disk in subjects with a pretreatment total disk displacement with or without reduction. The overall prevalence of signs of TMD was reduced from 48% before treatment to 24% one year posttreatment.

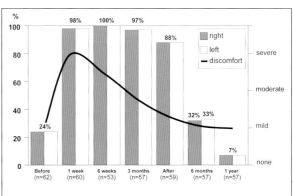

Fig. 16-4 Prevalence of a capsulitis of the lateral part of the inferior stratum of the posterior attachment in 62 consecutive Herbst patients. The number (n) of analyzed patients is given. The percentage (%) of affected joints is shown separately for the left and right TMJ. The level of discomfort (severe, moderate, mild and none) is indicated. *(Revised from Ruf and Pancherz 2000)*

8. Herbst appliance therapy and temporomandibular joint disc position: a prospective longitudinal magnetic resonance imaging study (Arruda Aidar et al. 2006)

The sample consisted of 20 Class II:1 patients (mean age 12.7 years) treated with the Herbst appliance for an average period of 12 months. A stepwise mandibular advancement procedure was used. MRIs were taken before treatment, during treatment (after 8-10 weeks) and after treatment.

Both before and after treatment all subjects presented a physiologic disk position. After 8-10 weeks of treatment a tendency towards a retrusive disk position was observed. This was due to the physiologic relative movement of disk and condyle upon mandibular protrusion. At the end of treatment, the disk had almost returned to its original pretreatment position. However, a slight retrusive disk position prevailed.

Interpretation of the results

In clinical terms the important questions with respect to the short- and long-term effects of the Herbst appliance on TMJ function are: (1) Does the Herbst appliance damage the TMJ? (2) Does the Herbst appliance improve TMJ function? (3) What kind of Class II patients may benefit from Herbst treatment in terms of improved TMJ function?

Does the Herbst appliance damage the TMJ?
The findings to be expected, in case of an adverse effect of the Herbst appliance on the TMJ or the masticatory musculature, would be an increase in the signs or symptoms of TMD compared to both pretreatment values and untreated controls.

After Herbst treatment, Pancherz and Anehus-Pancherz (1982) described a decrease in joint sounds by 100%, in joint tenderness by 25% and in muscle tenderness by 40%. Foucart et al. (1998) reported an increase in disk displacements by 30%. Ruf and Pancherz (2000), on the other hand, found a decrease in disk displacement by 45%, a decrease in structural bony changes by 41% and an increase in subclinical capsulitis by 64%. Finally, Arruda Aidar et al. (2006) described a physiologic disk position in all subjects before and after Herbst treatment.

A possible explanation for the contradictory results in terms of disk displacement might be that Foucart et al. (1998) used a removable instead of a fixed Herbst appliance and took sagittal instead of angulated sagittal MRIs. On straight sagittal MRIs of the TMJ, the posterior band of the articular disk is not imaged reliably, especially in the lateral and medial joint sections (Steenks et al. 1994), resulting in an overestimation of disk displacements. This explanation seems quite feasable, as Foucart et al. (1998) reported that two out of three disk displacement patients were clinically symptom-free over the entire observation period.

One year after treatment the prevalence of TMD in Herbst subjects was 24% compared to 48% pretreatment (Ruf and Pancherz 2000). Correspondingly a 20% reduction in muscle tenderness, a 50% reduction in joint tenderness and a 100% reduction in TMJ sounds was described by Pancherz and Anehus-Pancherz (1982).

An average of four years after Herbst treatment (Ruf and Pancherz 1998a) 35% of the former Herbst patients showed clinical or subclinical signs of TMD. The TMD prevalence four years after Herbst treatment was, however, less than in Class II patients before treatment (Ruf and Pancherz 2000, Henrikson and Nilner 2003). Even if the TMD prevalence four years after treatment was increased compared to one year after Herbst treatment (Ruf and Pancherz 2000), this increase might be explained by the fact that signs and symptoms of TMD increase with age (Magnusson 1986, Egermark-Eriksson et al. 1987, Motegi et al 1992, Henrikson and Nilner 2003) and have a multifactorial etiology (Okeson 1996). Furthermore, it was found (Hansen et al. 1990) that patients an average of seven years after Herbst treatment exhibit normal structural conditions of the condyle and fossa and their anamnestic and clinical TMD findings are in accordance with those of an orthodontically untreated population of young adults.

Thus, it can be concluded that the Herbst appliance does not seem to have an adverse effect on TMJ function, either on a short- or long-term basis.

Does the Herbst appliance improve TMJ function?
As elucidated above, the prevalence of TMD in Herbst-treated Class II subjects decreased by 50% from before to directly after therapy and by 27% from before to four years after therapy (Ruf and Pancherz 1998a, 2000). Thus, the frequency change was opposite to that found in untreated populations, where the TMD prevalence increases with age (Magnusson 1986, Egermark-Eriksson et al. 1987, Motegi et al 1992, Henrikson and Nilner 2003). However, the signs and symptoms of TMD could not be completely resolved by Herbst treatment, which, as mentioned above, might be due to the fact, that the etiology of TMD is multifactorial.

In summary, it can be said that TMJ function was in fact improved by Herbst appliance treatment, possibly due to the normalization of the occlusion.

What kind of Class II patients may benefit from Herbst treatment in terms of improved TMJ function? (1) Disk position

A slight retrusion of the disk compared to pretreatment values was seen at the end of Herbst treatment (Pancherz et al. 1999, Arruda Aidar et al. 2006) and prevailed even one year posttreatment (Ruf and Pancherz 2000). The disk retrusion after treatment was due to a slight anterior position of the condyle after treatment (Fig. 16-2). The reason for the prevailing disk retrusion one year posttreatment is unknown.

The effect of the Herbst appliance on the position of the articular disk was found to depend on the pretreatment disk position. The prognosis for disk repositioning depended on the degree of disk displacement existent pretreatment (Summer and Westesson 1997).

In patients with a physiologic pretreatment disk position, the position of the disk remained unchanged during Herbst treatment (Pancherz et al. 1999, Ruf and Pancherz 2000, Arruda Aidar et al. 2006). Similar results have been reported for other fixed or removable functional appliances (Chintakanon et al. 2000, Franco et al. 2002, Ruf et al. 2002, Kinzinger et al. 2006)

Partial disk displacements (Fig. 16-5) could be successfully repositioned and remained stable until the end of the observation period (Ruf and Pancherz 2000). In contrast to normal disk repositioning therapy (Lundh et al. 1985, Summer and Westesson 1997, Tallents et al. 1990), recapturing of the disk during Herbst treatment was achieved by a retrusion of the disk and not by a protrusion of the condyle. Corresponding success for repositioning of partial disk displacements has been reported for one other fixed functional appliance (Functional mandibular advancer) (Kinzinger et al. 2006). In contrast, for removable functional appliances no disk repositioning, irrespective of the degree of displacement, could be achieved (Chintakanon et al. 2000, Ruf et al. 2002). Total disk displacements with reduction could only be temporarily repositioned by means of Herbst treatment (Ruf and Pancherz 2000). Thus, with an increasing degree of displacement the retrusive effect of the Herbst appliance on the disk seems to be insufficient to stabilize the disk. Consequently and in concordance with previous findings (Lundh et al. 1985, Summer and Westesson 1997, Tallents et

al. 1990), the disk relapsed to a displaced position when the condyle moved backwards in the fossa during the treatment period.

Total disk displacement without reduction prevailed during and after Herbst treatment (Ruf and Pancherz 2000). However, a newly formed pseudo-disk due to extensive fibrotic adaptation of the posterior attachment (Scapino 1983, Isacsson et al. 1986, Luder 1993) was seen in some joints (Fig. 16-6). Furthermore, TMJ function in general improved in all subjects with a total disk displacement without reduction. Clinically these subjects were indistinguishable from healthy individuals after treatment.

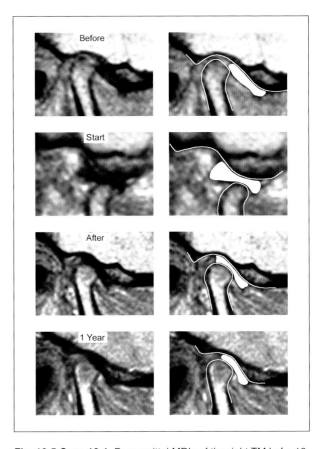

Fig. 16-5 Case 16-1 Parasagittal MRIs of the right TMJ of a 12-year-old male Class II:1 subject treated with the Herbst appliance. *Before* treatment. Note the partial disk displacement with reduction. *Start* of Herbst treatment. The disk was recaptured. Both *After* as well as *1 Year* after Herbst treatment, the recaptured disk is in a physiologic disk-condyle relationship. *(Revised from Ruf 2003)*

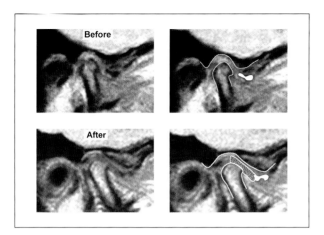

Fig. 16-6 Case 16-2 Parasagittal MRIs of the right TMJ of a 15- year-old male Class II:1 subject treated with the Herbst appliance. Before treatment. a total disk displacement without reduction is present. After treatment: A pseudo-disk (dotted area) has developed. Note also the improvement in condylar bony shape. After treatment the patient was free from pain and movement restrictions. *(Revised from Ruf 2003)*

(2) TMJ soft tissues

In general inflammatory conditions of the temporomandibular joint are subdivided into synovitis and capsulitis (Okeson 1996). In the following, capsulitis refers to an intracapsular inflammation primarily affecting the posterior attachment. The term posterior attachment is used as described by Scapino (1991a,b) and refers to the vascular and innervated tissue lying behind the articular disk.

The only intraarticular soft tissue structure affected by Herbst treatment was the inferior stratum of the posterior attachment, in which a temporary capsulitis was induced (Ruf and Pancherz 2000). It must, however, be stressed that already pretreatment a capsulitis of the inferior stratum of the bilaminar zone existed in 24% of the subjects and that the corresponding signs were both clinical and subclinical. However, during and after Herbst treatment all signs where solely subclinical, meaning that none of the patients was complaining about TMJ pain. Nevertheless, over the entire observation period from before treatment to one year posttreatment, the prevalence of a capsulitis of the inferior attachment was reduced from 24% to 7% of the subjects.

The induction of a temporary subclinical capsulitis of the inferior stratum of the posterior attachment is probably due to the advancement of the condyle during Herbst treatment which results in an expansion of the posterior attachment (Wilkinson and Crowley 1994). In contrast to normal mouth opening or protrusive jaw movement, during which this expansion prevails only for seconds, in Herbst treatment it remains 24 hours a day. Although, the soft tissue expansion does not seem to have a long-lasting effect on the synovial pressure (Ward et al. 1990), no doubt it will result in a mechanical irritation of the tissue leading to an inflammatory reaction (Pinals 1995, Carvalho et al. 1997), explaining the observed capsulitis of the inferior stratum of the posterior attachment. It should be mentioned that the induction of a capsulitis during functional appliance treatment not only is a side effect of Herbst treatment, but has also been reported for Activator treatment (Ruf et al. 2002), and must thus be expected to appear during any functional appliance therapy.

In summary it was found that Herbst treatment reduced the frequency of capsulitis from before treatment to one year posttreatment.

(3) TMJ bony structures

Normally the prevalence of structural TMJ bony changes increases with age (Dibbets and van der Weele 1992). However, a spontaneous disappearance of osseous condylar changes during adolescence has been reported (Dibbets and van der Weele 1992, Peltola et al. 1995). During Herbst therapy, the pretreatment prevalence of structural bony changes of the condyle (flattening, subchondral sclerosis, erosions, osteophytes) decreased from 14% to 3% of the subjects (Ruf and Pancherz 2000). Probably the modeling processes of the condyle induced by the Herbst appliance (Ruf and Pancherz 1998b, 1999) promoted the normalization of the condylar bony structures. For example, the disappearance of osteophytes might be explained by the anterior resorptive process (see Chapter 10: Effects on TMJ growth) taking place in the course of condylar modeling during Herbst treatment.

In all joints with a physiologic disk-condyle relationship, the signs of structural bony changes disappeared during the observation period from before to one year after Herbst treatment. In joints with a pretreatment disk displacement without reduction, a condition which in both clinical and animal studies has been shown to be more susceptible to the development of bony changes (Scapino 1983, Westesson and Rohlin 1984, Isacsson et al. 1986), the condylar bony structure improved (but was not normalized) during Herbst treatment.

(4) Masticatory musculature

The reaction of the masticatory musculature to Herbst treatment was analyzed by two different methods: muscle palpation (Pancherz and Anehus-Pancherz 1982, Hansen et al. 1990, Foucart et al. 1998) and isometric muscle contraction exercises (Foucart et al. 1998, Ruf and Pancherz 1998a, Ruf and Pancherz 2000). The results of these two different approaches are difficult to compare. Thus, in the assessment of myofascial pain isometric muscle contractions have been shown to exhibit less intra- and inter-examiner variability (Thomas and Okeson 1987, Malerba et al. 1993, Leggin et al. 1996, Lagerström and Nordgren 1998) than muscle palpation. Furthermore, in contrast to muscle palpation, myofascial pain provoked by means of isometric contractions is associated with morphologic changes of the muscle, in form of a muscle oedema detectable by means of MRI (Evans et al. 1998).

In using palpation to assess myofascial pain, it could be shown that during Herbst treatment (Pancherz and Anehus-Pancherz 1982) the percentage of patients exhibiting muscle tenderness increased from 25% before to 55% after 3 months Herbst treatment. Foucart et al. (1998) described an increase from 0% to 10% during treatment. After treatment, muscle tenderness was either absent (Foucart et al. 1998) or present in 15% of the subjects (Pancherz and Anehus-Pancherz 1982). One year after Herbst treatment (Pancherz and Anehus-Pancherz 1982) a total of 20% of the subjects exhibited tender muscle sites. This was identical to the after treatment percentage of Class II subjects treated with multibracket appliances and 24% less than in untreated Class II subjects (Henrikson and Nilner 2003). Seven and a half years after Herbst treatment (Hansen et al. 1990), 32% of the subjects showed tender muscle sites, which was still 12% less than in untreated Class II subjects after a 2-year control period (Henrikson and Nilner 2003).

On the other hand, using isometric contractions to assess myofascial pain, no pathologic findings were detected before, during, after, one year after or four years after Herbst treatment (Foucart el al. 1998, Ruf and Pancherz 1998a, Ruf and Pancherz 2000).

Conclusion and clinical implications

The only functionally compromising effect of the Herbst appliance is a temporary reduction of the lateral movement capacity of the mandible.

Herbst appliance treatment does not induce TMD. On the contrary, it improves TMJ function in certain patients with pretreatment TMD:

- *Partial disk displacement:* Good prognosis for disc repositioning with the Herbst appliance. The Herbst should be the appliance of choice to achieve maximum functional improvement during orthodontics even if the malocclusion could have been treated with other methods as well.
- *Total disk displacement with reduction:* Bad prognosis for disk repositioning but not for successful Class II correction with the Herbst appliance.
- *Total disk displacement without reduction:* No chance for disk repositioning with any orthodontic / orthopedic approach. However, good prognosis for tissue adaptation and functional improvement when using the Herbst appliance.
- *Capsulitis of posterior attachment:* The Herbst appliance should be considered for treatment in Class II cases with clinically manifest or subclinical capsulitis of the inferior stratum of the posterior attachment, as there is a 70% chance for adaptation during a period from before treatment to one year posttreatment.
- *Structural bony changes*: No contraindication for Herbst treatment. Due to the modeling processes taking place during therapy an improvement of the bony conditions is possible.
- *Musculature:* Herbst treatment resulted in a decrease in the prevalence of tender muscle sites existing pretreatment.

References

Arruda Aidar LA, Abrahao M, Yamashita HK, Dominguez GC. Herbst appliance therapy and temporomandibular joint disc position: a prospective longitudinal magnetic resonance imaging study. Am J Orthod Dentofac Orthop 2006;129:486-496.

Bumann A, Lotzmann U. TMJ disorders and orofacial pain. The role of dentistry in a multidisciplinary diagnostic approach. Stuttgart, New York: Georg Thieme; 2002.

Carlsson GE, Helkimo M. Funktionell undersökning av tuggapparaten. In: Holst JJ et al. (eds.) Nordisk Klinisk Odontologi, Forlaget for faglitteratur, Copenhagen, 1972:8-11.

Carvalho RS, Scott JE, Bumann A, Yen EHK. Connective tissue response to mechanical stimulation. In: McNeill C (ed) Science and practice of occlusion. Chicago: Quintessence, 1997:205-219.

Chintakanon K, Sampson W, Wilkinson T, Townsend G. A prospective study of Twin-block therapy assessed by magnetic resonance imaging. Am J Orthod Dentofac Orthop 2000;118:494-504.

Croft RS, Buschang PH, English JD, Meyer R. A cephalometric and tomographic evaluation of Herbst treatment in the mixed dentition. Am J Orthod Dentofac Orthop 1999;11:435-443.

Dibbets JMH, van der Weele LT. Prevalence of structural bony change in the mandibular condyle. J Craniomandib Disord 1992;6:254-259.

Egermark-Eriksson I, Carlsson GE, Magnusson T. A long-term epidemiologic study of the relationship between occlusal factors and mandibular dysfunction in children and adolescents. J Dent Res 1987;66:67-71.

Foucart JM, Pajoni D, Crapentier P, Pharaboz C. Étude I.R.M. du compartement discal de L'A.T.M. des enfants porteurs d'hyperpropulseur. Orthod Fr 1998;69:79-91.

Franco AA, Yamashita HK, Lederman HM, Cevidanes LH, Proffit WR, Vigorito JW. Fränkel appliance therapy and the temporomandibular disc: a prospective magnetic resonance imaging study. Am J Orthod Dentofac Orthop 2002;121:447-457.

Hansen K, Pancherz H, Petersson A. Long-term effects of the Herbst appliance on the craniomandibular system with special reference to the TMJ. Eur J Orthod 1990;12: 244-253.

Henrikson T, Nilner M. Temporomandibular disorders, occlusion and orthodontic treatment. J Orthod 2003;30:129-137.

Ingervall B. Range of movement of the mandible in children. Scand J Dent Res 1970;78:311-322.

Isacsson G, Isberg AM, Johansson AS, Larson O. Internal derangement of the temporomandibular joint: radiographic and histologic changes associated with severe pain. J Oral Maxillofac Surg 1986;44:771-778.

Kinzinger GS, Roth A, Gulden N, Bucker A, Diedrich PR. Effects of orthodontic treatment with fixed functional orthopaedic appliances on the disc-condyle relationship in the temporo mandibular joint: a magnetic resonance imaging study (Part II). Dentomaxillofac Radiol 2006;35:347-356.

Lagerström C, Nordgren B. On the reliability and usefulness of methods for grip strength measurements. Scand J Rehabil Med 1998;30:113-119.

Leggin BG, Neuman RM, Iannotti JP, Williams GR, Thompson EC. Intrarater and interrater reliability of three isometric dynamometers in assessing shoulder strength. J Shoulder Elbow Surg 1996;5:18-24.

Luder HU. Articular degeneration and remodeling in human temporomandibular joints with normal and abnormal disc position. J Orofac Pain 1993;7:391-402.

Lundh H, Westesson PL, Kopp S, Tillstrom B. Anterior repositioning splint in the treatment of temporomandibular joints with reciprocal clicking: comparison with a flat occlusal splint and an untreated control group. Oral Surg Oral Med Oral Pathol 1985;60:131-136.

Luther F. TMD and occlusion part I. Damned if we do? Occlusion: the interface of dentistry and orthodontics. Br Dent J 2007;202:E2.

Magnusson T. Five-year longitudinal study of signs and symptoms of mandibular dysfunction in adolescents. J Craniomand Pract 1986;4:338-344.

Malerba JL, Adam ML, Harris BA, Krebs DE. Reliability of dynamic and isometric testing of shoulder external and internal rotators. J Orthop Sports Phys Ther 1993;18:543-552.

Motegi E, Miyazaki H, Ogura I, Konishi H, Sebata M. An orthodontic study of temporomandibular joint disorders. Part 1: Epidemiological research in Japanese 6-18 year olds. Angle Orthod 1992;62:249-256.

Okeson JP. Orofacial pain: guidelines for assessment, diagnosis, and management. Chicago: Quintessence, 1996:32-34,116-127.

Pancherz H, Anehus-Pancherz M. The effect of continuous bite jumping with the Herbst appliance on the masticatory system: a functional analysis of treated Class II malocclusions. Eur J Orthod 1982;4:37-44.

Pancherz H, Ruf S, Thomalske-Faubert C. Mandibular articular disk position changes during Herbst treatment: a prospective longitudinal MRI study. Am J Orthod Dentofac Orthop 1999;116:207-214.

Peltola JS, Könönen M, Nyström M. A follow-up study of radiographic findings in the mandibular condyles of orthodontically treated patients and associations with TMD. J Dent Res 1995;74:1571-1576.

Pinals RS. Traumatic arthritis and allied conditions. In: McCarthy DJ (ed) Arthritis and allied conditions. Philadelphia: Lea & Febiger, 1995:1205-1222.

Popowich K, Nebbe B, Major PW. Effect of Herbst treatment on temporomandibular joint morphology: a systematic literature review. Am J Orthod Dentofac Orthop 2003;123:388-394.

Ruf S, Pancherz H. Long-term TMJ effects of Herbst treatment: a clinical and MRI study. Am J Orthod Dentofac Orthop 1998a;114:475-483.

Ruf S, Pancherz H. Temporomandibular joint growth adaptation in Herbst treatment. A prospective magnetic resonance imaging and cephalometric roentgenographic study. Eur J Orthod 1998b;20:375-388.

Ruf S, Pancherz H. Temporomandibular joint remodeling in adolescents and young adults during Herbst treatment: a prospective longitudinal magnetic resonance imaging and cephalometric radiographic investigation. Am J Orthod Dentofac Orthop 1999;115:607-618.

Ruf S, Pancherz H. Does bite-jumping damage the TMJ? A prospective longitudinal clinical and MRI study of Herbst patients. Angle Orthod 2000;70:183-199.

Ruf S. Short- and long-term effects of the Herbst appliance on temporomandibular joint function. Semin Orthol 2003;9: 70–86.

Ruf S, Wüsten B, Pancherz H. TMJ effects of activator treatment. A prospective longitudinal magnetic resonance imaging and clinical study. Angle Orthod 2002;72:527-540.

Scapino RP. Histopathology associated with malposition of the human temporomandibular joint disc. Oral Surg Oral Med Oral Pathol 1983;55:382-397.

Scapino RP. The posterior attachment: Its structure, function, and appearance in TMJ imaging studies. Part 2. J Craniomandib Disord 1991a;5:155-166.

Scapino RP. The posterior attachment: its structure, function, and appearance in TMJ imaging studies. Part 1. J Craniomandib Disord 1991b;5:83-95.

Steenks MH, Bleys RL, Witkamp TD. Temporomandibular joint structures: a comparison between anatomic and magnetic resonance findings in a sagittal and an angulated plane. J Orofac Pain 1994;8:120-135.

Summer JD, Westesson PL. Mandibular repositioning can be effective in treatment of reducing TMJ disk displacement. A long-term clinical and MR imaging follow-up. J Craniomand Pract 1997;15:107-120.

Tallents RH, Katzberg RW, Macher DJ, Roberts CA. Use of protrusive splint therapy in anterior disk displacement of the temporomandibular joint: a 1- to 3-year follow-up. J Prosthet Dent 1990;63:336-341.

Thomas CA, Okeson JP. Evaluation of lateral pterygoid muscle symptoms using a common palpation technique and a method of functional manipulation. J Craniomand Pract 1987;5:125-129.

Ward DM, Behrents RG, Goldberg JS. Temporomandibular synovial fluid pressure response to altered mandibular positions. Am J Orthod Dentofacial Orthop 1990;98:22-28.

Westesson PL, Rohlin M. Internal derangement related to osteoarthrosis in temporomandibular joint autopsy specimens. Oral Surg Oral Med Oral Pathol 1984;57:17-22.

Wilkinson TM, Crowley CM. A histologic study of retrodiscal tissues of the human temporomandibular joint in the open and closed position. J Orofac Pain 1994;8:7-17.

Chapter 17

Treatment of the retrognathic and prognathic facial type

Research

Class II malocclusions of the retrognathic facial type are said to be more difficult to treat successfully than those of the prognatic facial type (Bishara and Jakobsen 1985, Janson 1987, Zaher et al. 1994). Such a statement is mainly based on (1) clinical experience, (2) the use of removable functional or conventional multibracket appliances, (3) short-term evaluations and (4) the consideration of only the vertical dimension ("high-angle" or "low-angle") in the assessment of facial retrognathism and prognathism.

Herbst treatment of Class II:1 malocclusions of the retrognathic and prognathic facial type (Bock and Pancherz, 2006).

In Class II:1 subjects of different facial types the skeletofacial changes during and after Herbst treatment were assessed. In the characterization of facial retrognathism / prognathism both the sagittal (SNA and SNB angles) and the vertical (ML/NSL angle) dimensions were considered.

The screened Herbst sample of Class II:1 malocclusions with complete orthodontic records and a follow-up period of at least three years posttreatment comprised of 360 subjects. Of these, 26 fulfilled the requirements for being assigned to either the retrognathic (SNA < 76°, SNB < 72° and ML/NSL > 37°) or the prognathic (SNA > 83°, SNB > 80° and ML/NSL < 32°) facial type group.

Before treatment all 26 subjects had an overjet larger than 6 mm and a Class II molar relationship exceeding 0.5 cusp widths. In the vertical dimension 5 of the 10 retrognathic subjects had an open bite with overbite (Moyers, 1973), which in 4 subjects was closed during treatment and remained closed after treatment. None of the prognathic subjects had an open bite, either before or after treatment.

The average age of the subjects at start of treatment was 14 years (15 years for the retroganthic and 13 years for the prognathic subjects). The average treatment time with the Herbst appliance amounted to 7 months. After Herbst therapy, 18 of the 26 subjects received further treatment with a multibracket appliance for an average period of 12 months. No further treatment was performed in the other 8 subjects. The subjects were, on average, reinvestigated 39 months after Herbst treatment.

Lateral head films in habitual occlusion from before Herbst treatment (T1), immediately after (T2), 1 year after (T3) and 3 years after (T4) Herbst treatment were analyzed with respect to the mechanism of overjet correction using the SO-Analysis (see Chapter 6: Herbst research - subjects and methods). Skeletofacial treatment changes were visualized by superimposed facial polygons (Fig. 17-1).

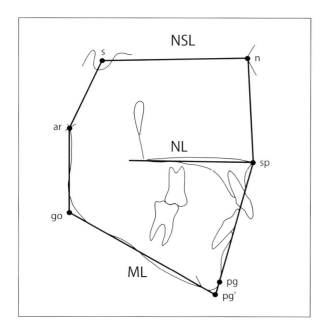

Fig. 17-1 Reference points and planes used in defining the facial polygon.

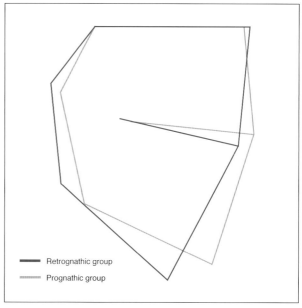

Fig. 17-2 Superimposed facial polygons of the retrognathic (n=10) and prognathic (n=16) groups at before treatment.

The **retrognathic facial type** group comprised of 10 subjects (5 males and 5 females). The cephalometric characteristics (mean values) were: SNA = 74.5°, SNB = 70.4° and ML/NSL = 41.1°.

The **prognathic facial type** group comprised 16 subjects (7 males and 9 females). The cephalometric characteristics (mean values) were: SNA = 86.7°, SNB = 81.5° and ML/NSL = 25.1°.

The difference in pretreatment skeletofacial morphology of the retrognathic and prognathic group is shown in Fig. 17-2.

Changes during 7 months of Herbst treatment (T2 – T1)

In all subjects treatment resulted in an overcorrection of overjet (incisor edge-to-edge position) and sagittal molar relationship (mild Class III).

Even if the amount of changes in the retrognathic and prognathic groups were statistically comparable there was a tendency for a relatively larger amount of skeletal changes contributing to overjet correction in the prognathic group than in the retrognathic group (Fig. 17-3).

Changes during 1 year after Herbst treatment (T3 – T2)

The occlusion settled into Class I in all subjects during the first year after treatment.

The amount of recovering overjet changes was somewhat larger in the retrognathic (3.2 mm) than in the prognathic (2.5 mm) group (Fig. 17-3). The maxillary base moved posteriorly in the retrognathic group (0.6 mm) and anteriorly in the prognathic group (0.7 mm). The mandibular base moved posteriorly in the retrognathic group (1.2 mm) and anteriorly in the prognathic group (0.2 mm).

Changes during 3 years after Herbst treatment (T4 – T2)

The amount of recovering overjet changes was somewhat larger in the retrognathic (3.8 mm) than in the prognathic (3.1 mm) group (Fig. 17-3). The maxillary base moved anteriorly in both groups, however, somewhat more in the prognathic (1.3 mm) than in the retrognathic (1.0 mm) group. The mandibular base moved posteriorly in the retrognathic (0.2 mm) and anteriorly in the prognatic (1.0 mm) group.

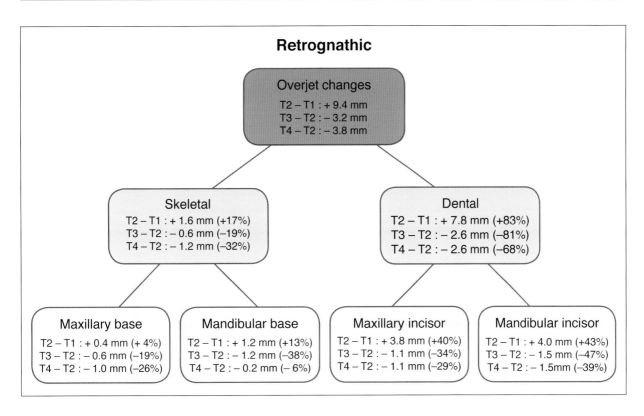

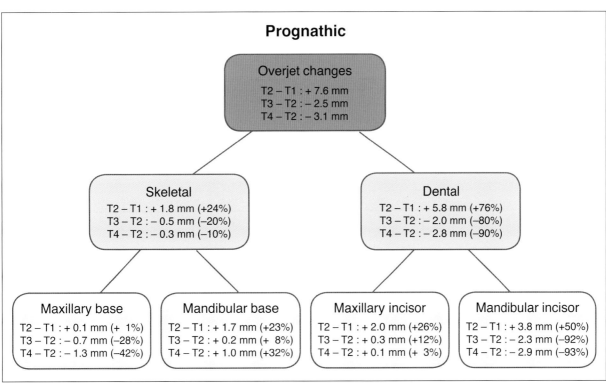

Fig. 17-3 SO-Analysis. Skeletal and dental components contributing to overjet changes in 10 **Retrognathic** and 16 **Prognathic** Class II:1 malocclusions treated with the Herbst appliance. Plus (+) means favorable changes contributing to an overjet reduction and minus (-) means unfavorable changes contributing to an overjet increase. **T1**: Before treatment; **T2**: After treatment; **T3**: 1 year after treatment; **T4**: 3 years after treatment.

When looking at treatment and posttreatment changes using the superimposed facial polygons, vertical changes dominate in the retrognathic group and horizontal changes dominate in the prognathic group (Fig. 17-4).

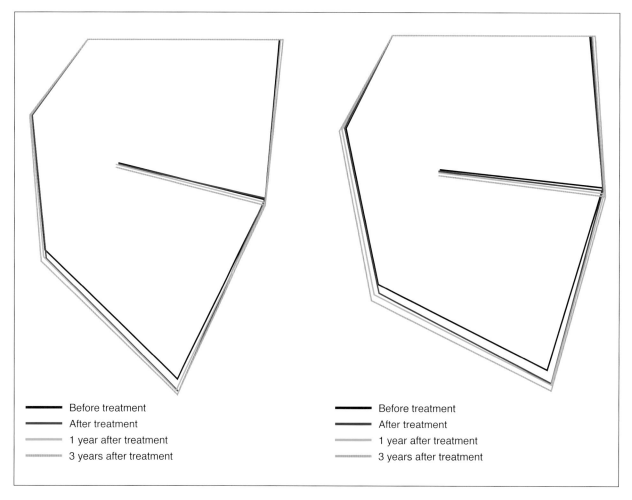

Before treatment
After treatment
1 year after treatment
3 years after treatment

Before treatment
After treatment
1 year after treatment
3 years after treatment

Fig. 17-4 Superimposed facial polygons visualizing changes in skeletofacial morphology of the retrognathic (n=10) group (left) and the prognathic (n =16) group (right) of Class II:1 malocclusions treated with the Herbst appliance.

Interpretation of the results

During treatment (T2 – T1), in all cases the overjet was overcorrected to an incisal edge-to-edge position and the molars to a mild Class III relationship. Therefore, when the occlusion settled (Pancherz and Hansen, 1986) to a stable Class I tooth interdigitation during the T3 – T2 period, the overjet increased to normal values. This will imply that later (after T3) unfavorable growth changes, as seen especially in the retrognathic subjects, could be buffered by the occlusion. This was confirmed by the fact that during the posttreatment period (T4 – T2) no clinically significant relapse in the overjet occurred in any of the retrognathic or prognathic subjects. With respect to the maxillary and mandibular growth changes, the small differences existing between the two facial type groups during treatment and posttreatment were certainly a result of the existing basic growth pattern (Pancherz and Fackel, 1990): vertical (unfavorable) growth in the retrognathic subjects and horizontal (favorable) growth in the prognathic subjects.

Clinical examples

Two Class II:1 subjects treated with the Herbst appliance, one retrognathic (Case 17-1) and one prognathic (Case 17-2) subject, are presented. Both subjects were treated successfully to a normal overjet and to a Class I dental arch relationship. The treatment result in both subjects was stable at the time of follow up 3 years after Herbst therapy.

Case 17-1 (Fig. 17-5)

A 12.5-year-old male with a Class II:1 malocclusion and a retrognathic facial morphology (SNA = 76°, SNB = 72°, ML/NSL = 39°) was treated with a banded Herbst appliance for 6 months. Posttreatment, no retention was performed.

Case 17-2 (Fig. 17-6)

A 14-year-old male with a Class II:1 malocclusion and a prognathic facial morphology (SNA = 86°, SNB = 79.5°, ML/NSL = 24.5°) was treated with a cast splint Herbst appliance for 9 months followed by a Multibracket (MB) appliance for 14 months. Posttreatment retention was carried out using bonded maxillary and mandibular cuspid-to-cuspid retainers.

Conclusion and clinical implications

Successful Herbst therapy seems to be independent of the facial type. On a long-term basis, however, retrognathic subjects are prone to exhibit more unfavourable mandibular growth changes than prognathic subjects and will thus, exhibit a greater risk for an occlusal relapse, if a stable Class I occlusion is not attained after treatment.

References

Bishara SE, Jakobsen JR. Longitudinal changes in three normal facial types. Am J Orthod 1985;88:466-502.

Bock N, Pancherz H. Herbst treatment of Class II:1 malocclusions of the retrognathic and prognathic facial type. Angle Orthod 2006;76:930-941.

Janson I. Bionator-Modifikationen in der kieferorthopädischen Therapie. München: Hanser Verlag, 1987:22-56.

Moyers RE. Handbook of Orthodontics. Chicago: Year Book Medical Publishers, 1973:292.

Pancherz H. The mechanism of Class II correction in Herbst appliance treatment. A cephalometric investigation. Am J Orthod 1982;82:104-113.

Pancherz H, Fackel U. The skeletofacial growth pattern pre- and postdentofacial orthopedics. A long-term study of Class II malocclusions treated with the Herbst appliance. Eur J Orthod 1990;12:209-218.

Pancherz H, Hansen K. Occlusal changes during and after Herbst treatment: a cephalometric investigation. Eur J Orthod 1986;8:215-228.

Zaher AR, Bishara SE, Jakobsen JR. Posttreatment changes in different facial types. Angle Orthod 1994;64:425-436.

Before Herbst   **After Herbst**   **Follow-up 3 years**

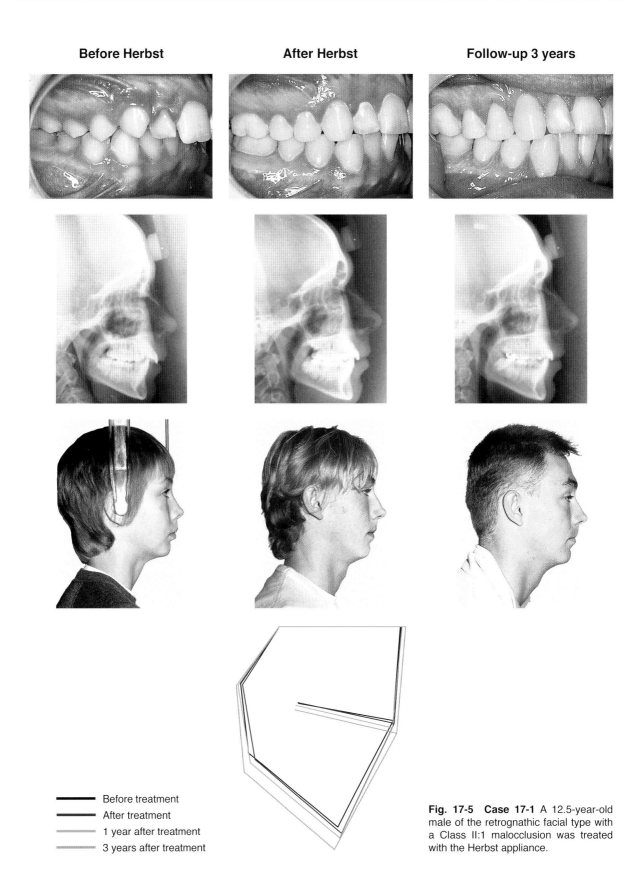

Before treatment
After treatment
1 year after treatment
3 years after treatment

Fig. 17-5   Case 17-1 A 12.5-year-old male of the retrognathic facial type with a Class II:1 malocclusion was treated with the Herbst appliance.

Before Herbst   **After Herbst /MB**   **Follow-up 3 years**

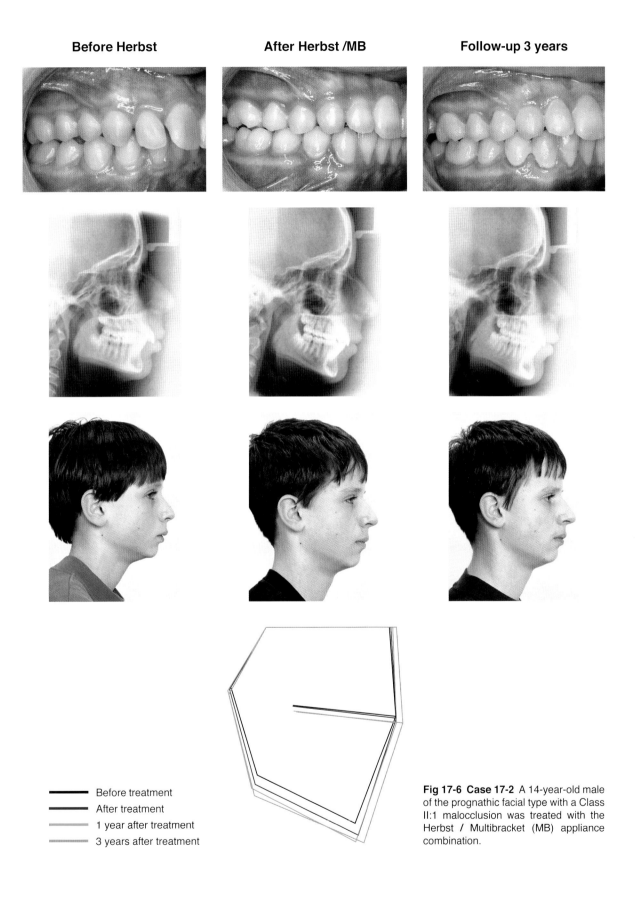

Before treatment
After treatment
1 year after treatment
3 years after treatment

Fig 17-6 Case 17-2 A 14-year-old male of the prognathic facial type with a Class II:1 malocclusion was treated with the Herbst / Multibracket (MB) appliance combination.

Chapter 18

Treatment of hyper- and hypodivergent Class II:1 malocclusions

Research

The success of Class II treatment is said to depend, among other things, on the vertical jaw base relationship (mandibular plane angle).

Treatment of hyperdivergent (large mandibular plane angle) Class II cases with removable functional appliances (Activator, Bionator, Fränkel) is not recommended, as the reaction to therapy is supposed to be unfavorable and the appliances will result in an unfavorable posterior mandibular growth rotation (Tulley 1972, Valinot 1973, Hirzel and Grewe 1974, Woodside 1974, Creekmore and Radney 1983, Bolmgren and Moshiri 1986), which consequently could detoriate facial esthetics.

Herbst appliance treatment of hyperdivergent Class II subjects has, on the other hand, been shown either not to alter the basic mandibular growth rotation or to enhance a more anterior directed mandibular rotation (Pancherz 1982, Hägg 1992, Schiavoni et al. 1992, Grobety 1999, Ruf and Pancherz 1996). Furthermore, it has been demonstrated that Herbst treatment is most efficient in hyperdivergent Class II malocclusions and that the skeletal treatment changes contributing to Class II correction are independent of the vertical jaw base relationship (Windmiller 1993, Ruf and Pancherz 1997). In the assessment of TMJ growth changes in Herbst subjects of different facial types, Pancherz and Michaelidou (2004) could demonstrate that condylar growth was directed more posteriorly in hyperdivergent than in hypodivergent subjects.

The effect of Herbst appliance treatment on the mandibular plane angle: a cephalometric roentgenographic study (Ruf and Pancherz, 1996)

The individual reaction pattern and the long-term effects of Herbst treatment on the mandibular plane angle (ML/NSL) were assessed. Longitudinal data derived from lateral head films of 80 Class II:1 subjects treated exclusively with the Herbst appliance were analyzed. The subjects were divided into three groups according to their pretreatment mandibular plane angle: hypodivergent (n=11), normodivergent (n=61) and hyperdivergent (n=8). The patients were treated for an average period of 7 months and followed for 4.5 - 5 years after therapy. The age of the subjects at start of treatment varied between 10-14 years. All cases were treated to Class I occlusal relationships.

The results of the study (Figs. 18-1 and 18-2) revealed that the ML/NSL angle was, on average, unaffected by Herbst therapy. Posttreatment, a continuous decrease in the ML/NSL angle took place. However, a large individual variation existed (Fig. 18-1). There was no statistically significant difference between hypo-, normo- and hyperdivergent subjects.

Interpretation of the results
The increase of the ML/NSL at start of treatment (T1-T2) was a result of the incisal edge-to-edge construction bite, which led to a posterior rotation of the mandible (Fig. 18-1). The decrease of the ML/NSL from start to after treatment (T2-T3) could be attributed to a anterior autorotation of the lower jaw due to the headgear effect of the appliance (Pancherz and Anehus-Pancherz 1993). The intrusion

of the maxillary molars, and intrusion of the lower incisors (Pancherz 1982) may facilitate a closing rotation of the mandible. The decrease of the ML/NSL during the first 6 months after treatment (T3-T4) was certainly a result of the settling of the occlusion (Pancherz and Hansen 1986), during which the incisal edge-to-edge position changed to a normal overjet and overbite, allowing the mandible to continue to autorotate anteriorly. The ML/NSL decrease during the follow-up period (T4-T5) could be interpreted as a result of normalized function (Moss 1968) that permitted normal growth and development (Bathia and Leighton 1993) (Fig. 18-2). The only difference between the growth standards of Bathia and Leighton (1993) and the three vertical jaw base relationship groups of Herbst patients was the absolute value of the ML/NSL angle (Fig. 18-2). The posttreatment development pattern of ML/NSL was identical.

The mechanism of Class II correction during Herbst therapy in relation to the vertical jaw base relationship: a cephalometric roentgenographic study (Ruf and Pancherz, 1997)

The sagittal skeletal and dental effects of Herbst treatment contributing to Class II correction in subjects with a small and large mandibular plane angle were assessed. Lateral head films of 16 hyperdivergent (ML/NSL > 39° and 15 hypordivergent (ML/NSL ≤ 26°) Class II:1 subjects were analyzed. The patients were treated for an average period of 7 months. The age of the subjects at the start of Herbst treatment varied between 11 and 14 years.

The results revealed that the amount of skeletal changes contributing to overjet and Class II molar (Fig. 18-3) correction during 7 months of Herbst treatment was larger in the hyperdivergent group (37% and 44%, respectively) than in the hypodivergent group (25% and 25%, respectively).

Temporomandibular joint growth changes in hyperdivergent and hypodivergent Herbst subjects. A long-term roentgenographic cephalometric study (Pancherz and Michaelidou 2004)

The amount and direction of "effective TMJ growth" (the sum of condylar modeling, glenoid fossa modeling and condylar position changes in the fossa) and glenoid fossa growth displacement (see Chap-

ter 6: Herbst research - subjects and methods) was assessed in 13 hyperdivergent (ML/NSL ≥ 37° degrees), 17 hypodivergent (ML/NSL ≤ 26°) and 38 normodivergent (ML/NSL 26.5°- 36.5°) subjects treated with the Herbst appliance during an average period of 7 months. Lateral head films from before, after and 5 years after treatment were scrutinized.

The results revealed that during Herbst treatment the amount of "effective TMJ growth" (Fig. 18-4) was comparable in the three facial type groups. Group differences existed, however, with respect to the direction of changes: hyperdivergent subjects exhibited more posterior-directed growth changes than hypodivergent subjects. Posttreatment, "effective TMJ growth" in all three groups was directed more vertically compared to the treatment changes.

The glenoid fossa (Fig. 18-5) was displaced anteriorly and inferiorly during Herbst treatment and posteriorly posttreatment. No statistical differences existed between the three facial type groups.

Interpretation of the results

Herbst treatment stimulates bone apposition, especially at the posterior pole of the condyle (Pancherz and Littmann 1989, Ruf and Pancherz 1998, Pancherz and Fischer 2003, Peterson and McNamara 2003). This is especially true in hyperdivergent subjects (Pancherz and Michaelidou 2004) in whom the therapeutic effect coincides with the inherited horizontal condylar growth direction (Björk 1969), and thus could explain the favorable skeletal effect in these cases (Fig. 18-4) when compared to hypodivergent subjects.

When interpreting the findings of the study of Pancherz and Michaelidou (2004) it must be remembered that during normal growth, the glenoid fossa is displaced in a posterior and inferior direction (Björk and Skieller 1972, 1983, Buschang and Santos-Pinto 1998). Furthermore, anterior-directed glenoid fossa displacement and posterior-directed "effective TMJ growth" are favorable changes in skeletal Class II treatment as they contribute to increase mandibular prognathism. On the other hand, posterior-directed fossa displacement and anterior-directed "effective TMJ growth" are unfavorable changes for Class II correction.

Herbst treatment seemed to have only a temporary effect on glenoid fossa displacement in an anterior direction during the active phase of therapy (T2-T1) (Fig. 18-5). Posttreatment (T3-T2), fossa displacement was in a posterior direction. Therefore, in the total observation period (T3-T1), the direction of fossa displacement posteriorly and inferiorly corresponded to that of normal growth changes. The amount and direction of fossa changes seemed to be independent of the vertical facial type of the patients.

Thus, when looking at the direction of "effective TMJ growth" during the different examination periods (Fig. 18-4), anterior and inferior fossa displacement changes during treatment (T2-T1) are added to posterior condylar growth, whereas posterior fossa displacement changes posttreatment (T3-T2) are subtracted from posterior condylar growth.

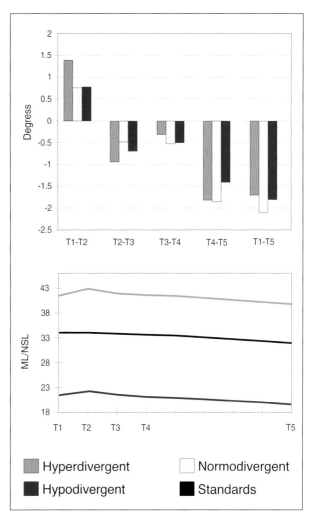

Fig. 18-2 Average changes (in degrees) of ML/NSL during different observation intervals. Analysis of 80 Class II:1 subjects treated with the Herbst appliance grouped according to their vertical jaw base relationship (hyperdivergent, normodivergent and hypodivergent). T1: Before treatment; T2: Start of treatment (after insertion of the Herbst appliance); T3: After treatment (after removal of the Herbst appliance); T4: Six months after removal of the Herbst appliance (at the time the occlusion has settled); T5: Follow-up (4.5-5 years after removal of the Herbst appliance). The growth standards (Standards) of normal untreated subjects (Bathia and Leighton 1993) are shown in the lower graph. *(Revised from Ruf and Pancherz 1996)*

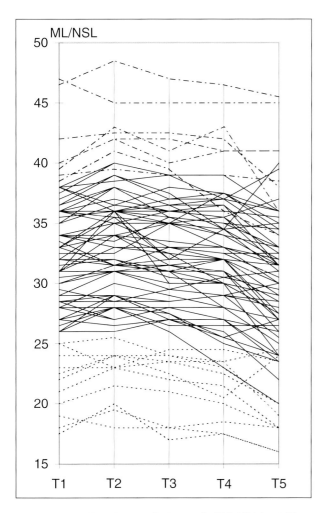

Fig. 18-1 Individual changes (in degrees) of ML/NSL in 80 Class II:1 subjects treated with the Herbst appliance grouped according to their vertical jaw base relationship (hyperdivergent –·–·–·–· normodivergent ———— and hypodivergent ······). T1: Before treatment; T2: Start of treatment (after insertion of the Herbst appliance); T3: After treatment (after removal of the Herbst appliance); T4: Six months after removal of the Herbst appliance (at the time the occlusion has settled); T5: Follow-up (4.5-5 years after removal of the Herbst appliance). *(Revised from Ruf and Pancherz 1996)*

155

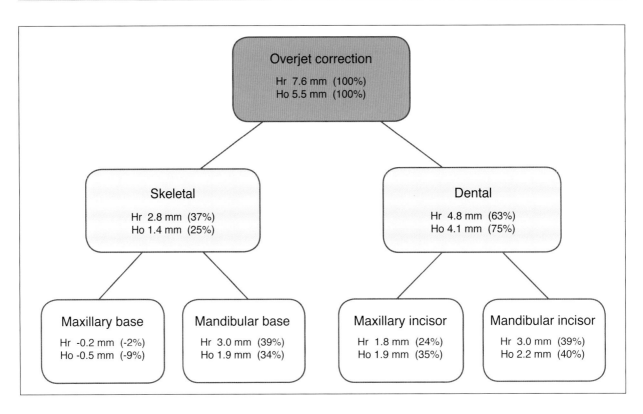

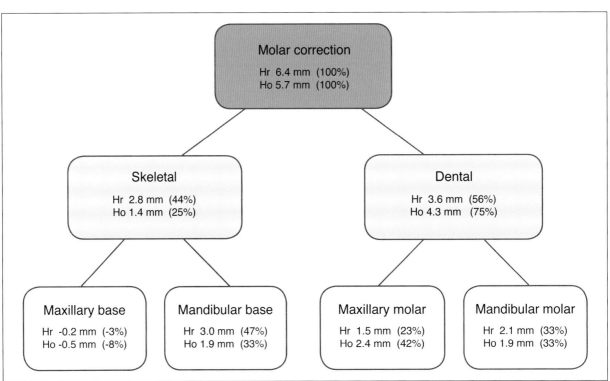

Fig. 18-3 Dental and skeletal changes contributing to the correction of overjet (above) and Class II molar relaton (below) in 16 hyperdivergent (Hr) and 15 hypodivergent (Ho) Class II:1 malocclusions treated with the Herbst appliance. Minus (-) implies unfavorable changes for overjet or molar correction. *(Revised from Ruf and Pancherz 1997)*

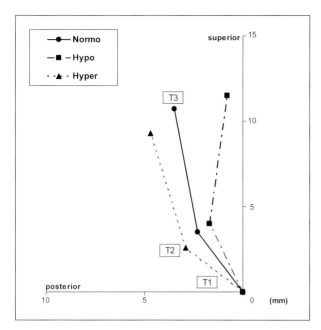

Fig. 18-4 "Effective TMJ growth" (mean changes) in 38 normodivergent (*Normo*), 17 hypodivergent (*Hypo*) and 13 hyperdivergent (*Hyper*) Herbst subjects. T1: Before treatment. T2: After treatment. T3: 5 years after treatment. *(Revised from Pancherz and Michaelidou 2004)*

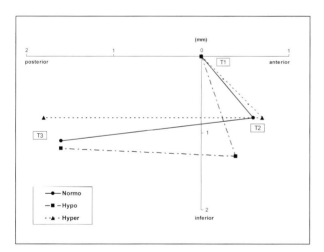

Fig. 18-5 Glenoid fossa displacement (mean changes) in 38 normodivergent (*Normo*), 17 hypodivergent (*Hypo*) and 13 hyperdivergent (*Hyper*) Herbst subjects. T1: Before treatment. T2: After treatment. T3: 5 years after treatment. *(Revised from Pancherz and Michaelidou 2004)*

Clinical examples

Two hyperdivergent Class II:1 subjects (Cases 18-1 and 18-2) treated with the Herbst appliance are presented. In both subjects, Herbst treatment was followed by a Multibracket appliance treatment phase. Due to severe mandibular anterior crowding, extraction of the four first premolars were performed in both subjects and retention after treatment was done with a maxillary plate and a mandibular cuspid-to-cuspid retainer.

Case 18-1 (Fig. 18-6)
A 14-year-old male with a mandibular plane angle of 41.5°. Pretreatment the overjet was 16 mm and the ANB angle 5.5°. Treatment was performed with a casted splint Herbst appliance for 7 months followed by a Multibracket appliance, with extractions of four first premolars, for 23 months.

Case 18-2 (Fig. 18-7)
A 13-year-old female with a mandibular plane angle of 42°. Pretreatment, the overjet was 8 mm and the ANB angle 7°. Treatment was performed with a casted splint Herbst appliance for 7 months followed by a Multibracket appliance, with- out extractions of teeth, for 12 months.

Conclusions and clinical implications

- Herbst treatment does not result in an undesired backward rotation of the mandible.
- A large mandibular plane angle will not affect the treatment response unfavorably.
- "Effective TMJ growth" and glenoid fossa displacement changes are only temporarily affected favorably in sagittal direction by Herbst therapy. However, "effective TMJ growth" is directed more posteriorly in hyperdivergent than in hypodivergent subjects during treatment and posttreatment.
- Hyperdivergent Class II subjects are good Herbst patients.

Before Herbst	**After Herbst**	**After Multibracket**

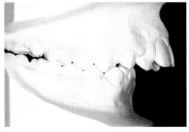 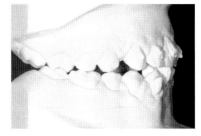 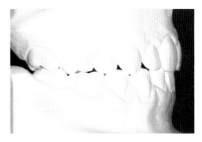

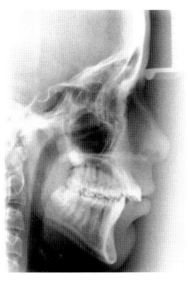 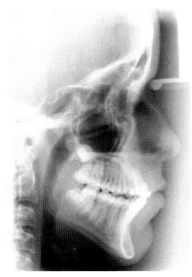 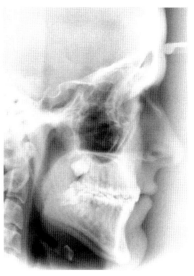

ML/NSL = 41.5°
SNA   = 76.5°
SNB   = 71.0°
ANB   = 5.5°

ML/NSL = 38.0°
SNA   = 77.5°
SNB   = 74.0°
ANB   = 3.5°

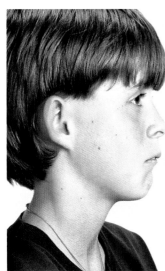 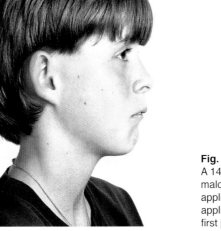 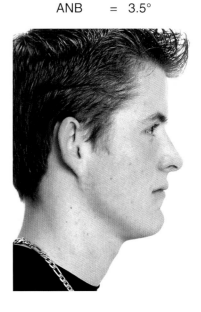

Fig. 18-6 Case 18-1
A 14-year-old male with a Class II:1 malocclusion treated with the Herbst appliance followed by a Multibracket appliance with extractions of four first premolars.

Before Herbst   **After Herbst**   **After Multibracket**

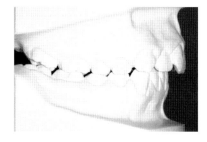
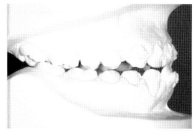
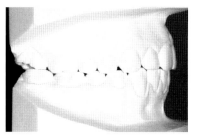

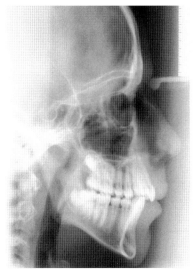
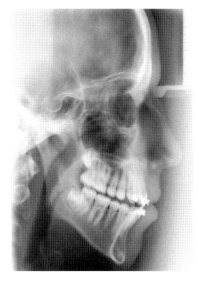
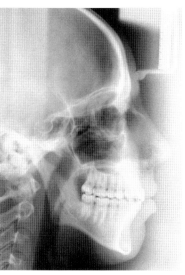

ML/NSL = 42.0°   ML/NSL = 41.5°
SNA   = 77.0°   SNA   = 74.0°
SNB   = 70.0°   SNB   = 68.5°
ANB   = 7.0°   ANB   = 5.5°

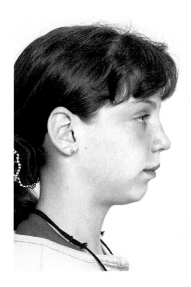

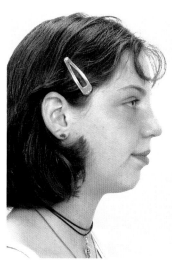

Fig. 18-7 Case 18-2
A 13-year-old female with a Class II:1 malocclusion treated with the Herbst appliance followed by a Multibracket appiance.

References

Bathia SN, Leighton BC. A manual of facial growth: a computer analysis of longitudinal cephalometric growth data. Oxford: Oxford University Press, 1993:337.

Björk A. Prediction of mandibular growth rotation. Am J Orthod 1969;55:585-599.

Björk A, Skieller V. Facial development and tooth eruption. An implant study at the age of puberty. Am J Orthod 1972;62:339-383.

Björk A, Skieller V. Normal and abnormal growth of the mandible. A synthesis of longitudinal cephalometric implant studies over a period of 25 years. Eur J Orthod 1983;5:1-46.

Bolmgren GA, Moshiri F. Bionator treatment in Class II, Division 1. Angle Orthod 1986;56:255-262.

Buschang P, Santos-Pinto A. Condylar growth and glenoid fossa displacement during childhood and adolescents. Am J Orthod Dentofac Orhop 1998;113:437-442.

Creekmore TD, Radney LJ. Fränkel appliance therapy: orthopedic and orthodontic? Am J Orthod 1983;83:89-108.

Grobety D. No management of facial height without mastering the mandibular growth. In Lagerström L (ed) Orthodontic Management of Facial height. Long Face and Short Face. München: Neuer Merkur GmbH, 1999:23-30.

Hägg U. Changes in mandibular growth direction by means of a Herbst appliance. A case report. Am J Orthod Dentofac Orthop 1992;102:456-463.

Hirzel HG, Grewe JM. Activators: a practical approach. Am J Orthod 1974;66:557-570.

Moss ML. The primacy of functional matrices in orofacial growth. Dent Practitioner 1968;19:65-73.

Pancherz H. Vertical dentofacial changes during Herbst appliance treatment. A cephalometric investigation. Swed Dent J (Suppl) 1982;15:189-196.

Pancherz H, Anehus-Pancherz M. The head-gear effect of the Herbst appliance. a cephalometric long-term study. Am J Orthod Dentofac Orthop 1993;103:510-520.

Pancherz H, Hansen K. Occlusal changes during and after Herbst treatment: a cephalometric investigation. Eur J Orthod 1986;8:215-228.

Pancherz H, Littmann C. Morphologie und Lage des Unterkiefers bei der Herbst-Behandlung. Eine kephalometrische Analyse der Veränderungen bis zum Wachstumsabschluss. Inf Orthod Kieferorthop 1989;20:493-513.

Pancherz H, Fischer S. Amount and direction of temporomandibular joint growth changes in Herbst treatment: a cephalometric long-term investigation. Angle Orthod 2003;73:493-501.

Pancherz H, Michaelidou C. Temporomandibular joint growth changes in hyperdivergent and hypodivergent Herbst subjects. A long-term roentgenographic cephalometric study. Am J Othod Dentofac Orthop 2004;126:153-161.

Peterson JE, McNamara JA. Temporomandibular joint adaptations associated with Herbst appliance treatment in juvenile Rhesus monkeys (Macaca Mulatta). Semin Orthod 2003;9:12-25.

Ruf S, Pancherz H. The effect of Herbst appliance treatment on the mandibular plane angle: a cephalometric roentgenographic study. Am J Orthod Dentofac Orthop 1996;110:225-229.

Ruf S, Pancherz H. The mechanism of Class II correction during Herbst therapy in relation to the vertical jaw base relationship. A cephalometric roentgenographic study. Angle Orthod 1997;67:271-276.

Ruf S, Pancherz H. Temporomanibular joint growth adaptation in Herbst treatment: a prospective magnetic resonance imaging and cephalometric roentgenographic study. Eur J Orthod 1998;20:375-388.

Schiavoni R, Grenga V, Macri, V. Treatment of Class II high angle malocclusionwith the Herbst appliance: a cephalometric investigation. Am J Orthod Dentofac Orthop 1992;102:393-409.

Tulley WJ. The scope and limitations of treatment with the activator. Am J Orthod 1972;61:562-577.

Valinot JR. The European activator: its basis and use. Am J Orthod 1973;63:561-580.

Windmiller EC. The acrylic Herbst appliance: a cephalometric evaluation. Am J Ortho Dentofac Orthop 1993;104:73-84.

Woodside DG. The activator. In Salzman JA, ed. Orthodontics in daily practice. Philadelphia: Lippincott, 1974:556-591.

Chapter 19

Anchorage problems

Research

The dental effects of the Herbst appliance are basically a result of anchorage loss. As a result of the forces excerted by the Herbst telescopes, the maxillary teeth are driven posteriorly and the mandibular teeth are driven anteriorly. The maxillary dental reaction is advantageous in Class II treatment and has been discussed in Chapter 9: The headgear effect of the Herbst appliance. The mandibular dental reaction, however, is most of the time unwanted, as it results in a proclination of the front teeth (Pancherz 1979, 1982, Pancherz and Hägg 1985, Pancherz and Hansen 1986, Hansen et al. 1997, Ruf et al. 1998). In order to reduce the proclination effect of the Herbst appliance on the mandibular incisors different attempts have been made to increase mandibular anchorage by incorporating an increasing number of dental units, soft tissue structures (Pancherz and Hansen 1988) or by using casted splints instead of bands to attach the telescope mechanism (Franchi et al. 1999, Weschler and Pancherz 2005, von Bremen et al. 2007). The influence of the amount of bite jumping, age and skeletal maturity of the patients on mandibular anchorage loss has been addressed in two publications (Pancherz and Hansen 1988, Martin and Pancherz 2007).

The scientific evidence on the topic of mandibular anchorage loss during Herbst treatment will be presented by scrutinizing three publications.

1. Mandibular anchorage in Herbst treatment (Pancherz and Hansen 1988)

In this study the treatment and early posttreatment effects of the Herbst appliance are evaluated by comparing 5 different anchorage forms. At the time of investigation, the original sample of consecutive Class II:1 malocclusions treated with the Herbst appliance at the Department of Orthodontics, University of Lund, Sweden, comprised 108 patients. Herbst therapy resulted in Class I or overcorrected Class I dental arch relationships in all 108 cases. Following Herbst treatment, a multibracket appliance was used in 37 patients. These 37 subjects were not included in this study. In 6 subjects the mandibular anchorage form had to be changed during Herbst treatment (see Pelott anchorage), and consequently these subjects were also excluded from the analysis. Thus the final sample comprised 65 subjects (48 males and 17 females) aged 10 to 16 years treated with the Herbst appliance for an average period of 7 months. According to the mandibular anchorage form used, the patients were divided into the following 5 groups:

Premolar anchorage (P). The first premolars were banded and connected with a lingual sectional arch wire touching the lingual surfaces of the front teeth (Fig. 19-1A). This type of anchorage was used in 16 subjects.

Premolar-Molar anchorage (PM). The first premolars and permanent first molars were banded and connected with a lingual arch wire touching the lingual surfaces of the front teeth (Fig. 19-1B). This type of anchorage was utilized in 20 subjects.

Pelotte anchorage. The lingual arch wire of a PM anchorage form was not in contact with the front teeth. The arch wire was furnished with an acrylic pelotte touching the lingual mucosa about 3 mm below the gingival margin (Fig. 19-1C). This type of anchorage was originally used in 12 subjects. In 6 subjects, however, severe ulcerations (Fig.19-2) occurred so that treatment had to be discontinued.

Labial-Lingual anchorage (LL). A labial premolar-to-premolar arch wire (first round, later rectangular) was added to a PM anchorage form. The labial arch-wire was attached to brackets on the front teeth and to tubes on the first premolar bands (Fig. 19-1D). This type of anchorage was used in 10 subjects.

Class III elastics (Cl III). Class III elastics (about 150 cN) were added to a LL anchorage form (the labial arch wire ended distal to the canines).

The Class III elastics were attached to the mandibular labial arch wire and to the screws on the maxillary molar bands (Fig. 19-1E). The patients were instructed to use the elastics full time. This type of anchorage was used in 13 subjects.

No statistical difference in age was found between the 5 anchorage groups. The patients were re-examined 6 months and 12 months after removal of the Herbst appliance. The lengths of the treatment period and the posttreatment periods were comparable in the different anchorage groups. No further treatment after Herbst therapy was performed in any of the subjects. Posttreatment retention (activator with and without a mandibular cuspid-to-cuspid retainer) was performed in 37 subjects and 28 subjects were not retained.

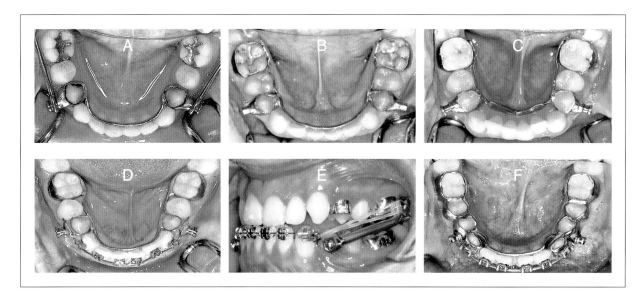

Fig. 7-1 Six mandibular anchorage forms of the Herbst appliance. **A**, Premolar anchorage (P). **B**, Premolar-Molar anchorage (PM). **C**, Pelotte anchorage. **D**, Labial-Lingual anchorage (LL). **E**, Class III elastics (CL III). **F**, Cast splint anchorage (S).

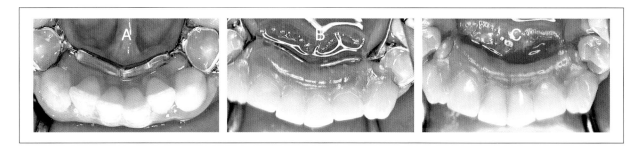

Fig. 7-2 Pelotte anchorage and damage of the lingual mucosa. **A**, Start of Herbst treatment when placing the appliance. **B**, Ulceration of the lingual mucosa after 2 months of treatment. **C**, After removal of the Pelotte.

162

2. Efficiency of three mandibular anchorage forms in Herbst treatment: a cephalometric investigation (Weschler and Pancherz 2005)

In this study the treatment and late posttreatment effects of the Herbst appliance on incisor tooth angulation were evaluated. Two of the mandibular banded anchorage forms (P anchorage and PM anchorage) from the study of Pancherz and Hansen (1988), were compared with a mandibular cast splint anchorage form.

Cast splint anchorage (S). Bilateral splints casted from cobalt cromium alloy covered the buccal and lingual surfaces of the teeth from the canines to the permanent first or second molars. The two splints were connected with each other by a lingual sectional arch wire resting on the lingual surfaces of the incisors (Fig 19-1F).

The S anchorage group comprised 34 subjects aged 10 to 17 years. They were treated with the Herbst appliance for 7 months. All patients had a subsequent multibracket appliance treatment phase for about another year after Herbst therapy. Thereafter, retention was performed for 1 to 2 years with either a positioner or an activator in combination with a mandibular cuspid-to-cuspid retainer. All patients were treated at the Department of Orthodontics, University of Giessen, Germany.

The patients of the three anchorage groups were re-examined 2 years and 4 years after Herbst treatment. The lengths of the treatment period and the posttreatment periods were comparable in the different anchorage groups. In both investigations (Pancherz and Hansen 1988, Weschler and Pancherz 2005), incisor tooth inclination changes were evaluated by means of lateral head films.

Mandibular tracings of the head films from before treatment, after treatment and posttreatment were superimposed on the anterior and inferior mandibular bone contours. The original mandibular line (ML) was used as a reference line for the registration of mandibular incisor inclination changes.

In the patients from both investigations no statistically significant difference existed between retention and no retention cases. Therefore, the retention and no retention samples were pooled in the final analysis. The results of the two studies revealed the following:

Treatment changes

The lower incisors proclined in all subjects independent of the anchorage form used (Figs. 19-3 and 19-4). The average proclination, for all anchorage forms, was 9.4° A large individual variation existed, however. Incisor proclination was least in the Pelotte group. Subjects with P anchorage exhibited significantly less tooth proclination than subjects with LL, Class III and S anchorage.

Short-term posttreatment changes (Fig. 19-3)

In the 65 subjects (Pancherz and Hansen 1988) investigated 12 months posttreatment, recovery in incisor tooth inclination had occurred in all cases. About 80% of the incisor movements during treatment recovered after treatment. Most of these tooth movements took place during the first 6 months posttreatment. On average, the largest recovery 12 months posttreatment was seen in subjects with the Pelotte (100%) and LL (97%) anchorage, while the smallest recovery was seen in subjects with the P (62%) anchorage.

Fig. 19-3 Diagram illustrating the average changes (degrees) in mandibular incisor inclination in 65 Class II:1 malocclusions treated with the Herbst appliance using 5 anchorage forms: Premolar (P) anchorage (n=16), Premolar-Molar (PM) anchorage (n=20), Pelotte anchorage (n=6), Labial-Lingual (LL) anchorage (n=10), Class III (Cl III) elastics (n=13). Registrations before and after Herbst treatment, 6 months and 12 months posttreatment. (*Revised from Pancherz and Hansen 1988*)

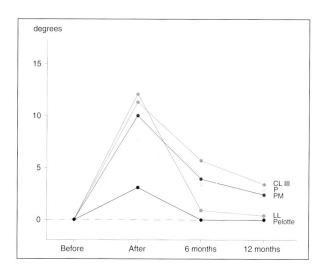

Interdependence between treatment and short-term posttreatment changes

In the 65 subjects (Pancherz and Hansen 1988), a significant moderate correlation (r=0.73) existed between the treatment and 12 months posttreatment changes. This means that a large proclination of the incisors during treatment was followed by a corresponding large retroclination (recovery) after treatment.

Long-term posttreatment changes (Fig. 19-4)

In the 70 subjects (Weschler and Pancherz 2005) investigated 4 years after Herbst treatment, 89% of the proclination seen during treatment had recovered in the P group, 88% in the PM group and 53% in the S group. No statistically significant difference existed when comparing the three anchorage groups. When comparing the 4-year findings with the 2-year findings, lower incisor inclination in all three anchorage groups was, on average, almost stable. No statistically significant difference existed between the three anchorage groups.

caused by the pressure of the acrylic pelott on the soft tissue (Fig.19-2). Surprisingly, anchorage loss was more pronounced in subjects with the most comprehensive anchorage systems (LL, Class III and S). This could be due to (1) the difference in the severity of the malocclusion (=overjet) existing in the patient groups, putting a different load on the dentition by the telescope mechanism, or (2) that the front teeth were deliberately proclined by the labial sectional arch wires (attached to the LL, Class III and S anchorage systems) for tooth alignment in crowded cases. It could be expected that by combining the LL anchorage system with Class III elastics, the pull of the elastics would counteract the push of the telescope mechanism, thus preventing the proclination of the incisors. This was, however, not the case. A possible explanation could be that the force (150 cN) of the Class III elastics was too weak for sufficient anchorage control and /or that the patients did not use the elastics on a full-time basis as they were instructed.

Fig. 19-4 Diagram illustrating the average changes (degrees) in mandibular incisor tooth inclination in 70 Class II:1 malocclusions treated with the Herbst appliance using 3 anchorage forms: Premolar (P) anchorage (n=16), Premolar-Molar (PM) anchorage (n=20), Cast splint (S) anchorage (n=34). Registrations before and after Herbst treatment, 2 years and 4 years posttreatment. (*Revised from Weschler and Pancherz 2004*)

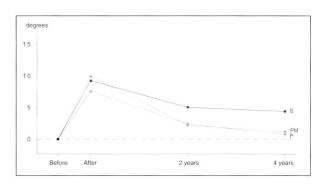

Interpretation of the results

Treatment changes

None of the 6 anchorage forms investigated could withstand the strain placed on the anterior portion of the mandibular dentition by the Herbst telescope mechanism. Even when using a cobalt chromium cast framework (S anchorage), incorporating into anchorage the permanent first molar and the second and first premolars on both sides of the mandibular arch, anchorage loss was pronounced. At first glance the Pelotte anchorage seemed to be better (less anchorage loss) than any of the other anchorage forms. It must be remembered, however, that this group consisted of only 6 finished cases selected from an original group of 12 subjects. In the other 6 subjects treatment had to be discontinued due to severe ulcerations of the lingual mucosa

Short-term posttreatment changes

As mentioned above, 80% of the incisor tooth movements during treatment (proclination) recovered after treatment (retroclination). This was especially the case during the first 6 months after therapy. When comparing the 5 banded anchorage groups, most of the recovering incisor tooth movements occurred in the LL group. This was certainly due to the fact that this group had the largest overjet pre-treatment and exhibited the largest treatment change. As an association existed between the treatment and posttreatment tooth movements, the LL group also exhibited the largest posttreatment change. Furthermore, it must be noted that no retention was used in any of the LL subjects after the Herbst appliance was removed.

Long-term posttreatment changes

The lower incisors continued to upright insignificantly during the period 2 years posttreatment to 4 years posttreatment. In comparison to before treatment, the lower incisors in all three anchorage groups investigated (P, PM and S) , still had a slightly proclined position 4 years posttreatment. This could be the result of an incomplete recovery or due the dentoalveolar compensatory mechanism in connection with normal mandibular anterior growth rotation described by Björk and Skieller (1972). A net proclined incisor position 4 years posttreatment was especially obvious in the S group because these subjects had a subsequent multibracket treatment phase for about another year after Herbst therapy and posttreatment retention was performed in all cases. On the other hand, in the banded Herbst appliance groups (P and PM) every second patient was not retained, allowing an unrestricted recovery in incisor position.

3. Position changes of the mandibular incisors in Herbst / Multibracket appliance treatment in relation to the amount of bite jumping, age and skeletal maturation (Martin and Pancherz 2007)

In this study an assessment was made of the effect of different amounts of mandibular advancement (bite jumping) at start of Herbst therapy on the inclination changes of the mandibular incisors. In the evaluation, the age and skeletal maturity of the patients was considered. The subject material comprised 67 male and 66 female Class II:1 subjects treated with a cast splint Herbst appliance for 7 months (6-13 months) followed by a multibracket appliance (MB) for 12 months (6-15 months). Total treatment time was 19 months (18-30 months). All patients were treated at the Department of Orthodontics, University of Giessen, Germany. With respect to the amount of bite jumping at start of Herbst treatment, the subjects were divided into three groups:

Group I   Bite jumping   ≤ 7.0 mm
Group II   Bite jumping   7.5 mm to 9.5 mm
Group III   Bite jumping   > 9.5 mm

Lateral head film in habitual occlusion from three occasions were evaluated: (1) before Herbst treatment, (2) after Herbst treatment / start of MB treatment, (3) after MB treatment.

Mandibular tracings of the three head films from each patient were superimposed on the stable reference structures of the mandible. The original occlusal line was used as a reference line for the registration of the inclination changes of the mandibular incisors. Skeletal maturation of the subjects was assessed using hand-wrist radiographs. The maturity stages proposed by Hägg and Taranger (1980) were used.

Herbst treatment changes (Fig. 19-5)

During the Herbst treatment phase the mandibular incisors proclined in all 133 subjects investigated. Incisor proclination was significantly larger in bite jumping group III than in bite jumping group I. Furthermore, a significantly larger incisor proclination

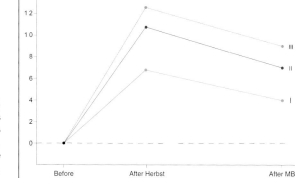

Fig. 19-5 Diagram illustrating the average changes (degrees) in mandibular incisor inclination in 133 Class II:1 malocclusions treated with the Herbst appliance. Division of the subjects into 3 bite jumping groups. **Group I**: Bite jumping ≤ 7.0 mm (n= 49). **Group II**: Bite jumping: 7.5 mm to 9.5 mm (n=44), **Group III**: Bite jumping > 9.5 mm (n=40). Registrations before Herbst treatment, after Herbst treatment and after MB treatment.

was seen in bite jumping group II when compared to group I. In the total subject material (n=133) a significant moderate correlation (r=0.44) existed between the amount of bite jumping and incisor proclination.

MB treatment changes (Fig.19-5)
During the MB treatment phase a rebound in incisor inclination (retroclination) occurred in all 133 subjects. Incisor retroclination was significantly smaller in bite jumping group I than in bite jumping group III. Other group comparisons were statistically not significant. In the total subject material a significant but weak correlation (r=0.18) existed between the amount of bite jumping during the Herbst treatment phase and incisor retroclination during the MB treatment phase.

Total (Herbst+MB) treatment changes (Fig.19-5)
During the total examination period the mandibular incisors became proclined in all 133 subjects. Incisor proclination was significantly larger in bite jumping group III than in bite jumping group I. No statistically difference was found when comparing groups III and II. The comparison of groups I and II revealed a significant larger proclination in group II. In the total subject material a significant but weak correlation (r=0.32) existed between the amount of bite jumping during the Herbst treatment phase and incisor proclinaton during the total examination period.

Age and skeletal maturation
No association existed between mandibular incisor inclination changes during the different examination periods and the age or skeletal maturity of the subjects in any of the three bite jumping groups.

Interpretation of the results
In interpreting the present findings it must be pointed out that bite jumping in all subjects was performed to an incisal edge to edge position of the maxillary and mandibular incisors. Thus, the amount of bite jumping reflects the severity of the malocclusion in the frontal region (=overjet). An association existed between the amount of bite jumping at the start of treatment and the amount of incisor proclination (anchorage loss) during treatment. A similar finding was seen in the study by Pancherz and Hansen (1988). As mentioned before, an increased load on the anterior front teeth upon larger mandibular advanced could be an explanation. Perhaps a stepwise mandibular advancement instead of a single step advancement (as was done in the present Herbst

subjects) would reduce the strains on the mandibular incisors, thus resulting in less incisor proclination. Du et al. (2002) could, however, not verify this.

A stepwise advancement would possibly have the advantage of producing more skeletal effects (larger bone formation in the condyle and glenoid fossa) than a single step advancement as has been shown experimentally in rats (Rabie et al 2003). Finally, when looking at the outcome of Class II treatment using different bite jumping appliances, in Twin-block patients no advantage of incremental bite jumping in comparison to maximum jumping was found (Banks et al. 2004), while in Herbst subjects a direct relationship existed between the amount of bite jumping at the start of treatment (single step advancement) and the improvement in occlusal relationships (Pancherz 1982).

During the MB treatment phase, a rebound occurred in the incisor proclination. However, in all bite jumping groups a net proclination remained after MB treatment, which, on average, was larger in subjects with a larger amount of bite jumping then in subjects with a smaller amount of bite jumping. This phenomenon, which is difficult to explain, was also observed on a long-term basis (Weschler and Pancherz 2005) when comparing the S anchorage group (in which a MB phase was following the Herbst phase) with the two banded (P and PM) anchorage groups (Fig. 19-4). Perhaps the findings have something to do with the efficiency of incisor buccal root torque during the MB treatment phase.

Clinical examples

Lateral head films of 4 patients are presented to demonstrate mandibular incisor anchorage loss (tooth proclination) during Herbst appliance treatment and recovery (tooth retroclination) after appliance removal. None of the 4 subjects had any active treatment after Herbst therapy.

Case 19-1 (Fig. 19-6)
A 13.9-year-old female treated with the Herbst appliance for 7 months using a mandibular LL anchorage form (see Fig.19-1D). Posttreatment retention with an activator was performed for 2 years. Mandibular incisor inclination (in relation to the mandibular line) was 104.5° before treatment, 113.5° after treatment, 105.5° 6 months posttreatment and 107.5° 5 years posttreatment.

Case 19-2 (Fig. 19-6)

A 12.6-year-old male treated with the Herbst appliance for 7 months using a mandibular LL anchorage form (see Fig. 19-1D). Posttreatment retention with an activator was performed for 2 years. Mandibular incisor inclination (in relation to the mandibular line) was 87.0° before treatment, 94.0° after treatment, 94.5° 6 months posttreatment and 95.5° 5 years posttreatment.

Case 19-3 (Fig. 19-6)

A 12.2-year-old male treated with the Herbst appliance for 6 months using a mandibular PM anchorage form (see Fig.19-1B). No posttreatment retention was performed. Mandibular incisor inclination (in relation to the mandibular line) was 96.5° before treatment, 104.0° after treatment, 99.0° 6 months posttreatment and 99.0° 5 years posttreatment.

Case 19-4 (Fig. 19-6)

A 13.7-year-old male treated with the Herbst appliance for 7 months using a mandibular LL anchorage form (see Fig.19-1D). No posttreatment retention was performed. Mandibular incisor inclination (in relation to the mandibular line) was 92.0° before treatment, 107.5° after treatment, 98.0° 6 months posttreatment and 96.0° 5 years posttreatment.

Conclusions and clinical implications

- Mandibular anchorage is an unsolved problem in Herbst treatment. Anchorage loss is a reality with which the orthodontist has to live.
- None of the 6 anchorage forms investigated could withstand the strains placed on the anterior portion of the lower dentition by the Class II mechanism of the Herbst appliance. Irrespective of the anchorage form, a proclination of the lower incisors (anchorage loss) occurred in all subjects.
- Even if the cast splint anchorage form of the Herbst appliance was not superior to the different banded anchorage forms, it is still recommended as the complication prevalence (breakages) is less (see Chapter 24: Complications).
- The Pelott anchorage form should not be used, as the risk of soft tissue damage is high.

- An association existed between the amount of bite jumping at the start of Herbst treatment and the amount of incisor proclination (anchorage loss) during treatment. In order to reduce any possible strains on the mandibular front teeth by the telescope mechanism, especially when a large advancement of the mandible jaw is necessary to correct the malocclusion (=overjet), it could be advantageous to jump the mandible forward in successive small steps instead of one single large step. This hypothesis needs, however, to be investigated more closely.
- In the individual patient, anchorage loss during Herbst treatment can not be predicted. Irrespective of age, skeletal maturity, the anchorage form, amount of bite jumping, skeletal morphology and growth pattern, a large individual variation in incisor proclination (anchorage loss) has to be expected (Fig. 19-7).

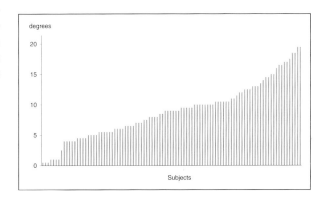

Fig. 19-7 Individual registrations of mandibular incisor proclination (anchorage loss) in 98 subjects treated with the Herbst appliance. The changes (in increasing order) during 6-8 months of treatment are shown. (*Based on the subject material from Ruf et al. 1998*)

Case 19-1   Case 19-2

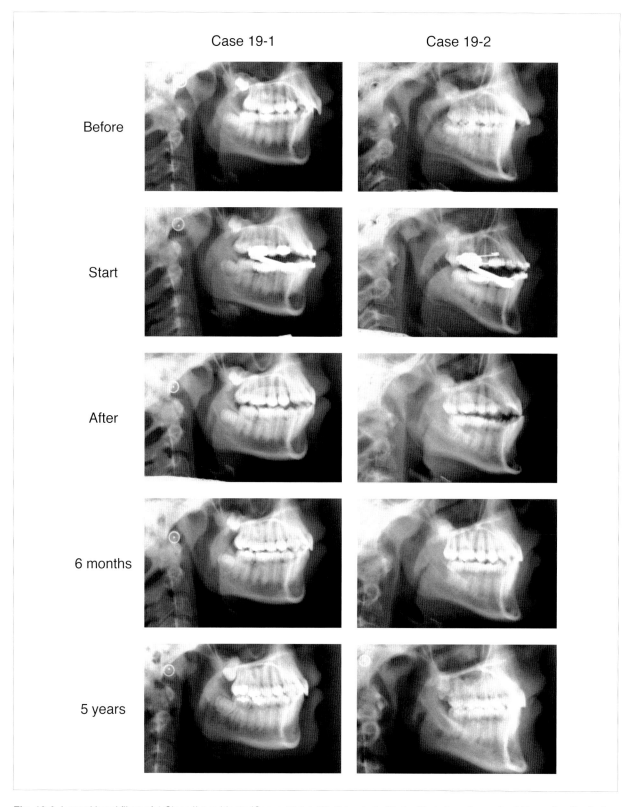

Before

Start

After

6 months

5 years

Fig. 19-6 Lateral head films of 4 Class II:1 subjects (Cases 19-1 to19-4) treated with the Herbst appliance for 6-7 months, illustrating the changes in mandibular incisor inclination at the different times of examination. Note that in the start picture of Case 19-3 the telescope mechanism is not yet attached to the teeth. The dental casts of the 4 subjects are presented as Cases 8-2 to 8-5 in Figs.8-11 to 8-14 (Chapter 8).

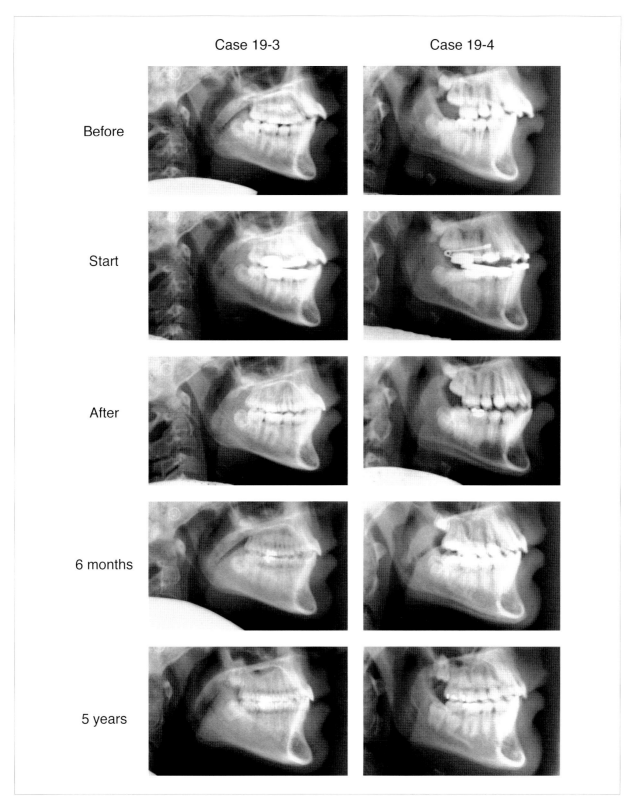

Case 19-3   Case 19-4

Before

Start

After

6 months

5 years

Fig. 19-6 (continued)

References

Banks P, Wright J, O`Brian K. Incremantal versus maximum bite advancement during Twin-block therapy: a randomized controlled clinical trial. Am J Orthod Dentofac Orthop 2004;126:583-588.

Björk A, Skieller V. Facial development and tooth eruption. Am J Orthod 1972;62:339-383.

Du Xi, Hägg V, Rabie ABM. Effects of headgear Herbst and mandibular step-by-step advancement versus conventional Herbst appliance and maximal jumping of the mandible. Eur J Orthod 2002; 24:167-174.

Franchi L, Baccetti T, McNamara JA. Treatment and posttreatment effects of acrylic splint Herbst appliance therapy. Am J Orthod Dentofac Orthop 1999;115:429-438.

Hägg U, Taranger J. Skeletal stages of the hand and wrist as indicators of the pubertal growth spurt. Acta Odont Scand 1980;38:187-200.

Hansen K, Koutsonas TG, Pancherz H. Long-term effects of Herbst treatment on the mandibular incisor segment: a cephalometric and biometric investigation. Am J Orthod Dentofac Orthop 1997;112:92-103.

Martin J, Pancherz H. Position changes of the mandibular incisors in Herbst / Multibracket appliance treatment in relation to the amount of bite jumping, age and skeletal maturation of the patients. Am J Orthod Dentofac Orthop 2007 (accepted for publication).

Pancherz H. Treatment of Class II malocclusions by jumping the bite with the Herbst appliance. A cephalometric investigation. Am J Orthod 1979;76:423-442.

Pancherz H. The mechanism of Class II correction in Herbst appliance treatment. A cephalometric investigation. Am J Orthod 1982;82:104-113.

Pancherz H, Hägg U. Dentofacial orthopedics in relation to somatic maturation. An analysis of 70 consecutive cases treated with the Herbst appliance. Am J Orthod 1985;88:273-287.

Pancherz H, Hansen K. Occlusal changes during and after Herbst treatment: a cephalometric investigation. Eur J Orthod 1986;8:215-228.

Pancherz H, Hansen K. Mandibular anchorage in Herbst treatment. Eur J Orthod 1988;10:149-164.

Rabie ABM, Chayanupatkul A, Hägg U. Stepwise advancement using fixed functional appliances: experimental perspective. Semin Orthod 2003;9:41-46.

Ruf S, Hansen K, Pancherz, H. Does orthodontic proclination of lower incisors in children and adolescents cause gingival recession? Am J Orthod Dentofac Orthop 1998;114:100-106.

von Bremen J, Pancherz H, Ruf S. Reduced mandibular cast splints - an alternative in Herbst therapy ? A prospective multicenter study Eur J Orthod 2007 (in press)

Weschler D, Pancherz H. Efficiency of three mandibular anchorage forms in Herbst treatment: a cephalometric investigation. Angle Orthod 2005;75:23-27.

Chapter 20

Effects on anchorage teeth and tooth-supporting structures

Research

Controversy exists whether excessive orthodontic forces applied on the teeth, will result in periodontal breakdown (Zachrisson and Alnaes 1973, 1974, Kloen and Pfeifer 1974, Dorfman 1978, Alstad and Zachrisson 1979, Coatoam et al. 1981, Hollender et al. 1980, Busschop et al. 1985, Artun and Krogstad 1987, Artun and Grobety 2001, Allais and Melsen 2003, Melsen and Allais 2005, Litsas et al. 2005) or root resorption (Killany 1999, Brezniak and Wasserstein 2002a, 2002b, Krishnan 2005).

Despite the fact that no scientific proof has been presented, the Herbst appliance has been said to increase the risk for (1) gingival recession, (2) marginal bone loss, and (3) root resorptions. Addressing these topics, two publications will be reviewed.

1. Does orthodontic proclination of lower incisors in children and adolescents cause gingival recession? (Ruf et al. 1998)

This study is concerned with mandibular incisor proclination during Herbst treatment with respect to the possible development of gingival recession.

The patient sample investigated comprised 98 children and adolescents (67 males and 31 females) with Class II:1 malocclusion treated with the Herbst appliance for an average period of 7 months. The mean age of the subjects at start of therapy was 12.8 years (SD=1.4 years). All patients were treated to Class I or overcorrected Class I dental arch relationships. All subjects exhibited acceptable oral hygiene throughout treatment. A total of 392 incisors were screened. The following analyses were performed. (1) Lateral head films from before and after Herbst treatment (when the appliance was removed) with respect to the degree of mandibular incisor proclination. (2) Dental casts and intraoral photographs from before treatment and 6 months after removal of the Herbst appliance (when any gingival irritation caused by treatment had healed), with respect to crown height and gingival status, respectively. An assessment was made separately for each of the four incisors. Gingival recession was recorded if the labial cemento-enamel junction was exposed or the vestibolo-gingival margin was markedly below the marginal level of the adjacent teeth. As no gender differences existed, the male and female samples were pooled.

In the 98 subjects, the lower incisors proclined an average of 8.9° (minimum=0.5°, maximum=19.5°) during treatment (Fig.20-1). On average, crown height in the 392 teeth remained unchanged during the observation period from before treatment to 6 months posttreatment. Gingival condition was unaffected or improved during the observation period in 380 teeth (97%), and gingival recession developed or was aggravated in 12 teeth (3%). No statistically significant difference in the amount of gingival recessions existed when comparing before and 6 months posttreatment registrations. In none of the teeth examined did an interrelation exist between the degree of incisor tooth inclination before treatment or incisor inclination changes during treatment and changes in crown height or the incidence of gingival recession.

To analyze the effect of excessive tooth proclination on the gingival status, the sample was divided into two subsamples with high (Mean+SD) and low (Mean−SD) mandibular incisor proclination (Fig. 20-2). The high-proclination group consisted of 16 subjects (64 teeth) with an average proclination of 16.4° (Fig. 20-3A). The low-proclination group comprised 17 subjects (68 teeth) with a mean proclination of 2.7° (Fig. 20-3B).

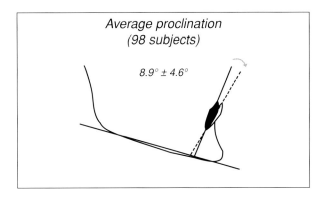

Fig. 20-1 Proclination (Mean and SD) of mandibular incisors in 98 Class II:1 malocclusions treated with the Herbst appliance.

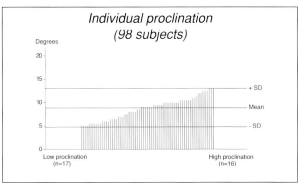

Fig. 20-2 Proclination (Individual registrations arranged in increasing order) of mandibular incisor proclination in 98 Class II:1 malocclusions treated with the Herbst appliance. The high (n=16) and low (n=17) proclination groups are marked in Light blue.

A

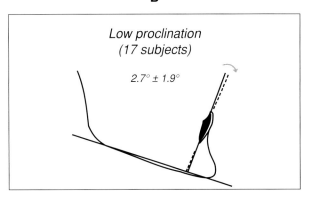

B

In the high-proclination group, recession was found in five teeth (8%) before treatment and in six teeth (9%) 6 months posttreatment. During the observation period, recession diminished in four teeth (6%) and remained unchanged in one tooth (1.5%). In one tooth (1.5%), new recession developed (Fig. 20-4A).

In the low-proclination group, eight teeth (12%) exhibited recession, before and 6 months after treatment. Recession improved in one tooth (1.5%) and remained unchanged in 7 teeth (10.5%). No new recession developed in any tooth (Fig. 20-4B).

In summary, only one tooth (high-proclination group) developed recession during Herbst treatment.

In 70 of the present 98 Herbst patients (280 teeth) with available intraoral photos from 5 years posttreatment, the long-term effects of mandibular incisor proclination on the gingival condition were assessed. The analysis showed newly developed recession or slightly deteriorated gingival recession in only 7 teeth (2.5%). This development was, however, independent of the amount of lower incisor proclination during Herbst treatment.

Fig. 20-3 Proclination (Mean and SD) of mandibular incisors in the high- (A) and low- (B) proclination groups.

A

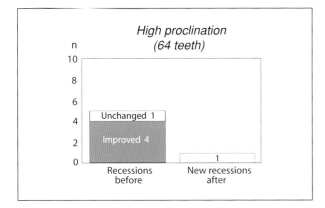

B

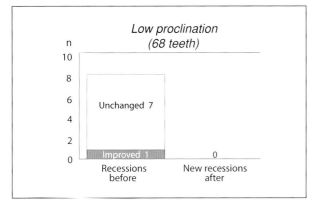

Fig. 20-4 Number of gingival recessions before Herbst treatment and 6 months posttreatment in the high- (A) and low- (B) proclination groups.

Interpretation of the results

In the sample investigated, the frequency of teeth with pretreatment recession (13%) lay within the reported range (1% to 19%) of mucogingival problems on single or multiple teeth found in children and adolescents (Parfitt and Mjör 1964, Dorfman 1978, Stoner and Mazdyasna 1980). The present findings did not support the view that mandibular incisor proclination affects the gingival status. This is in agreement with the results of several other studies (Pearson 1968, Kloen and Pfeifer 1974, Karring et al. 1982, Busschop et al. 1985, Andlin-Sobocki and Persson 1994, Artun and Grobety 2001, Allais and Melsen 2003, Melsen and Allais 2005). However, some studies have yielded contrasting findings (Dorfman 1978, Alstad and Zachrisson 1979, Artun and Krogstad 1987). The inconsistency of results may be due to differences in subject selection (e.g.

adults) or the analysis of other tooth movements than the labial tipping of incisors (e.g. closure of extraction spaces). Finally, when interpreting the present long-term results it must be remembered that an approximately 80% spontaneous reversal of the incisor proclination after Herbst treatment occurs (Pancherz and Hansen 1986).

2. Position changes and loading damage of the anchorage teeth during Herbst treatment (Pietz 2000) [Thesis in German]

This study deals with two questions with respect to the impact of Herbst treatment on the main anchorage teeth (=maxillary permanent first molars and mandibular first premolars). (1) To what extent does Herbst treatment affect the sagittal and vertical position of the anchorage teeth? (2) Will the load on the anchorage teeth result in marginal bone loss and/or apical root resorption?

The subject material comprised 58 consecutive Class II:1 malocclusions (36 males and 22 females) treated with the banded type of Herbst appliance (see Chapter 3: Design, construction and clinical management of the Herbst appliance). The average age of the subjects at start of treatment was 12.5 years. Herbst treatment was performed during an average time period of 7.5 months. The patients were examined before and after Herbst treatment as well as 3 years posttreatment.

Sagittal (Fig. 20-5) and vertical (Fig. 20-6) changes of the anchorage teeth were assessed on lateral head films from before and after Herbst therapy. The possible occurrence of marginal bone loss and/or apical root resorptions were determined by analysing orthopantomograms (OPG) from before and after Herbst treatment as well as 3 years posttreatment. The results of the investigation revealed the following changes:

- During treatment the maxillary first molars were moved distally (maximum 5.5 mm) in 81% of the subjects and the teeth were intruded (maximum 3.0 mm) in 19% of the cases. The mandibular first premolars were moved mesially (maximum 4.5 mm) in 55% of the subjects and the teeth were extruded (maximum 3.0 mm) in 28% of the subjects, while vertical premolar position was unchanged in the remaining 72% of the cases.
- Neither during Herbst treatment nor posttreatment, did any of the maxillary and mandibular anchorage teeth experience marginal bone loss or apical root resorptions, as seen on the OPGs.

173

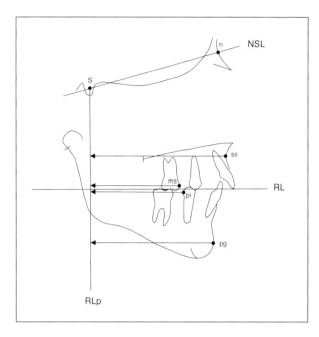

Fig. 20-5 Method for the assessment of sagittal changes of the anchorage teeth (maxillary first molar and mandibular first premolar). A modification of the SO-Analysis was used. Before and after treatment differences of ms/RLp – ss/RLp represent the sagittal movement of the maxillary molar and of pi/RLp – pg/RLp represent the sagittal movement of the mandibular premolar.

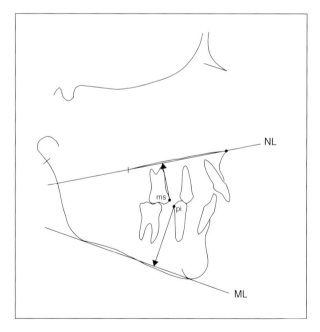

Fig. 20-6 Method for the assessment of vertical changes of the anchorage teeth (maxillary first molar and mandibular first premolar). Before and after treatment differences of ms/NL represent the vertical movement of the maxillary molar, and of pi/ML represent the vertical movement of the mandibular premolar.

Interpretation of the results

It has been shown that apical root resorptions are a general finding in orthodontic treatment, especially in adult patients and when using multibracket appliances, with heavy continuous forces over a long period of time (Linge and Ohm Linge 1983, 1991, Harris and Baker 1990, Levander et al. 1994, Owman-Moll 1995, Acar et al. 1999, Maltha et al. 2004, Chan and Darendeliler 2005).

The telescope mechanism of the Herbst appliance exerts a disto-cranially directed force on the maxillary anchorage teeth (first molars) and a mesio-caudally directed force on the mandibular anchorage teeth (first premolars). These forces will result in corresponding molar and premolar movements. However, due to the measuring method used, the intrusive movement of the premolar was masked to a large extent as the vertical distance of the reference point at the crown to the mandibular line (ML) increased when the tooth moved mesially (Fig. 20-6). Thus, the premolar erroneously seemed to extrude.

Although movements of the anchorage teeth were extensive during Herbst treatment, it seemed as if therapy did not harm the teeth (no apical root resorptions) or their supporting bone structures (no marginal bone loss). This was in accordance with Athanasios et al. (2006) but still surprising as the appliance force could be rather high. Investigations of Nasipoulos (1992) and Sander et al. (1993), in which the Herbst appliance was used, showed that the forces transmitted to the anchorage teeth varied between 0-10 N and with peaks up to 30 N (Sander et al. 1993). An explanation for the absence of harmful effects could be that the treatment period with the Herbst appliance was relatively short (on average 7.5 months) and the forces worked intermittantly on the dentition (only upon biting). Thus, when comparing before and after treatment OPGs, the marginal and apical conditions were comparable. No blunt roots (the first sign of a apical root resorption) were seen in any of the after treatment OPGs. Even if the OPG provides a good overview of the teeth in the lateral segments (premolars and molars), it must be pointed out, that it is a rather rough tool in the evaluation of marginal bone loss and apical root resorptions. Furthermore, with this radiographic technique, possible lateral root damage on the buccal and lingual tooth surfaces will remain undetected.

Clinical examples

Three adolescent Class II:1 malocclusions (Case 20-1 to Case 20-3) treated with the banded type of Herbst appliances are presented in order to illustrate the treatment and posttreatment changes with respect to: (1) mandibular incisor position, (2) gingival status and (3) marginal bone and root status of the anchorage teeth (maxillary first molars and mandibular first premolars). From each case, lateral head films, intraoral photographs and OPGs from before treatment, immediately after treatment, 6 months posttreatment and 5 years posttreatment are shown (Figs. 20-7 to 20-9).

Case 20-1 (Fig. 20-7)

A 12.5-year-old female was treated with the Herbst appliance for 7 months. No retention was instituted after treatment. The mandibular incisors were proclined 15° during treatment (from 101° before treatment to 116° after treatment). During the first 6 months posttreatment the teeth uprighted spontaneously by 7° to 109°.

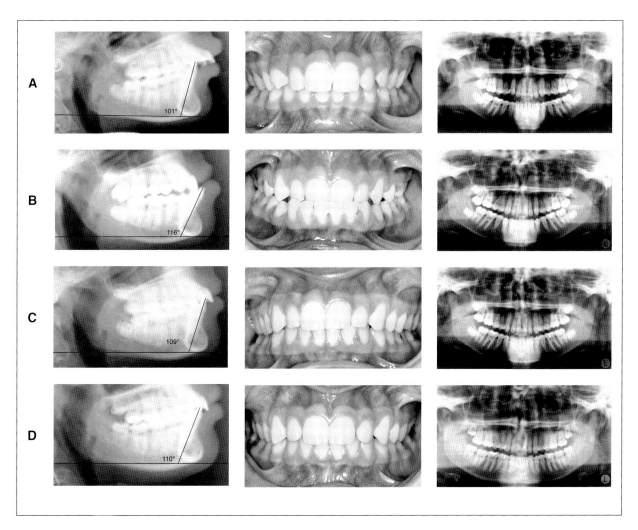

Fig. 20-7 Case 20-1 A 12-year-old female was treated with the Herbst appliance. **A**. Before treatment. **B**. Immediately after treatment. **C**. 6 months posttreatment. **D**. 5 years posttreatment. No gingival recession developed during the treatment period or during the follow-up period of 5 years. No root resorptions or marginal bone loss of the anchorage teeth (maxillary first molars and mandibular first premolars) occurred.

Case 20-2 (Fig. 20-8)

A 14-year-old male was treated with the Herbst appliance for 6 months. No retention occurred after treatment. The mandibular incisors were proclined 8° during treatment (from 112° before treatment to 120° after treatment). During the first 6 months posttreatment the teeth uprighted spontaneously to their original inclination (112°).

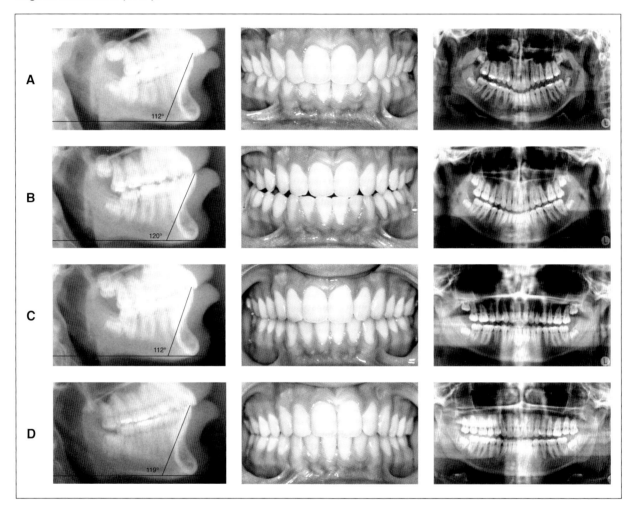

Fig. 20-8 Case 20-2 A 14-year-old male was treated with the Herbst appliance. **A**. Before treatment. **B**. Immediately after treatment. **C**. 6 months posttreatment. **D**. 5 years posttreatment. No gingival recession developed during the treatment period or during the follow-up period of 5 years. No root resorptions or marginal bone loss of the anchorage teeth (maxillary first molars and mandibular first premolars) occurred.

Case 20-3 (Fig. 20-9)

A 13-year-old male was treated with the Herbst appliance for 7 months. Activator retention for 2 years was performed after treatment. The mandibular incisors were proclined 11° during treatment (from 115° before treatment to 126° after treatment). During the first 6 months posttreatment the teeth uprighted spontaneously to their original inclination (115°).

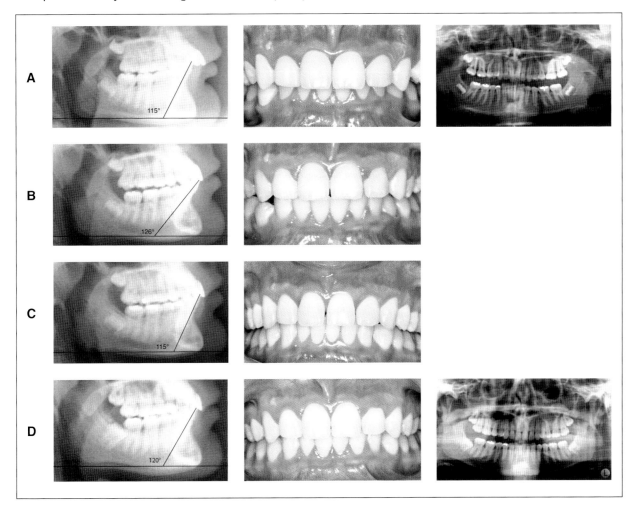

Fig. 20-9 Case 20-3 A 13-year-old male was treated with the Herbst appliance. **A**. Before treatment. **B**. Immediately after treatment. **C**. 6 months posttreatment. **D**. 5 years posttreatment. No gingival recession developed during the treatment period or during the follow-up period of 5 years. No root resorptions or marginal bone loss of the anchorage teeth (maxillary first molars and mandibular first premolars) occurred.

Conclusions and clinical implications

In children and adolescents treated with the Herbst appliance:
- proclination of mandibular incisors seems not to result in gingival recession;
- strong forces acting on the anchorage teeth seem not to result in damage such as marginal bone loss and / or root resorption.

In adults treated with the Herbst appliance, no current scientific data exist with respect to tooth proclination and appliance forces and their effects on the status of the gingiva, marginal bone and tooth roots. Clinical experience, however, indicates no problems in young adult Herbst subjects with healthy periodontal conditions (see Chapter 23: Treatment of adults - an alternative to orthognathic surgery).

References

Acar A, Canyurek U, Kocaaga M, Erverdi N. Continuous vs. discontinuous force application and root resorption. Angle Orthod 1999;69:159-164.

Allais D, Melsen B. Does labial movement of lower incisors influence the level of the gingival margin? A case-control study of adult orthodontic patients. Eur J Orthod 2003;25:343-352.

Alstad S, Zachrisson BU. Longitudinal study of periodontal condition associated with orthodontic treatment. Am J Orthod 1979;76:277-286.

Andlin-Sobocki A, Persson M. The association between spontaneous reversal of gingival recession in mandibular incisors and dentofacial changes in children: a 3-year longitudinal study. Eur J Orthod 1994;16:229-239.

Artun J, Krogstad O. Periodontal status of mandibular incisors following excessive proclination: a study in adults with surgical treated mandibular prognathism. Am J Orthod Dentofac Orthop 1987;91:225-232.

Artun J, Grobety D. Periodontal status of mandibular incisors after pronounced advancement during adolescence: a follow up evaluation. Am J Orthod Dentofac Orthop 2001;119:2-10.

Athanasios TN, Afanasios EA, Moschos A, Papadopoulos GK, Joulia J. Premolar root changes following treatment with the banded Herbst appliance. J Orofac Orthop 2006; 67: 261-271.

Brezniak N, Wasserstein A. Orthodontically induced inflammatory root resorption. Part I: The basic science aspect. Angle Orthod 2002a;72:175-179.

Brezniak N, Wasserstein A. Orthodontically induced inflammatory root resorption. Part II: The clinical aspect. Angle Orthod 2002b;72:180-184.

Busschop JL, Van Vlierberghe M, De Boever J, Dermaut L. The width of the attached gingiva during orthodontic treatment: a clinical study in human patients. Am J Orthod 1985;87:224-229.

Chan EKM, Darendeliler MA. Volumetric analysis of root resorption craters after application of light and heavy orthodontic forces. Am J Orthod Dentofac Orthop 2005;127:186-195.

Coatoam GW, Baerents RG, Bissada NF. The width of the keratinized gingival during orthodontic treatment: its significance and impact on periodontal status. J Periodontol 1981;52:307-313.

Dorfman HS. Mucogingival changes resulting from mandibular incisor tooth movement. Am J Orthod 1978;74:286-297.

Harris EF, Baker WC. Loss of root length and crestal bone hight before and during treatment of adolescent and adult orthodontic patients. Am J Orthod Dentofac Orthop 1990;98:463-469.

Hollender L, Rönnerman A, Thilander B. Root resorption, marginal bone support and clinical crown length in orthodontically treated patients. Eur J Orthod 1980;2:197-205.

Killany DM. Root resorption caused by orthodontic treatment: an evidence-based review of literature. Semin Orthod 1999;5:128-133.

Kloen JS, Pfeifer JS. The effect of orthodontic treatment on the periodontium. Angle Orthod 1974;44:127-134.

Karring T, Nyman S, Thilander B, Magnusson I. Bone regeneration in orthodontically produced alveolar bone dehiscences. J Period Res 1982;17:309-315.

Krishnan V. Critical issues concerning root resorption: a contemporary review. World J Orthod 2005;6:30-40.

Levander E, Malmgren O, Eliasson S. Evaluation of root resorption in relation to two orthodontic treatment regimes. A clinical experimental study. Eur J Orthod 1994;10:30-38

Linge L, Ohm Linge B. Apical root resorption in upper anterior teeth. Eur J Orthod 1983;5:173-183.

Linge L, Ohm Linge B. Patient characteristics and treatment variables associated with apical root resorption during orthodontic treatment. Am J Orthod Dentofac Orthop 1991;99:35-43.

Litsas GM, Acar A, Everdi N, Athanasiou AE. Mucogingival considerations and labial movement of lower incisors inorthodontic patients: a comprehensive review. Hell Orthod Rev 2005;8:33-42.

Maltha LA, van Leeuwen EJ, Dijkman GEHM, Kuijpers-Jagtman AM. Incidence and severity of root resorption in orthodontically moved premolars in dogs. Orthod Craniofac Res 2004;7:115-121.

Melsen B, Allais D. Factors of importance for the development of dehiscences during labial movement of mandibular incisors: a retrospective study of adult orthodontic patients. Am J Orthod Dentofac Orthop 2005;127:552-561.

Nasiopoulos A. Biomechanics of the Herbst Scharnier orthopaedic treatment method and head posture. A synchronozed EMG and dynamographic study. Academic Diss. (Thesis). Faculty of Odontology, University of Lund, Malmö 1992.

Owman-Moll P. Orthodontic tooth movement and root resorption with special reference to force magnitude and duration. A clinical and histological investigation in adolescents. Swed Dent J 1995;Suppl 105:1-45.

Pancherz H, Hansen K. Occlusal changes during and after Herbst treatment: a cephalmetric investigation. Eur J Orthod 1986;8:215-228.

Pearson LE. Gingival height of lower central incisors, orthodontically treated and untreated. Angle Orthod 1968;38:337-339.

Parfiit GJ, Mjör IA. A clinical evaluation of local gingival recession in children. J Dent Child 1964;31:257-262.

Pietz E. Positionsveränderungen und Belastungsschäden der Ankerzähne bei der Herbst-Behandlung. Diss. med. dent. (Thesis), Giessen 2000.

Ruf S, Hansen K, Pancherz, H. Does orthodontic proclination of lower incisors in children and adolescents cause gingival recession? Am J Orthod Dentofac Orthop 1998;114:100-106.

Sander FG, Ruppert W, Wichelhaus A. Biomechanische Untersuchungen bei der Anwendung des Herbstscharniers während des Nachtschlafes. Kieferorthop Mitteil 1993;6:23-34.

Stoner JE, Mazdyasna S. Gingival recession in the lower incisor region of 15 year old subjects. J Periodontol 1980;51:74-76.

Zachrisson BU, Alnaes L. Periodontal condition in orthodontically treated and untreated individuals. II. Loss of attachment, gingival pocket depth and clinical crown height . Angle Orthod 1973:43:402-411.

Zachrisson BU, Alnaes L. Periodontal condition in orthodontically treated and untreated individuals. II. Alveolar bone loss: radiographic findings. Angle Orthod 1974:44:48-55.

Chapter 21

Treatment indications

Original indications given by Emil Herbst

In the publication from 1934, Herbst recommended his "Retentionsscharnier" in the following instances:

1. Patients with a retrognathic mandible.
2. Asymmetric Class II malocclusions with mandibular midline deviation.
3. Postsurgery after condylar or hemimandibular resections. According to Herbst, the telescope mechanism works as an artifical joint in these cases. The device is removed after about two years when a new "condyle" had developed (after condylar resection) and muscular adaptation (after hemimandibular resection) had occurred.
4. Mandibular ramus fracture. According to Herbst, pain is relieved immediately after insertion of the appliance.
5. Prevention of bruxism. According to Herbst the bruxing stops when the mandible is advanced 1 mm.
6. "Diseases" of the TMJ. According to Herbst, the appliance relieves the pressure on the damaged articular structures and enhances the healing process. He even reported that clicking stopped.

Furthermore, Herbst mentioned the following advantages of his appliance:

1. Immediate improvement of facial appearance.
2. No damage to periostium and pulp.
3. Painless and comfortable.
4. Reduction in the number of appointments. Herbst reported about two patients which he had not seen for a whole year after placing the appliance. Treatment was successful in both cases.
5. In subjects with well developed tooth cusps, treatment can be as short as 6 months and no retention will be necessary.

6. No age limit for treatment. According to Herbst an adaptation of the TMJ takes place even in adult subjects. However, treatment will take longer (9-15 months) than in younger subjects.
7. Normalization of the intra- and extra-oral muscle activity as well as of the chewing function.

Current indications

Although the indications given and the advantages mentioned by Emil Herbst about 70 years ago were solely clinically based, research has confirmed most of Herbst´s findings.

In current evidence-based dentofacial orthopedics, the indications for the Herbst appliance are the following:

General indications

- The Herbst appliance is most useful in both Class II:1 and Class II:2 malocclusions. For an optimum treatment result, however, a tooth and dental arch alignment phase with a conventional multibracket appliance after Herbst therapy will be necessary. Few patients can be finished, with the teeth in a stable Class I occlusion, using the Herbst appliance alone.
- As treatment is aimed at enhancing mandibular growth, the Herbst appliance is especially indicated during the active growth period. However, with respect to treatment efficiency (i.e. a better result in a shorter period of time) and posttreatment stability, a "late" treatment approach (in the permanent dentition after the pubertal peak of growth) is recommended (see Chapter 18: Treatment timing).

- Many "extraction cases" can be treated non-ex-traction with the Herbst appliance, as removal of teeth is not necessary for Class II correction.
- In Class II:1 subjects with mandibular crowding, extractions of teeth (four premolars or one man-dibular incisor) may be necessary. The tooth re-moval can be done either before (less frequent procedure) or after (more frequent procedure) the Class II correction phase with the Herbst appliance. In Class II:2 cases with mandibular crowding, on the other hand, dental arch expan-sion has priority as extractions in these patients should be avoided whenever possible.
- In both Class II:1 and Class II:2 subjects with maxillary incisor or canine crowding, the problem can frequently be solved without extractions, due to the pronounced "headgear effect" of the Herbst appliance (see Chapter 9: The headgear effect of the Herbst appliance).

Specific indications
The following Class II patients which would not re-spond favorably to removable functional appliances (e.g. Activator, Bionator, Fränkel), are good candi-dates for the Herbst appliance:

- Subjects with nasal airway obstructions (mouth breathers).
- Uncooperative patients.
- Postadolescent subjects.
- Young adult borderline Class II malocclusions, as an alternative to mandibular advancement surgery (see Chapter 23: Treatment of adults – an alternative to orthognathic surgery).

Treatment of Class II:1 malocclusions

Class II:1 treatment is generally performed in two steps. In the first step, Class II correction is achie-ved using the Herbst appliance, and in the second step the teeth are aligned and the occlusion settled in Class I using a multibracket appliance.

Non-extraction treatment
Several clinical examples of non-extraction treat-ment have been given earlier (Cases 7-1, 7-2, 8-1, 13-1, 13-2, 17-1, 17-2, 18-2). Two additional patients (Cases 21-1 and 21-2) will be presented to show the great potential of the Herbst appliance in correcting a Class II malocclusion.

Case 21-1 (Fig. 21-1)
An 11-year-old male in the preadolescent growth period (MP3-F skeletal maturity stage) exhibiting an extreme Class II:1 malocclusion with an overjet of 20 mm and an overbite of 15 mm. The SNB angle was 70.0° and the ANB 6.5°. There was no space for the mandibular canines. Treatment was started with a mandibular multibracket appliance (in com-bination with a maxillary bite-raising plate) for the alignment of the mandibular teeth. At the age of 13 years, Herbst treatment was instituted. After 8 months of therapy the occlusion was overcorrected Class I with an overbite of 2 mm. After a further 11 months of final tooth alignment with a multibracket appliance, Class I occlusal conditions with a normal overjet and overbite were present. Long-term reten-tion was performed with an activator and a mandi-bular cuspid-to-cuspid retainer. At the follow-up 1.5 years posttreatment, at the age of 16 years, the pa-tient presented a stable treatment result.

Case 21-2 (Fig. 21-2)
An 11-year-old male in the preadolescent growth period (MP3-F skeletal maturity stage) showing a severe Class II:1 malocclusion with an overjet of 12 mm and an overbite of 8 mm. The SNB angle was 71.5° and the ANB 6.0°. At birth the boy had a microgenia and an isolated cleft of the soft and posterior part of the hard palate. He was suggested to have a Pierre Robin syndrome, but the absence of glossoptosis, feeding problems and blockage of the airway negated such a diagnosis. The cleft was repaired at the age of 9 months. At the age of 7 years, functional orthopedics with an activator was tried, but failed because of repeated ear, nose, and throat problems that caused obstruction of nose breathing. At the age of 11 years, Herbst treatment was started and lasted for 8 months. After Herbst therapy, overcorrected Class I dental arch relation-ships, overjet, and overbite conditions were seen. Active retention with an activator was performed for 1.5 years. At the follow-up, 6 years after Herbst treatment, at the age of 18 years, a stable treatment result was seen. However, the mandibular incisors were crowded. The growth changes in this patient have been analyzed in detail by Sarnäs et al. (2000).

Extraction treatment
Previously, a clinical example (Case 18-1) of a four premolar extraction case has been shown. In this patient, Class II correction (Herbst appliance) pre-ceeded the extractions and final tooth alignment (multibracket appliance).

Two additional extraction cases (Cases 21-3 and 21-4) will be presented. In Case 21-3, extractions of four premolars were performed before Class II correction. In Case 21-4, one lower incisor was extracted after Class II correction.

Case 21-3 (Fig.21-3)

A 14-year-old female in the postadolescent growth period (MP3-H skeletal maturity stage) exhibiting a Class II:1 malocclusion with severe maxillary crowding. The SNB angle was 70.5° and the ANB angle 3.5°. The girl had a large mandibular plane angle (ML/NSL = 44.0°)and a lateral tongue dysfunction habit. Herbst treatment was preceded by rapid maxillary expansion, extractions of 14, 24, 35, 45, and preliminary maxillary tooth alignment with a multibracket appliance. Herbst therapy was instituted at the age of 17 years and lasted for 11 months. The treatment was followed by a multibracket appliance phase for final tooth alignment lasting 11 months. At the end of treatment, Class I occlusal conditions with a normal overjet and overbite were present. A lateral open bite tendency existed. Long-term retention was performed with maxillary and mandibular bonded retainers. At the follow-up 1.5 years posttreatment, at the age of 20.5 years, the patient exhibited a stable treatment result.

Case 21-4 (Fig. 21-4)

A 15-year-old female in the late postadolescent growth period (R-I skeletal maturity stage) exhibiting a full Class II malocclusion, an overjet of 9 mm, and severe mandibular incisor crowding. The SNB angle was 71.5° and the ANB angle 5.5°. Herbst treatment was performed in combination with rapid maxillary expansion. After 7 months of Herbst therapy, tooth 41 was extracted and the maxillary and mandibular teeth were aligned using a multibracket appliance for 2 years. After treatment, acceptable Class I occlusal conditions with a normal overjet and overbite were attained. Long-term retention was performed with maxillary and mandibular bonded retainers. At follow-up 2 years posttreatment, at the age of 20 years, a stable treatment result was present except for a minor relapse in overjet.

183

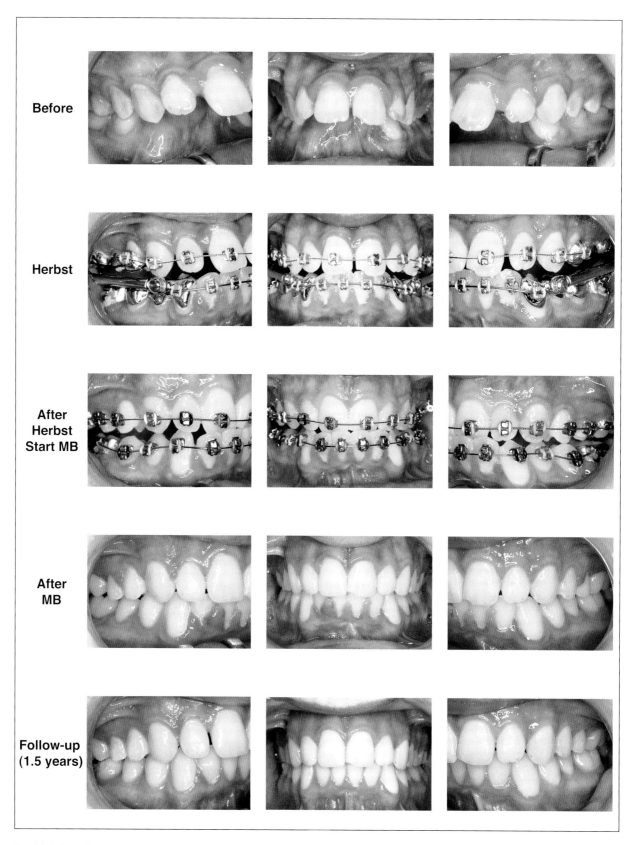

Fig. 21-1 Case 21-1 Herbst/Multibracket (MB) appliance treatment of an 11-year-old male with an extreme Class II:1 malocclusion.

Before	After Herbst / MB	Follow-up (1.5 years)

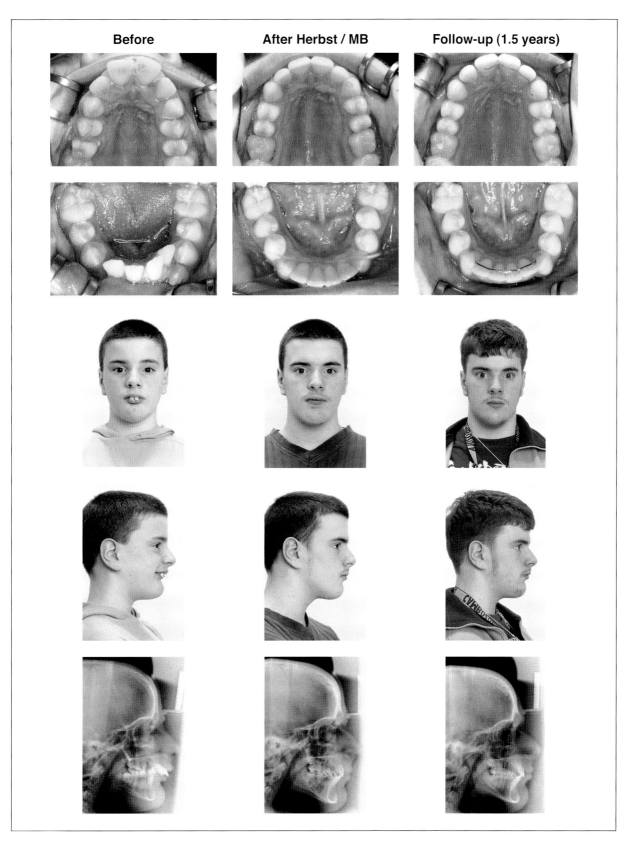

Fig. 21-1 Case 21-1 (continued)

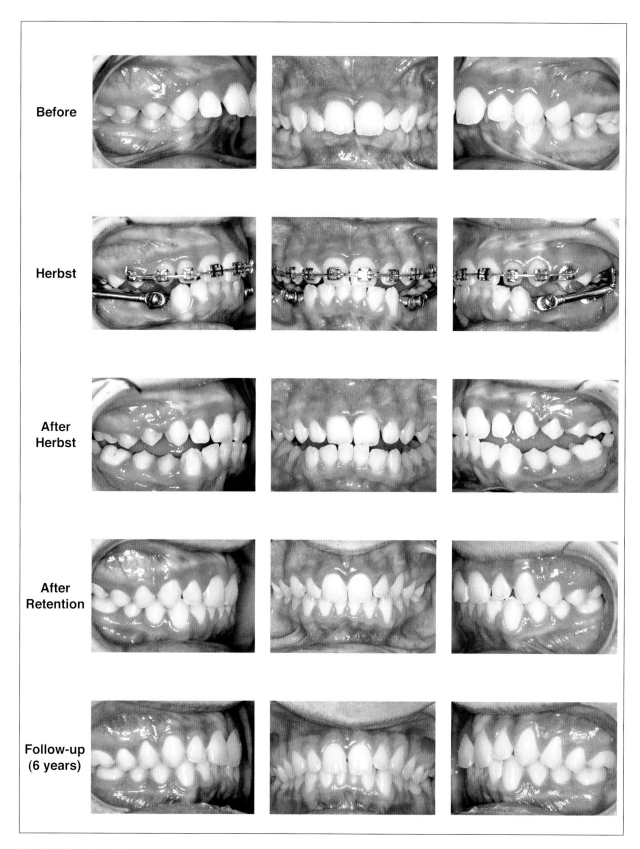

Before

Herbst

After Herbst

After Retention

Follow-up (6 years)

Fig. 21-2 Case 21-2 Herbst treatment of an 11-year-old male with a severe Class II:1 malocclusion.

Before	After Herbst / Retention	Follow-up (6 years)

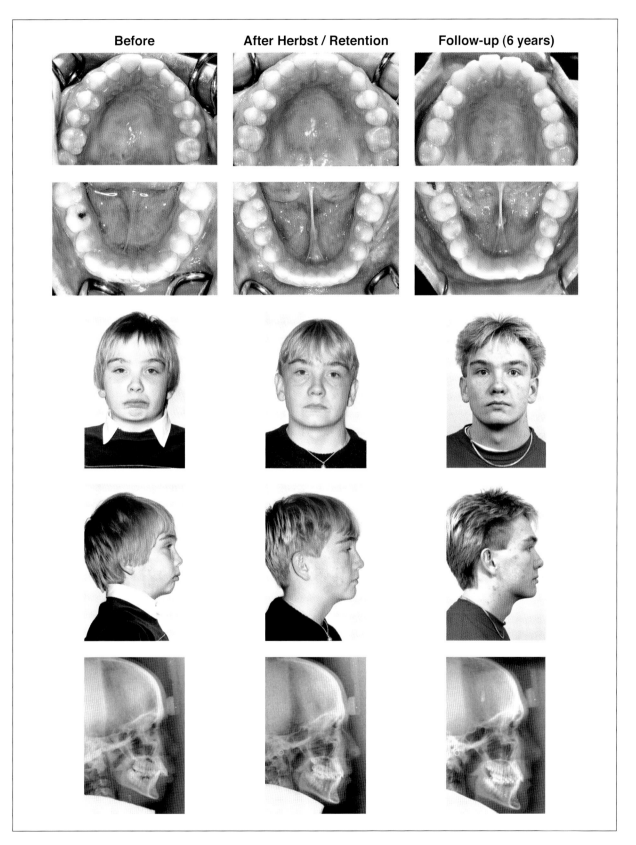

Fig. 21-2 Case 21-2 (continued)

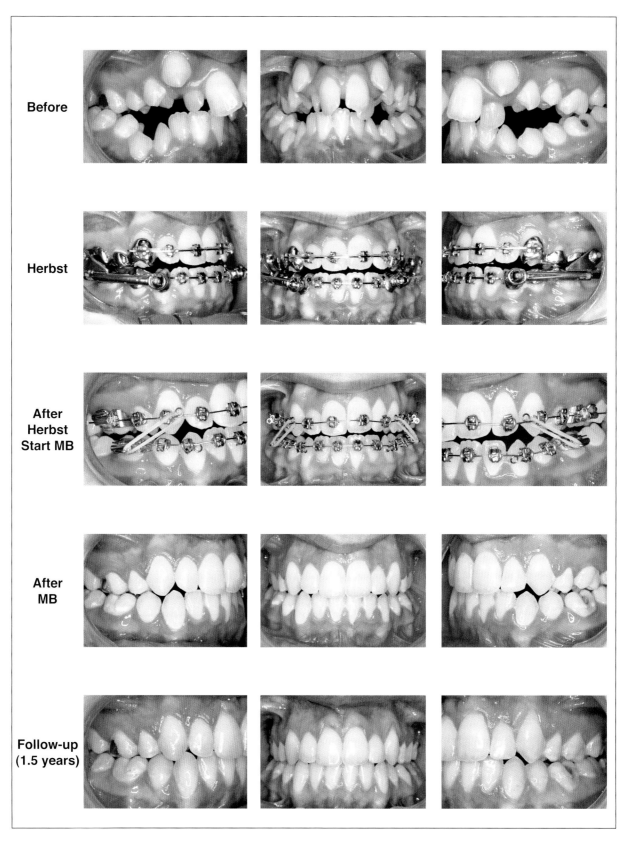

Fig. 21-3 Case 21-3 Herbst/Multibracket (MB) appliance treatment of a 14-year-old female with a Class II:1 malocclusion and maxillary and mandibular crowding. Extractions of four premolars were performed before the Herbst treatment phase.

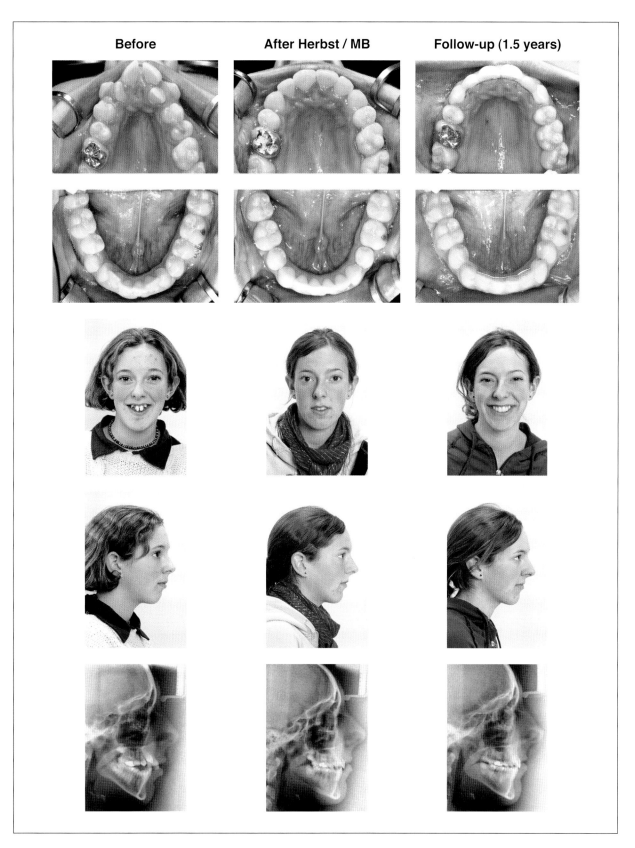

| Before | After Herbst / MB | Follow-up (1.5 years) |

Fig. 21-3 Case 21-3 (continued)

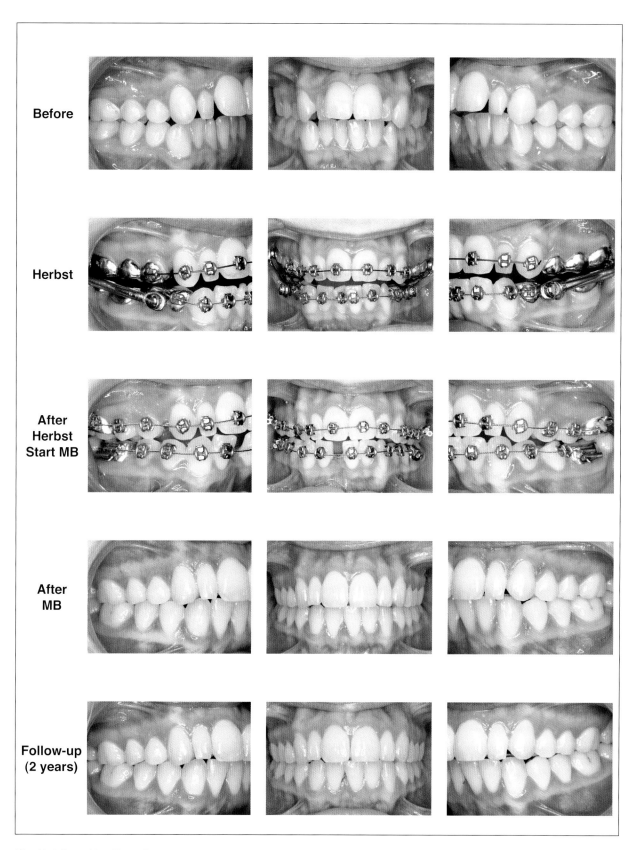

Fig. 21-4 Case 21-4 Herbst/Multibracket (MB) appliance extraction treatment of a 15-year-old female with a Class II:1 malocclusion and mandibular incisor crowding. Extraction of one mandibular incisor was performed after the Herbst treatment phase.

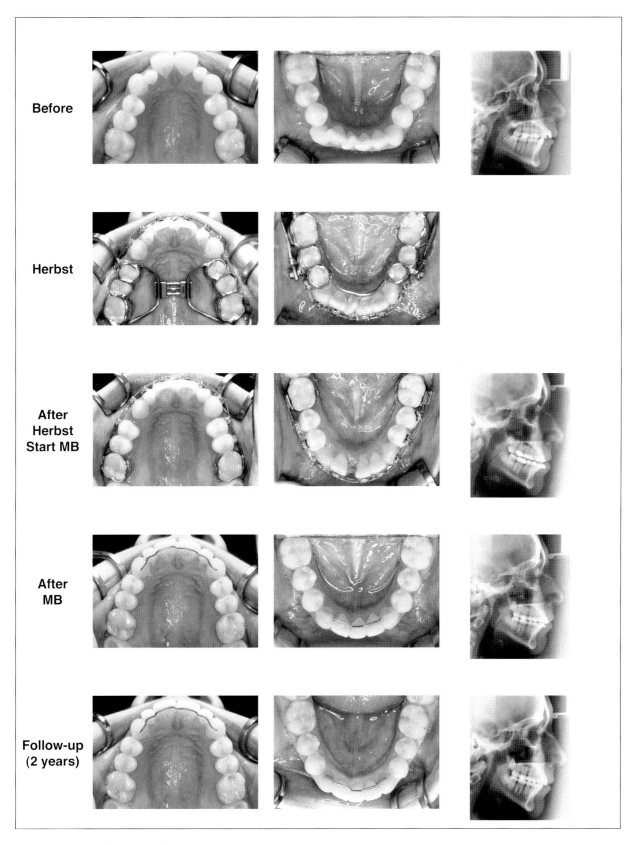

Before

Herbst

After
Herbst
Start MB

After
MB

Follow-up
(2 years)

Fig. 21-4 Case 21-4 (continued)

Treatment of Class II:2 malocclusions

Class II:2 treatment is generally performed in three steps. In the first step the maxillary incisors are proclined (the Class II:2 is converted to a Class II:1 malocclusion) using a maxillary plate or a multibracket appliance. In the second step the mandible is advanced with the Herbst appliance and in the third step final tooth alignment is done with a multibracket appliance.

As mentioned above, whenever possible Class II:2 treatment should be performed non-extraction, even in cases with crowding. Mandibular incisor crowding is corrected by proclination of the front teeth and maxillary incisor and canine crowding by the "headgear effect" of the Herbst appliance.

Class II:2 research

With respect to the effects of the Herbst appliance in Class II:2 malocclusions, to our knowledge there exist only four publications dealing with this topic. Three investigations consider preadolescent and adolescent patients (Obijou and Pancherz 1997, Schweitzer and Pancherz 2001, von Bremen and Pancherz 2003) and one study adult subjects (Marku 2006).

With respect to the mode of action of the Herbst appliance and the outcome of treatment in Class II:2 subjects, the existing scientific evidence will be presented by reviewing two of the above publications.

1. Herbst appliance treatment of Class II, Division 2 malocclusions (Obijou and Pancherz 1997)

A quantitative analysis of sagittal skeletal and dental changes contributing to occlusal correction in Class II:2 treatment using the Herbst appliance was assessed by the use of the SO-Analysis (see Chapter 6: Herbst research - subjects and methods).

Fourteen Class II:2 subjects (6 males and 8 females) treated with the cast splint Herbst appliance for an average period of 7.5 months were compared to 40 Class II:1 Herbst subjects (Pancherz and Hansen 1986). The patients in both groups were treated before or at the maximum of pubertal growth.

All Class II:2 and II:1 subjects were successfully treated to Class I or overcorrected Class I molar and edge-to-edge incisor relationships. The results of the SO-analysis are presented in Figs. 21-5 (overjet) and 21-6 (molar relation).When comparing the Class II:2 and Class II:1 pa-tients, for natural reasons overjet correction (= overjet reduction) was significantly larger in the Class II:1 patients. In the Class II:2 subjects the upper incisors were proclined (mean = 3.0 mm), whereas in the Class II:1 subjects, the incisors were retroclined (mean = 2.3 mm). The mandibular incisors were, on average, proclined significantly more in the Class II:2 subjects (mean = 3.4 mm) than in the Class II:1 subjects (mean = 2.4 mm). For sagittal molar correction, no differences were found between the two malocclusion groups.

Interpretation of the results

Due to definition, the maxillary incisors are retroclined in Class II:2 and proclined in Class II:1 malocclusions, and the goal of any orthodontic treatment is to corrected the inclination of these teeth.

However, the clinically important difference between the Class II:2 and Class II:1 malocclusion groups treated with the Herbst appliance was the behaviour of the mandibular incisors during therapy. In the Class II:2 patients the incisors were proclined significantly more than in the Class II:1 patients. This may be due to the difference in maxillary incisor tooth position changes. As the maxillary incisors in the Class II:1 subjects were retroclined during treatment, this movement will hinder the anterior movement of the mandibular incisors. In 12 of the 14 Class II:2 subjects, on the other hand, the maxillary incisor teeth were proclined with a multibracket appliance before the Herbst appliance was placed, in order to make a mandibular advancement possible. This decompensation of incisor position consequently will allow free mandibular incisor proclination during the mandibular advancement procedure with the telescope mechanism. Fortunately, the mandibular incisor tooth movements are advantageous in Class II:2 therapy to create a favorable small interincisal angle that will contribute to posttreatment overbite stability (Schweitzer and Pancherz 2001).

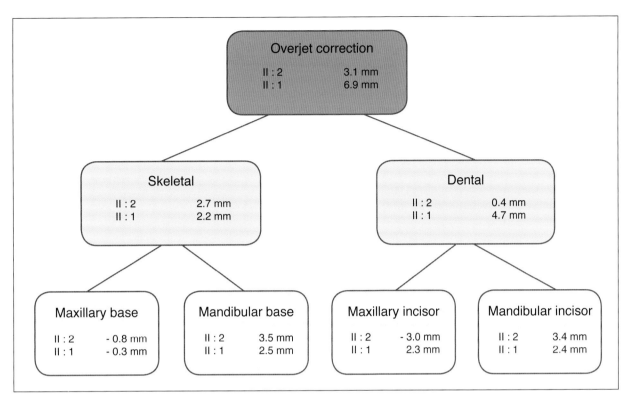

Fig. 21-5 SO-Analysis. Mechanism of overjet correction (= overjet reduction). Mean changes in 14 Class II:2 and 40 Class II:1 malocclusions treated with the Herbst appliance. The minus (-) sign implies disadvantageous changes that increase the overjet.

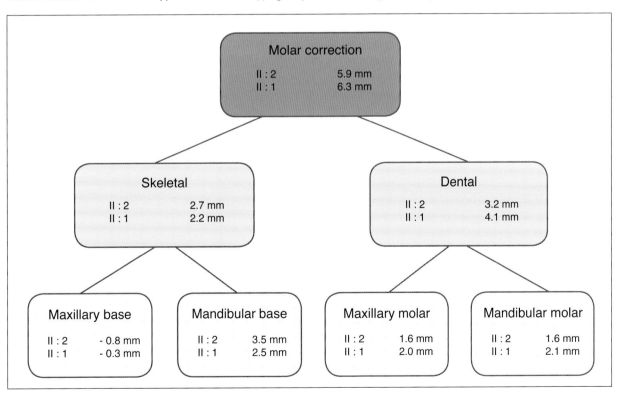

Fig. 21-6 SO-Analysis. Mechanism of Class II molar correction. Mean changes in 14 Class II:2 and 40 Class II:1 malocclusions treated with the Herbst appliance. The minus (-) sign implies disadvantageous changes that counteract Class II molar correction.

2. The incisor-lip relationship in Herbst/Multibracket appliance treatment of Class II, Division 2 malocclusions (Schweitzer and Pancherz 2001)

This study deals with the treatment and posttreatment effects of Herbst/Multibracket appliance treatment on the upper incisor-lower lip relationship in the management of adolescent Class II:2 malocclusions. The patient sample comprised 19 subjects (11 males and 8 females) treated for an average period of 1.8 years with a banded (n=4) or cast splint (n=14) Herbst appliance followed by a multibracket appliance. The average pretreatment age was 13 years and each patient had a bilateral Class II molar relationship, retroclined upper incisors, and a deep overbite. After treatment, all subjects exhibited Class I dental arch relationships with a normal overjet and overbite. Posttreatment retention was performed in all subjects using either a maxillary Hawley plate in combination with a mandibular cuspid-to-cuspid retainer (n=12) or an activator (n=7). Lateral head films were analyzed (Fig. 21-7) on three occasions: before treatment (T1), after Herbst/Multibracket appliance treatment (T2), and 1 year posttreatment (T3).

During the treatment period (T1-T2) the following significant changes were found (Figs. 21-8 and 21-9): (1) the lower lip overlap on the maxillary incisors was reduced by an average of 1.8 mm, (2) the maxillary incisors were proclined 15.3°, and (3) the mandibular incisors were proclined 9.6°. During the posttreatment period (T2-T3) the upper incisor-lower lip relationship remained stable, while relapsing tooth position changes occurred (Figs. 21-8 and 21-9): (1) the maxillary (0.6°) and mandibular (2.3°) incisors retroclined, and (2) the overbite increased (1.2 mm).

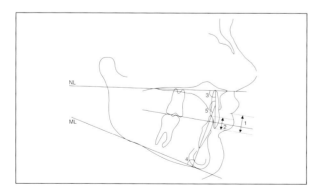

Fig. 21-7 Measuring variables. 1: Lower lip position; 2: Overbite; 3: maxillary incisor angulation; 4: mandibular incisor angulation; 5: Interincisal angle. (*Revised from Schweitzer and Pancherz 2001*)

Interpretation of the results

In several investigations (Mills 1973, van der Linden and Boersma 1988), a significant correlation was found between the lower lip overlap and the upper incisor position, the interincisal angle, and the overbite. In explaining the development of the Class II:2 incisor relationship, it has been claimed that the high positioned lip reclines the maxillary and mandibular incisors and the resulting large interincisal angle then causes the deep overbite, due to the missing incisal support, allowing the front teeth to erupt freely.

Long-term stability of treated Class II:2 malocclusions is, among other things, said to be related to a relative decrease of the lower lip cover on the maxillary incisors (Nicol 1964, Mills 1973, Luffingham 1982, van der Linden and Boersma 1988, Selwyn-Barnett 1991). Upon Herbst/Multibracket appliance treatment of the present Class II:2 subjects, the lower lip overlap on the maxillary incisors was reduced by 29% (from 5.9 mm to 4.2 mm). During the 1-year posttreatment period, the lip position remained stable. Postretention follow-up studies are, however, necessary to assess the long-term effect of the Herbst approach on the incisor-lower lip relationship (Binda et al. 1994).

Furthermore, in the present subjects the net overbite reduction (T1-T3) was 2.9 mm (59%), which is relatively high in comparison with other studies (Berg 1983, Fuhrmann 1989). The overbite reduction was mainly accomplished by the proclination of the maxillary and mandibular incisors, with the resulting reduction of the interincisal angle.

Relapse in overbite has been found to be significantly correlated with relapse of the interincisal angle (Nicol 1964, Schudy 1968, Simons and Joondeph 1973, Houston 1989). The large proclination of the mandibular incisors, as had occurred in the present subjects, would therefore result in a sufficient large reduction of the interincisal angle, which will contribute to overbite stability (Simons and Joondeph 1973). Berg (1983) considered an interincisal angle of less than 140° after treatment to be favorable for long-term stability. In the present sample, the interincisal angle was reduced from 150° to 125° during treatment and increased only 4° posttreatment.

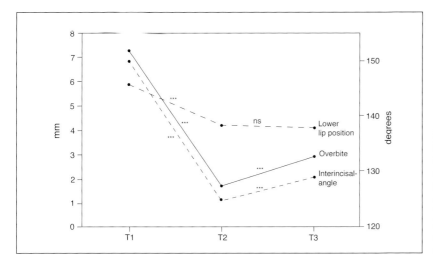

Fig. 21-8 Mean changes of lower lip position (mm), Overbite (mm), and Interincisal angle (degrees) in 19 Class II:2 malocclusions treated with the Herbst/Multibracket appliance. T1: Before treatment; T2: After treatment; T3: 1 year posttreatment. *** indicates significant changes at 0.1% level; ns indicates not significant changes. (*Revised from Schweitzer and Pancherz 2001*)

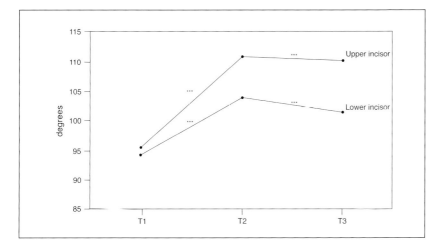

Fig. 12-9 Mean changes of maxillary and mandibular incisor inclination in 19 Class II:2 malocclusions treated with the Herbst/Multibracket appliance. T1: Before treatment; T2: After treatment; T3: 1 year posttreatment. *** indicates significant changes at 0.1% level. (*Revised from Schweitzer and Pancherz 2001*)

Clinical examples / Class II:2

Case 21-5 (Fig.21-10)

A 13-year-old male in the adolescent growth period (MP3-FG skeletal maturity stage) exhibiting a full Class II:2 malocclusion and a deep bite. The SNB angle was 70.0° and the ANB angle 5.5°. Herbst treatment was instituted after proclination of the maxillary incisors with a multibracket appliance. After 7 months of Herbst treatment overcorrected sagittal dental arch relationships were achieved. Final tooth alignment for 1 year was performed with a multibracket appliance. After treatment, Class I occlusal conditions with a normal overjet and overbite were present. Long-term retention was carried out using maxillary and mandibular bonded retainers. At the follow-up 6 years posttreatment, at the age of 21 years, a stable treatment result was present.

Case 21-6 (Fig. 21-11)

A 15-year-old male in the adolescent growth period (MP3-FG skeletal maturity stage) showing an extreme Class II:2 malocclusion. The overbite was 11 mm with palatal and labial soft tissue impingement of the lower and upper incisors, respectively. The SNB angle was 76.5° and the ANB angle 6.0 °. Herbst treatment was instituted after proclination of the maxillary incisors with a multibracket appliance and lasted for 7 months. After treatment, overcorrected Class I dental arch relationships were accomplished. Laterally, an extreme open bite existed which was closed during the final tooth alignment treatment phase with a multibracket appliance during a period of 22 months. Long-term retention was performed using an activator and a mandibular cuspid-to-cuspid retainer. At the follow-up 3.5 years posttreatment, at the age of 21 years, a stable treatment result was present, except for a minor increase in overbite.

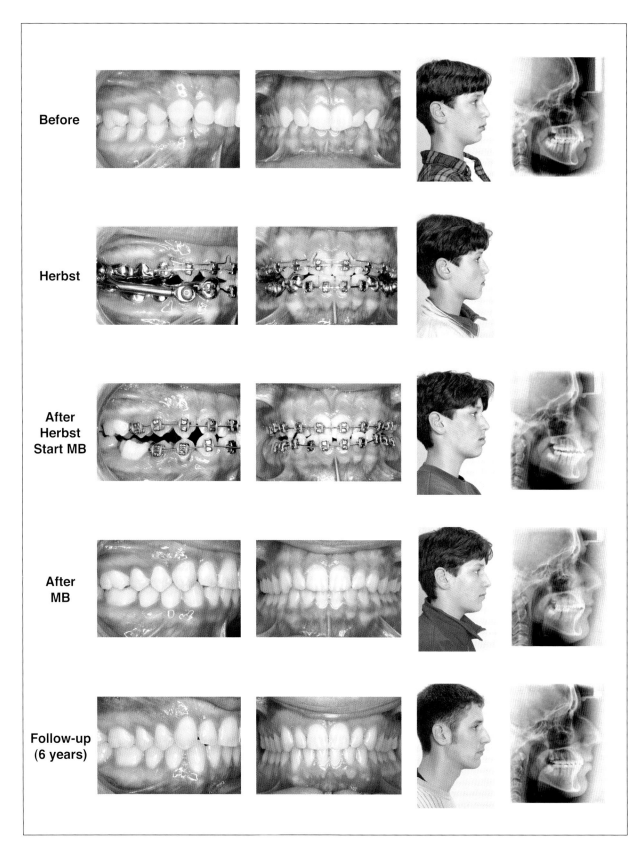

Fig. 21-10 Case 21-5 Herbst/Multibracket (MB) appliance treatment of a 13-year-old male with a Class II:2 malocclusion.

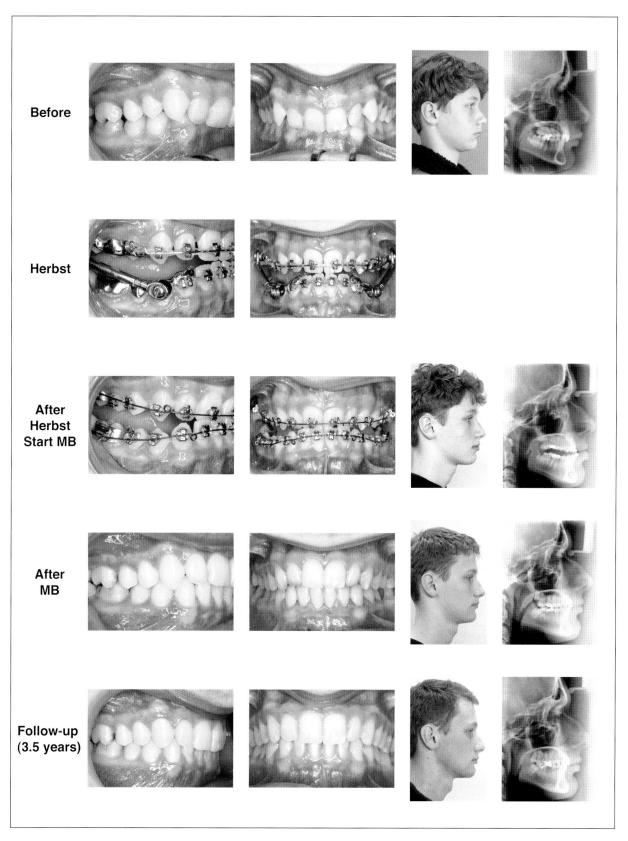

Before

Herbst

After Herbst Start MB

After MB

Follow-up (3.5 years)

Fig. 21-11 Case 21-6 Herbst/Multibracket (MB) appliance treatment of a 15-year-old male with an extreme Class II:2 malocclusion.

Class II:2 - Conclusions and clinical implications

- Class II:2 malocclusions are most suitable for treatment with the Herbst appliance.
- While proclination of the mandibular incisors usually is undesirable in orthodontics, it is advantageous in the correction of the deep bite in Class II:2 malocclusions.
- Furthermore, due to mandibular incisor proclination the interincisal angle is reduced, which will favour posttreatment overbite stability.

Treatment of specific problems in Class II malocclusions

- *Negligence*: Neglected cases (non-extraction and extraction) in which the Class II problem was not solved by treatment with removable or fixed appliances (Cases 21-7 and 21-8) at an earlier age.
- *Unilateral Class II / Midline deviation* (Case 21-9).
- *Lateral cross bite (Case 21-10 and 21-11).*
- *Lateral scissors bite (Case 21-12).*
- *Crowding of maxillary incisors (Cases 9-1 to 9-3).*
- *Lack of space for impacted maxillary canines (Case 9-4).*
- *Hemifacial microsomia (Sarnäs et al. 1982).*

Case 21-7 (Fig. 21-12)

A 15-year-old female in the postadolescent growth period (MP3-H skeletal maturity stage) showing a full Class II malocclusion with an overjet of 9 mm. The SNB angle was 74.0° and the ANB angle 6.5°. The girl had been previously treated unsuccessfully with removable functional appliance for 3.5 years. She was very disappointed with orthodontics in general, but wanted to give the Herbst appliance a try as she did not want either maxillary extractions (which actually would have spoiled her facial profile) or mandibular advancement surgery (which she considered too dangerous). After 7 months of Herbst treatment the Class II malocclusion was overcorrected. Final tooth alignment and settling of the occlusion in Class I was done with a multibracket appliance during a period of 7 months. After treatment, Class I occlusal conditions with a normal overjet and overbite existed. Retention was carried out for 2 years with a positioner only. At the follow-up 7 years posttreatment, at the age of 23 years, the treatment result was stable, except for a relapse in mandibular crowding (no mandibular incisor retention).

Case 21-8 (Fig. 21-13)

A 14.5-year-old male in the adolescent growth period (MP3-FG skeletal maturity stage). Three years earlier, at the age of 11 years, the four first premolars were extracted but no orthodontic treatment was performed. At the time of examination, the patient exhibited a full Class II:1 malocclusion, a deep bite, maxillary and mandibular incisor crowding and the extraction spaces closed. The SNB angle was 72.0° and the ANB angle was 8.5°. Herbst treatment was instituted and after 8 months of therapy the Class II malocclusion was overcorrected. After 1.5 years of final tooth alignment with a multibracket appliance, Class I occlusal conditions with a normal overjet and overbite were attained. Long-term retention was carried out with a maxillary Hawley plate and a mandibular cuspid-to-cuspid retainer. At follow-up 2 years posttreatment, at the age of 19 years, the treatment result was stable, except for a relapse in mandibular incisor crowding. This was in spite of the cuspid-to-cuspid retainer which was still in place.

Case 21-9 (Fig.21-14)

A 14-year-old female in the postadolescent growth period (MP3-I skeletal maturity stage) exhibiting a unilateral Class II:1 malocclusion with a mandibular midline deviation. The SNB angle was 70.0°, the ANB angle 3.0° and the mandibular plane angle was increased (ML/NSL = 40°). An atypical swallowing habit with an open bite tendency was present. During the 9 months period of Herbst treatment, the mandible was advanced more on the left than on the right side. After treatment, overcorrected Class I dental arch relationships on both sides and a corrected midline was present. Final tooth alignment and settling of the occlusion in Class I was performed during a period of 7 months, using a multibracket appliance with unilateral Class II elastics. Long-term retention was carried out with maxillary and mandibular bonded retainers. At the time of follow-up 3.5 years posttreatment, at the age of 19.5 years, the treatment result was stable, except for an anterior open bite relapse tendency due to a persisting tongue dysfunction habit (see Chapter 25: Relapse and Retention).

Case 21-10 (Fig. 21-15)

A 13-year-old female in the adolescent growth period (MP3-FG skeletal maturity stage) exhibiting a unilateral Class II:1 malocclusion with a unilateral cross bite due to a constricted maxilla. The SNB angle was 74.0° and the ANB angle 4.5°. Herbst treatment, in combination with rapid maxillary expansion (12 days) was performed during a period of 7 months. After treatment, overcorrected sagittal and corrected transverse dental arch relationships were present. Final tooth alignment and settling of the occlusion was accomplished during 10 months, using a multibracket appliance. Long-term retention was carried out with a maxillary bonded retainer in combination with a modified Hawley plate and a mandibular cuspid-to-cuspid retainer. At the time of follow-up 5 years posttreatment, at the age of 18 years, the treatment result was stable.

Case 21-11 (Fig. 21-16)

A 14-year-old female in the postadolescent growth period (MP3-H skeletal maturity stage) exhibiting a Class II:1 malocclusion with a bilateral crossbite due to a restricted maxilla. The SNB angle was 80° and the ANB angle 5°.

The four persisting second deciduous molars were extracted to enhance eruption of the second premolars. Rapid maxillary expansion (2 months) preceded the placement of the Herbst appliance which was furnished with a quad helix to retain the transversal expansion. After 7.5 months of Herbst treatment, overcorrected sagittal and corrected transversel dental arch relationships existed. Final tooth alignment and settling of the occlusion was accomplished during 10 months using a multibracket appliance. Long-term retention was carried out with maxillary and mandibular bonded retainers. At the time of follow-up 3.5 years posttreatment, at the age of 19 years, the patient exhibited a stable treatment result.

Case 21-12 (Fig. 21-17)

A 15-year-old male in the adolescent growth period (MP3-G skeletal maturity stage) exhibiting a severe Class II:1 malocclusion with a deep bite and a bilateral scissors bite. The SNB angle was 76.5° and the ANB angle 7.5°. Herbst treatment was preceded by mandibular lateral expansion using a quad helix in combination with a maxillary bite rising plate to facilitate the expansion. Herbst treatment was started at the age of 16 years and performed during a period of 8 months. After treatment, overcorrected sagittal and corrected transversal relationships were present. Final tooth alignment and settling of the occlusion in Class I was accomplished after 2 years of therapy with a multibracket appliance. Long-term retention was performed with maxillary and mandibular bonded retainers in combination with an activator. At the time of follow-up 2 years posttreatment, at the age of 21 years, the treatment result was stable.

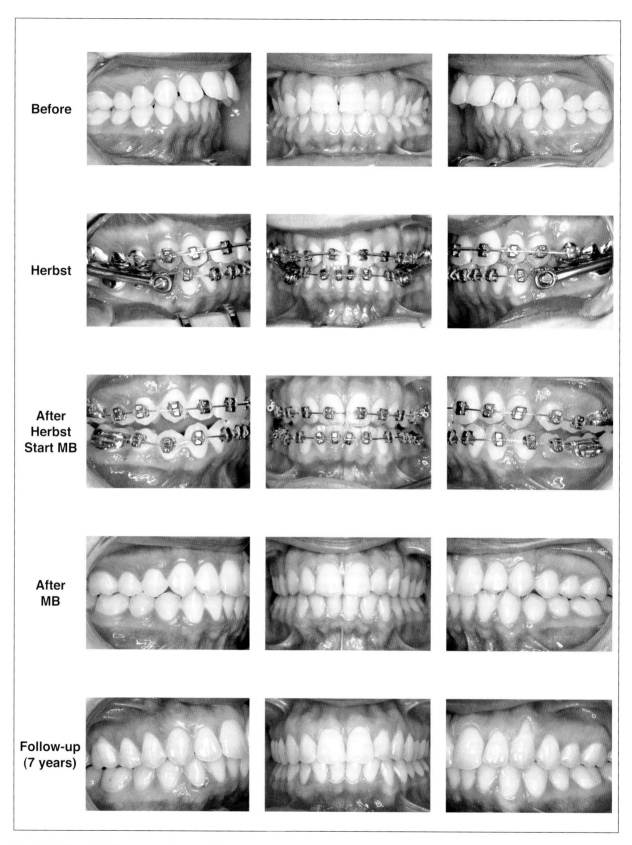

Fig. 21-12 Case 21-7 Herbst/Multibracket (MB) appliance treatment of a 15-year-old female with a Class II:1 malocclusion, previously treated unsuccessfully with an activator.

| Before | After Herbst / MB | Follow-up (7 years) |

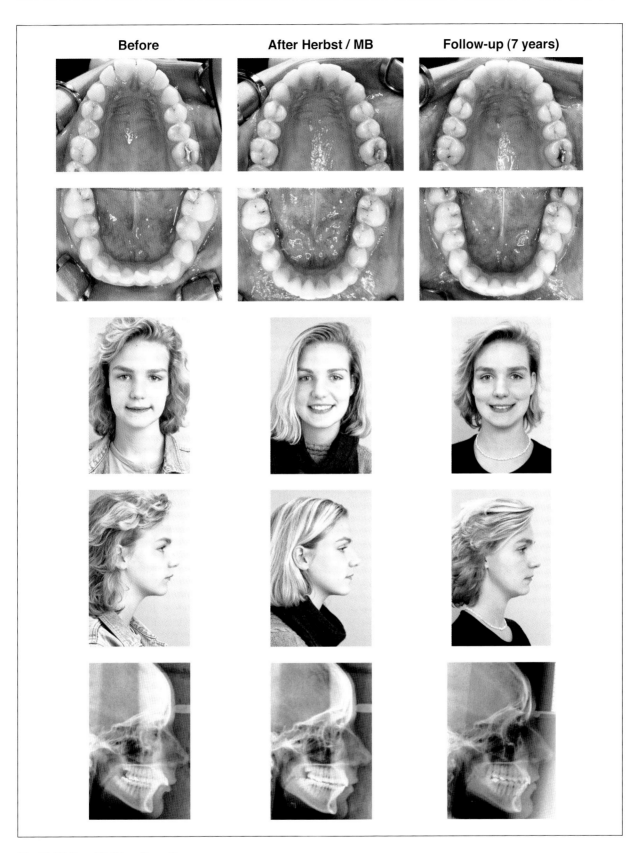

Fig. 21-12 Case 21-7 (continued)

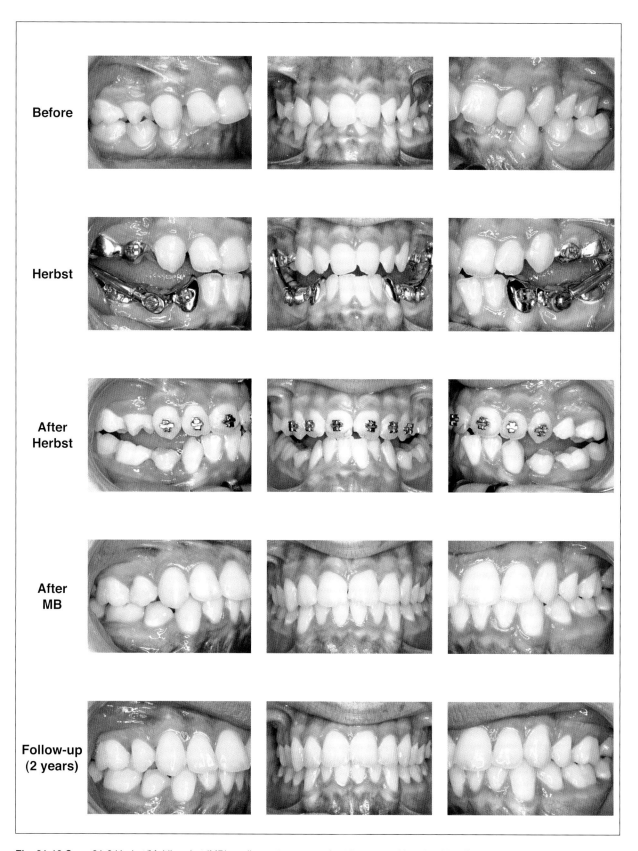

Fig. 21-13 Case 21-8 Herbst/Multibracket (MB) appliance treatment of a 14.5- year-old male with a Class II:1 malocclusion, previously "treated" by extractions of four premolars only.

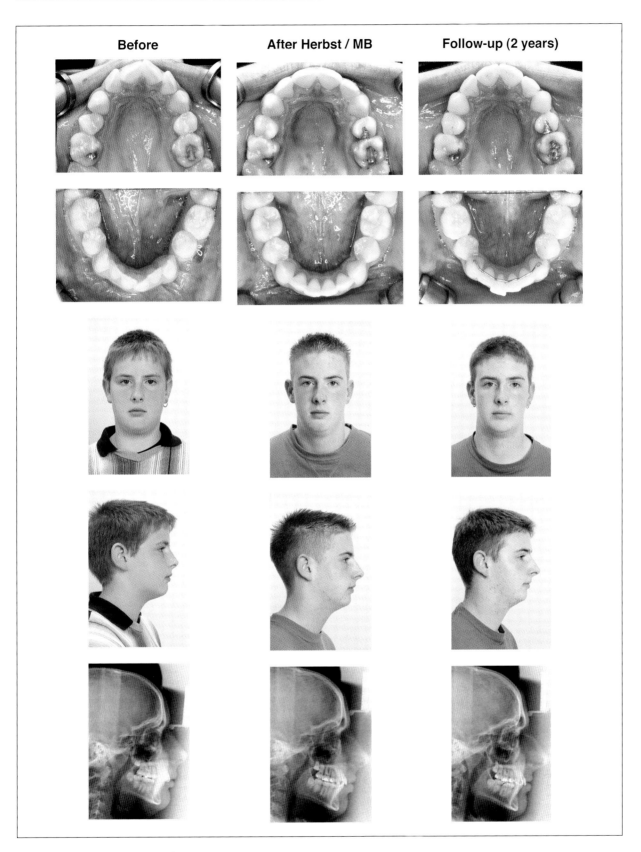

Before   **After Herbst / MB**   **Follow-up (2 years)**

Fig. 21-13 Case 21-8 (continued)

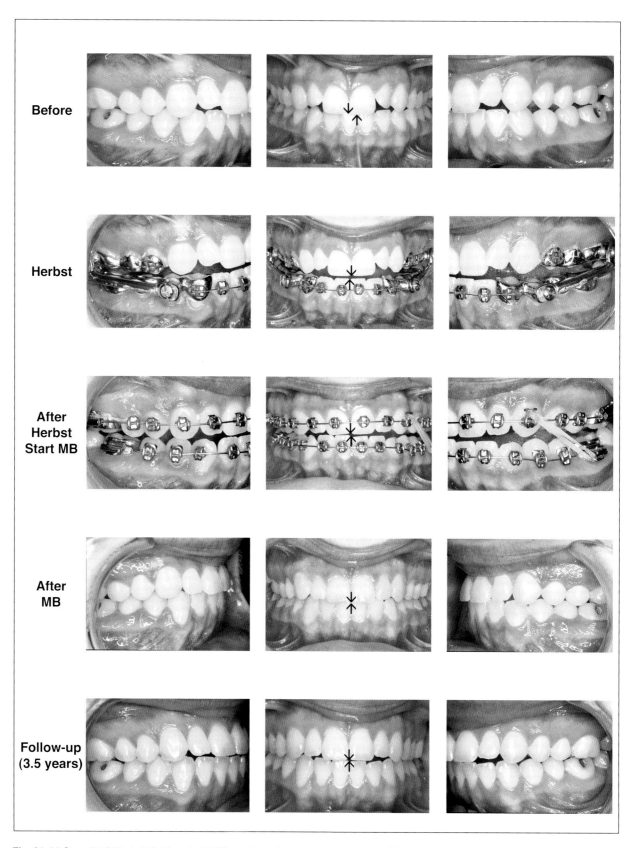

Before

Herbst

After Herbst Start MB

After MB

Follow-up (3.5 years)

Fig. 21-14 Case 21-9 Herbst/Multibracket (MB) appliance treatment of a 14-year-old female with a unilateral Class II:1 malocclusion.

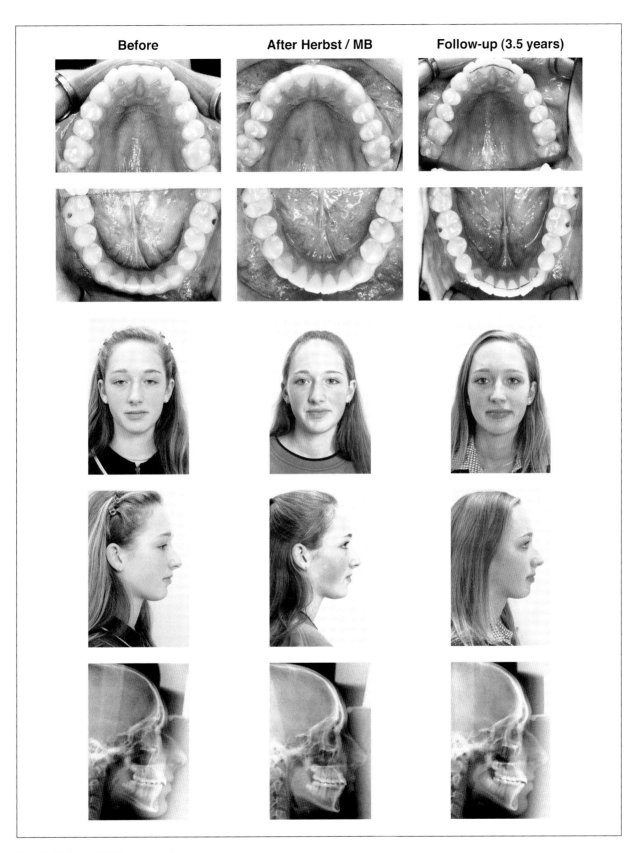

| Before | After Herbst / MB | Follow-up (3.5 years) |

Fig. 21-14 Case 21-9 (continued)

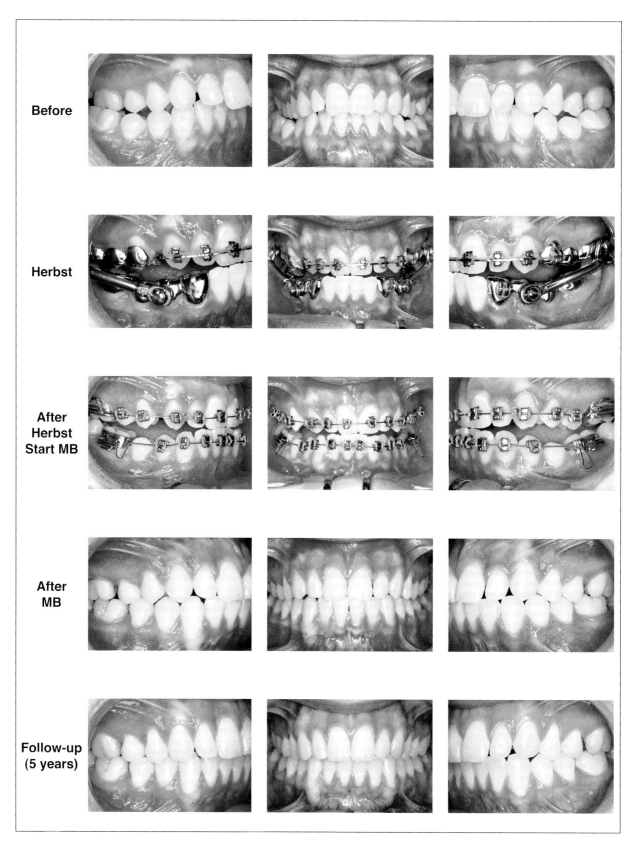

Before

Herbst

After Herbst Start MB

After MB

Follow-up (5 years)

Fig. 21-15 Case 21-10 Herbst/Multibracket (MB) appliance treatment of a 13-year-old female with a Class II:1 malocclusion and a unilateral cross bite.

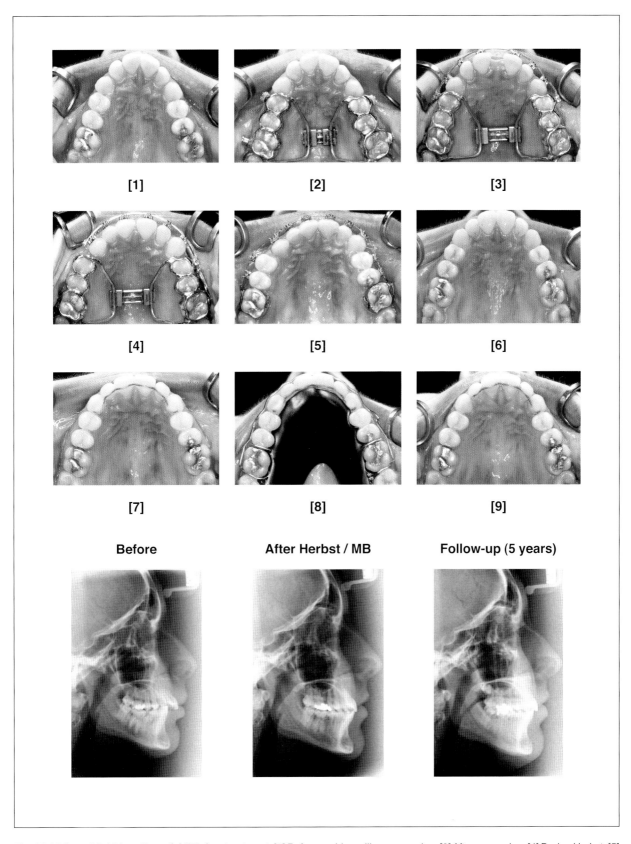

Before   **After Herbst / MB**   **Follow-up (5 years)**

Fig. 21-15 Case 21-10 (continued) [1] Before treatment; [2] Before rapid maxillary expansion; [3] After expansion; [4] During Herbst; [5] After Herbst/Start MB; [6] After MB; [7] Bonded retainer; [8] Bonded retainer in combination with retention plate; [9] Follow-up (5 years).

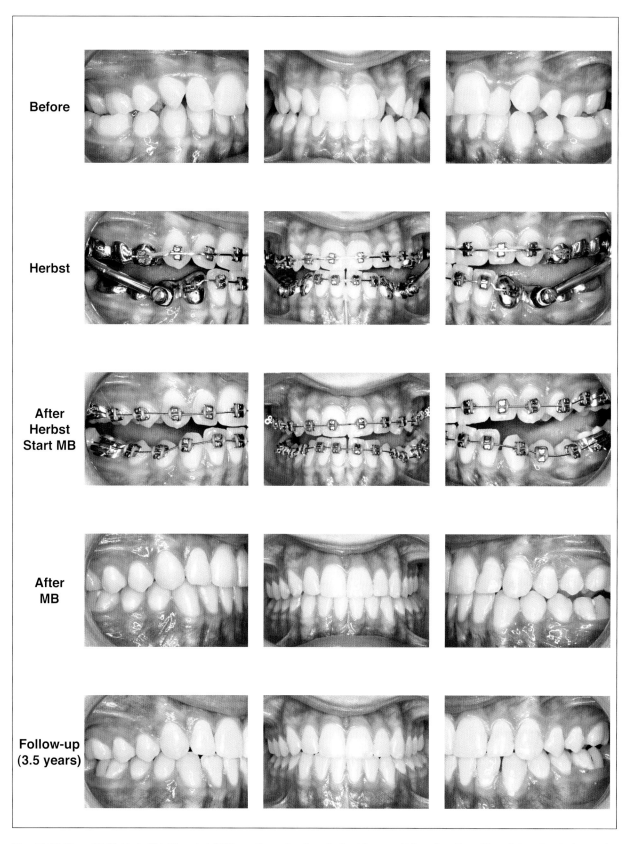

Fig. 21-16 Case 21-11 Herbst/Multibracket (MB) appliance treatment of a 14-year-old female with a Class II:1 malocclusion and a bilateral cross bite.

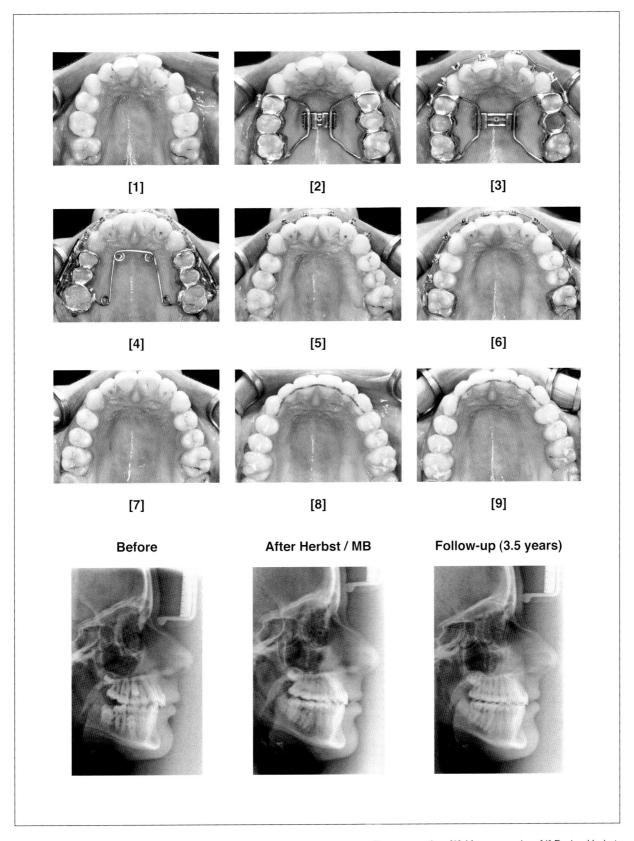

Fig. 21-16 Case 21-11 (continued) [1] Before treatment; [2] Before rapid maxillary expansion; [3] After expansion; [4] During Herbst; [5] After Herbst; [6] Start MB; [7] After MB; [8] Bonded retainer; [9] Follow-up (3.5 years).

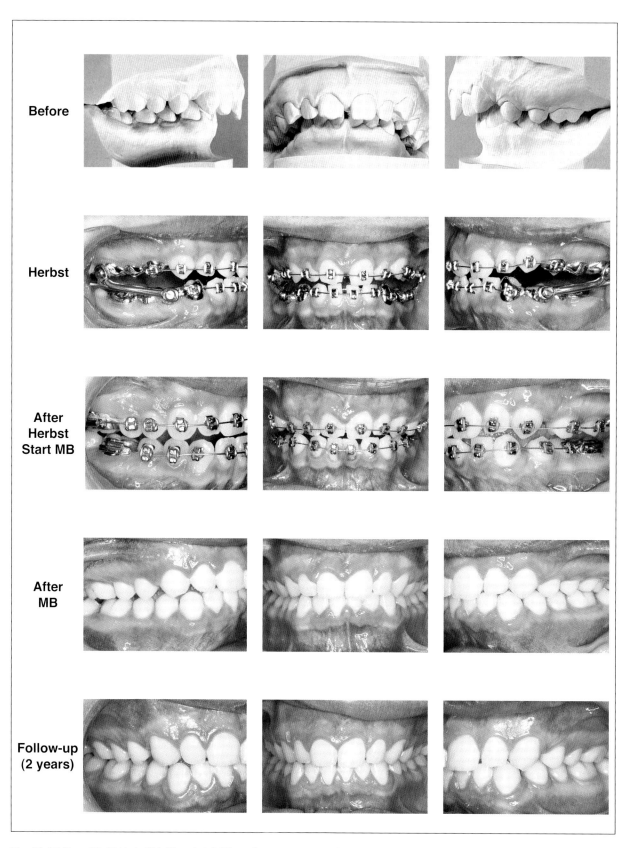

Fig. 21-17 Case 21-12 Herbst/Multibracket (MB) appliance treatment of a 15-year-old male with an extreme Class II:1 malocclusion and a bilateral scissors bite.

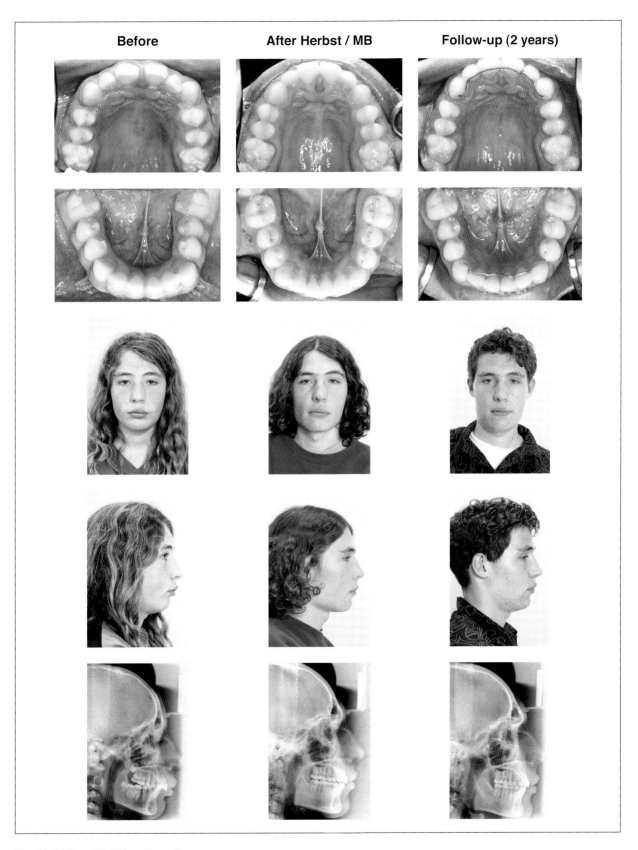

| Before | After Herbst / MB | Follow-up (2 years) |

Fig. 21-17 Case 21-12 (continued)

References

Berg R. Stability of deep overbite correction. Eur J Orthod 1983;5:75-83.

Binda SKR, Kuijpers-Jagtman AM, Maertens JKM, van Hoff MA. A long-term cephalometric evaluation of treated Class II, division 2 malocclusions. Eur J Orthod 1994;16:301-308.

Fuhrmann R. Kieferorthopädische Behandlung der Klasse II,2 Malokklusion. Nachuntersuchung von 17 Patienten unter besonderer Berücksichtigung der Unterlippenhöhe und der Bisshebung. Diss. med. dent. (Thesis), Homburg/Saar 1989.

Herbst E. Dreißigjährige Erfahrungen mit dem Retentions-Scharnier. Zahnärztl Rundschau 1934;43:1515-1524, 1563-1568, 1611-1616.

Houston WJB. Incisor edge–centroid relationships and overbite depth. Eur J Orthod 1989;11:139-143.

Luffingham JK. The lower lip and the maxillary central incisors. Eur J Orthod 1982;263-268.

Marku K. Die Klasse II/2 Behandlung bei Postadoleszenten und jungen Erwachsenen mit der Herbst-/Multibracket-Apparatur. Diss. med. dent. (Thesis), Giessen 2006.

Mills JR. The problem of overbite in Class II, Division 2 malocclusion. Br J Orthod 1973;1:34-48.

Nicol WA. The lower lip and the upper teeth in Angle´s Class II, division 2 malocclusion. Dent Pract 1964;14:179-182.

Obijou C, Pancherz H. Herbst appliance treatment of Class II, Division 2 malocclusions. Am J Orthod Dentofac Orthop 1997; 112:287-291.

Pancherz H, Hansen K. Occlusal changes during and after Herbst treatment: a cephalometric investigation. Eur J Orthod 1986;8:215-228.

Sarnäs KV, Pancherz, H Rune B, Selvik G. Hemifacial microsomia treated with the Herbst appliance. Report of a case analyzed by means of roentgen stereometry and metallic implants. Am J Orthod 1982;82:68-74.

Sarnäs KV, Rune B, Aberg M. Facial growth in a cleft palate patient treated with the Herbst appliance: a long-term profile roentgenographic and roentgen stereometric analysis of profile changes and displacement of the jaws. Cleft Palate Craniofac J 2000;37:71-77.

Schudy FF. The control of vertical overbite in clinical orthodontics. Angle Orthod 1968;38:19-39.

Schweitzer M, Pancherz H. The incisor-lip relation in Herbst/ Multibracket appliance treatment of Class II, Division 2 malocclusions. Angle Orthod 2001;71:358-363.

Selwyn-Barnett BJ. Rationale of treatment for Class II division 2 malocclusion. Br J Orthod 1991;18:173-181.

Simons ME, Joondeph DR. Change in overbite: a ten year postretention study. Am J Orthod 1973;64:349-367.

van der Linden F, Boersma H. Diagnose und Behandlungsplanung in der Kieferorthopädie. Band 3. Berlin: Quintessenz Verlag; 1988.

von Bremen J, Pancherz H. Efficiency of Class II, Division 1 and Class II, Division 2 treatment in relation to different treatment approaches. Semin Orthod 2003:9:87-92.

Chapter 22

Treatment timing

Research

In Class II malocclusions the optimal timing of growth modification therapy has for many years been a controversial topic.

When using removable functional appliances (Bionator, Fränkel, Twin-Block), several randomized controlled clinical trials (Tulloch et al. 1998, 2004, Keeling et al. 1998, Ghafari et al. 1998, O´Brian et al. 2003) have been performed. However, they could not give a reliable and universally accepted answer to the question of optimal treatment timing. Considering the Herbst appliance there are a number of well designed prospective and retrospective studies published, addressing the problem of treatment timing, both with respect to treatment efficiency and long-term stability (Pancherz and Hägg 1985, Hägg and Pancherz 1988, Pancherz and Littmann 1988, Hansen et al. 1991, Wieslander 1993, Pancherz 1994, 1997, Konik et al. 1997, von Bremen and Pancherz 2002, Pancherz and Ruf 2000, Ruf and Pancherz 2003). The scientific evidence on optimal treatment timing with the Herbst appliance will be presented by scrutinizing three publications.

1. Dentofacial orthopedics in relation to somatic maturation. An analysis of 70 consecutive cases treated with the Herbst appliance (Pancherz and Hägg 1985)

Sagittal mandibular condylar growth changes and sagittal incisor position changes were related to somatic maturation in 70 consecutive Class II malocclusion cases (52 males and 18 females, aged 10

to 16 years) treated with the Herbst appliance for an average period of 7 months. No posttreatment evaluation was performed. Twenty-three untreated Class II subjects, all males aged 9 to 14 years, were used as a control group. All patients were treated at the Department of Orthodontics, University of Lund, Sweden.

Mouth-open profile roentgenograms were analyzed. Longitudinal growth records of standing height over a 5-to 10-year-period were used for the assessment of somatic maturation at the time of Herbst treatment. From the growth records, individual velocity curves of standing height were constructed. By visual inspection, the peak height velocity was identified on the growth curves and three growth periods were established (Fig. 22-1): Prepeak, Peak and Postpeak.

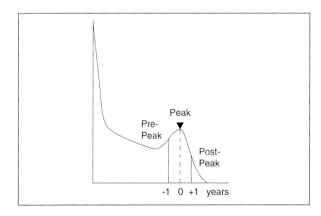

Fig. 22-1 Division of the velocity growth curve of standing height into three growth periods: Peak (the period at peak hight velocity ± 1 year), Prepeak (the period before Peak), and Postpeak (the period after Peak). (*Revised from Pancherz and Hägg 1985*)

The examination period in each subject was assigned to one of the three growth periods. The distribution of the Herbst and control subjects in relation to peak height velocity is shown in Fig. 22-2.

Herbst treatment resulted in Class I dental arch relationships in all 70 patients investigated. Sagittal condylar growth was increased and the mandibular incisors were moved anteriorly. When the mandibular skeletal and dental changes were related to the subjects' somatic maturation, significant differences

between the different growth periods existed in males (Fig. 22-3): (1) in the Prepeak period sagittal condylar growth and anterior incisor position changes were about equally large, (2) in the Peak period sagittal condylar growth was relatively more pronounced, and (3) in the Postpeak period anterior incisor position changes were relatively more extensive. However, for the skeletal and dental changes in all three growth periods, a large individual variation existed (Fig. 22-4).

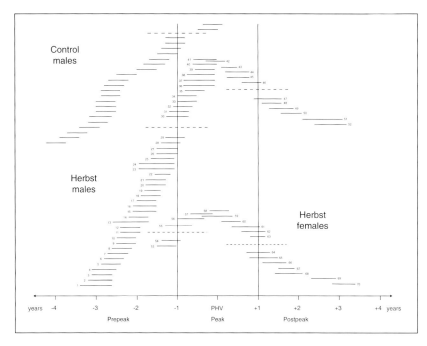

Fig. 22-2 Distribution of the 70 Herbst subjects (cases 1-70) and 23 control subjects in relation to the peak hight velocity (PHV). Division of the subjects into the three growth periods: Prepeak, Peak and Postpeak. The length of the examination period (——) is shown. (*Revised from Pancherz and Hägg 1985*)

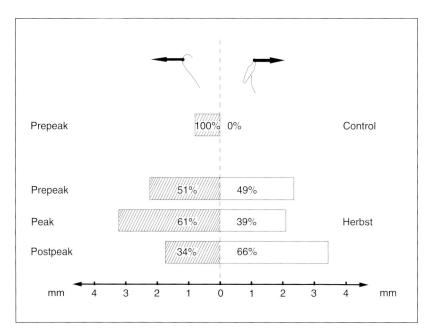

Fig. 22-3 Average mandibular condylar and incisor changes in 52 male Herbst subjects and 23 untreated male control subjects. Division of the subjects into the three growth periods: Prepeak, Peak and Postpeak.

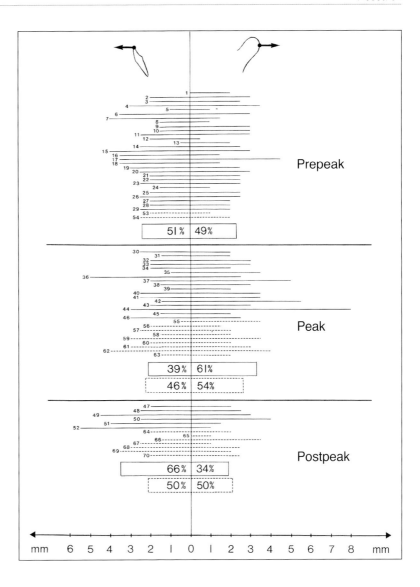

Fig. 22-4 Individual mandibular condylar and incisor changes in 52 males (——) and 18 females (-----) treated with the Herbst appliance. The subjects were arranged in relation to the peak hight velocity (PHV) in the order given in Fig. 22-2. (*Revised from Pancherz and Hägg 1985*)

Interpretation of the results

The level of somatic development influenced the outcome of Herbst therapy. Sagittal condylar growth changes dominated, on average, in the Peak treatment period and tooth movements in the Postpeak treatment period. These findings are in agreement with those from studies in monkeys fitted with mandibular protrusion splints or a Herbst appliance. In animals in the early growth period, condylar growth was increased in relation to untreated controls (McNamara and Carlson 1979, Peterson and McNamara 2003). In animals in the late growth period, on the other hand, the overall amount of condylar growth was reduced (McNamara et al. 1982) and the quantity of compensatory tooth movements was increased (McNamara 1975). In the Herbst subjects, the differences in the amount of condylar growth

seen, when comparing the various maturity groups, could be explained by the difference in the amount of basic condylar growth existing, which is larger in Peak than in Prepeak and Postpeak subjects (Hägg et al. 1987). Thus, the increase in sagittal condylar growth accomplished with the Herbst appliance will result in an equal addition to basic condylar growth, irrespective of the maturation of the subjects (Hägg et al. 1987).The dental changes during Herbst treatment were basically a result of anchorage loss (see Chapter 19: Anchorage problems). Since it is thought that neuromuscular adaptation will occur less easily in older than in younger subjects, and general muscle strength increases with maturation, the forces excerted upon the dentition by the appliance will be larger in older than in younger subjects.

2. Long-term effects of the Herbst appliance in relation to the treatment growth period: a cephalometric study (Hansen et al. 1991)

An analysis was performed on the long-term effects of the Herbst appliance on the dentofacial complex with special reference to the growth period in which the patients were treated.

At the time of examination the original sample of consecutive Class II:1 patients treated with the Herbst appliance at the Department of Orthodontics, University of Lund, Sweden, comprised 170 subjects. Herbst therapy resulted in a Class I or overcorrected Class I dental arch relationship in all 170 patients. The first 40 male subjects treated, who fulfilled the following criteria, were selected for this study: (1) no extractions of teeth, (2) a follow-up of at least 5 years posttreatment, until the end of growth defined by a complete fusion of the epiphysis of the radius (stage R-J; Hägg and Taranger 1980) as seen on hand-wrist radiographs.

The patient sample was divided into three groups according to the growth period in which they were treated (Pancherz and Hägg 1985): Prepeak (n=19), Peak (n=15) and Postpeak (n=6). The average length of the treatment period was 7 months. The subjects were re-examined, on average 6 months and 6.6 years posttreatment. For the length of the treatment and posttreatment periods no differences existed between the three maturity groups.

Lateral head films in habitual occlusion were analyzed at three stages: before treatment, 6 months posttreatment when the occlusion had settled (Pancherz and Hansen 1986) and at the time of follow-up 6.6 years posttreatment. Standard cephalometrics and the SO-Analysis (see Chapter 6: Herbst research - Subjects and methods) were used. The cephalometric changes during the following three examination periods were considered: P1 (treatment/settling period) - from before treatment to 6 months posttreatment. P2 (postsettling period) - from 6 months posttreatment to the end of growth. P3 (total examination period) - from before treatment to the end of growth.

Composite tracings of the three growth period groups at the three times of examination are shown in Fig. 22-5. The results of the SO-analysis are presented in Figs. 22-6 to 22-8.

P1 - treatment/settling period (Fig. 22-6)

The reduction in overjet was insignificantly larger in the Peak and Postpeak groups than in the Prepeak group.

The amount of maxillary and mandibular jaw growth was higher in the Peak and Postpeak groups than in the Prepeak group. The improvement in maxillary to mandibular jaw base relationship (skeletal changes) was, however, similar in all three groups. Mandibular growth exceeded maxillary growth: Prepeak group 2.2 mm, Peak group 2.1 mm and Postpeak group 2.6 mm.

P2 - postsettling period (Fig. 22-7)

The overjet recovered insignificantly in all three groups.

The amount of maxillary and mandibular growth was highest in the Prepeak group followed by the Peak and Postpeak groups. The improvement in maxillary to mandibular jaw base relationship (skeletal changes) was larger in the Prepeak and Peak groups in comparison to the Postpeak group. Mandibular growth exceeded maxillary growth: Prepeak group 2.4 mm, Peak group 2.2 mm and Postpeak group 1.3 mm.

P3 - total examination period (Fig. 22-8)

The reduction in overjet was insignificantly larger in the Peak and Postpeak groups than in the Prepeak group.

The amount of maxillary and mandibular growth was highest in the Prepeak group followed by the Peak and Postpeak groups. The improvement in maxillary to mandibular jaw base relationship (skeletal changes) was larger in the Prepeak group followed by the Peak group and Postpeak group. Mandibular growth exceeded maxillary growth: Prepeak group 4.8 mm, Peak group 4.2 mm and Postpeak group 3.9 mm.

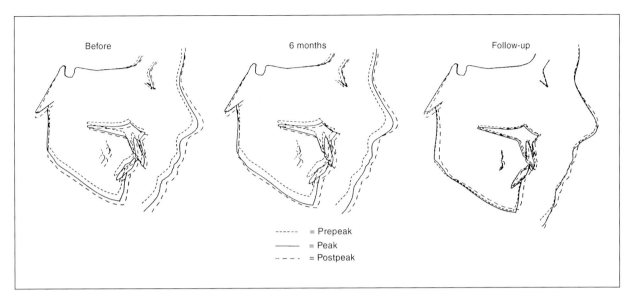

Fig. 22-5 Computer calculated composite tracings of 40 male Class II:1 malocclusions treated with the Herbst appliance. The distance between the hard and soft tissue profile is enlarged. Nineteen patients were treated during the Prepeak period, 15 during the Peak period and 6 during the Postpeak period. (*Revised from Hansen et al. 1991*)

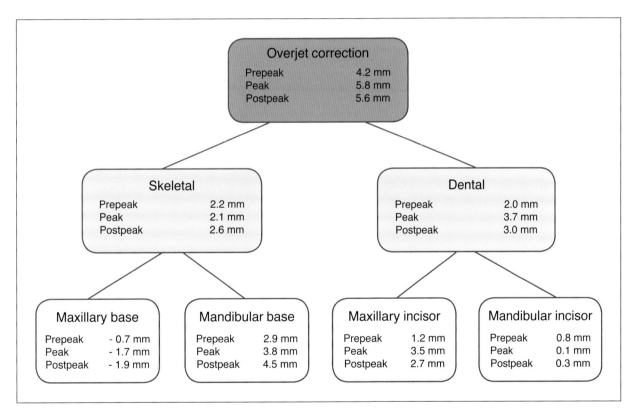

Fig. 22-6 The mechanism of overjet change in the treatment/settling period (P1). Analysis of 40 male Class II:1 malocclusions treated with the Herbst appliance. Nineteen patients were treated during the Prepeak period, 15 during the Peak period and 6 during the Postpeak period. The mean values are given. Minus (-) implies unfavorable changes for overjet correction.

217

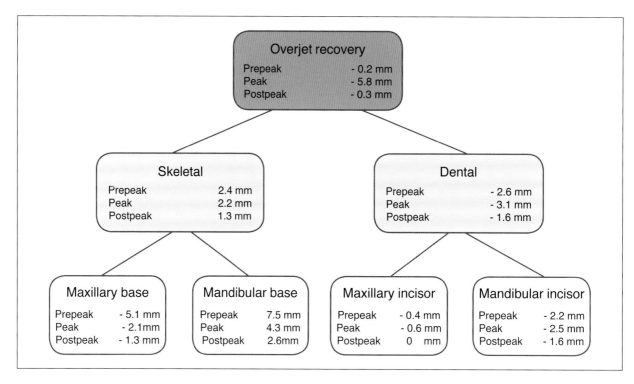

Fig. 22-7 The mechanism of overjet change in the postsettling period (P2). Analysis of 40 male Class II:1 malocclusions treated with the Herbst appliance. Nineteen patients were treated during the Prepeak period, 15 during the Peak period and 6 during the Postpeak period. The mean values are given. Minus (-) implies unfavorable changes for overjet correction.

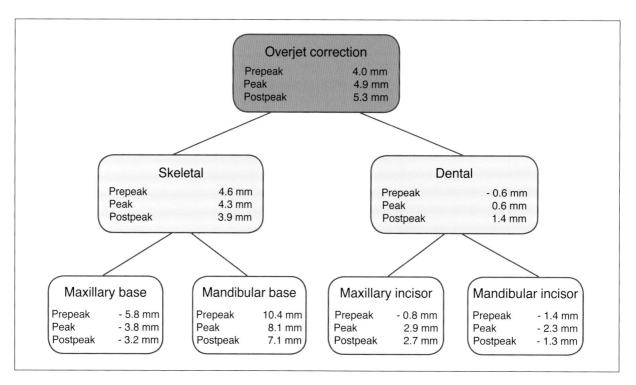

Fig. 22-8 The mechanism of overjet change in the total examination period (P3). Analysis of 40 male Class II:1 malocclusions treated with the Herbst appliance. Nineteen patients were treated during the Prepeak period, 15 during the Peak period and 6 during the Postpeak period. The mean values are given. Minus (-) implies unfavorable changes for overjet correction.

Interpretations of the results

The maxillary to mandibular growth inter-relationship during the three observation periods was favorable and comparable in all three growth groups. The relative increase in mandibular prognathism seen during the P1 period was certainly a result of the treatment (Pancherz 1979, 1982). As mentioned before, the Herbst appliance obviously increases sagittal condylar growth by the same amount, irrespective of the period of somatic maturation in which the patients are treated (Hägg et al. 1987). In other words, an equal amount of stimulated condylar growth is added to normal growth. The latter of which, of course, will vary with the subjects´ growth period.

Even if the amount of condylar (mandibular) growth is more pronounced in patients treated around the peak of pubertal growth (Pancherz and Hägg 1985), this does not imply that a maxillary/mandibular malrelationship is more effectively treated during the peak period, as growth of the maxilla also is increased during that period. Therefore, the net effect of Herbst treatment is the same irrespective of the growth period in which treatment is performed.

During the postsettling (P2) period, the relative increase in mandibular prognathism was most likely a result of normal growth changes. Thus, for natural reasons the amount of maxillary and mandibular jaw growth during this period was larger in the subjects treated before the maximum of pubertal growth than in the subjects treated at a later stage.

3. Early or late treatment with the Herbst appliance – stability or relapse? (Pancherz 1994) [Article in German]

In order to find the optimal time of Herbst treatment with respect to posttreatment stability, the long-term effects of Herbst treatment were assessed in Class II:1 subjects treated "early" and "late". Using the hand-wrist radiographic stages of Hägg and Taranger (1980) "early" treatment was defined by the stages MP3-E and F (= prepeak growth period) and "late" treatment by the stages MP3-H and I (= post-peak growth period).

From the original sample of 118 Class II:1 subjects treated with the Herbst appliance at the Department of Orthodontics, University of Lund, Sweden, those 31 "early" and 24 "late" treated subjects were selected in which a follow-up period of at least 5 years existed and no other treatment was performed after Herbst therapy. Dental casts and lateral head films from before treatment, 6 months after treatment, when the occlusion had settled and at follow-up, 5-10 years posttreatment, were analyzed. Furthermore, a clinical examination of the function of the masticatory system was performed at the time of follow-up.

With respect to long-term stability or relapse of overjet and sagittal molar relationship at the time of follow-up the total sample of 55 subjects was divided into three groups, separately for overjet and molar relationship:

Stable
- Overjet unchanged or reduced (n=35)
- Molar relation Class I (n=38)

Insignificant relapse
- Overjet increased ≤ 1.5 mm (n=7)
- Molar relation Class I or Class II tendency of less than one quarter premolar width (n=8)

Relapse
- Overjet increased ≥ 2 mm (n=13)
- Molar relation Class II of at least half premolar width (n=9)

For the assessment of the possible causes of the relapse the following "*relapse promoting factors*", in addition to "early" treatment (**E**), were considered:
- Persisting oral habits (tongue dysfunction, atypical swallowing) - **H**
- No posttreatment retention - **R**
- Mixed dentition treatment - **M**
- Occlusal instability posttreatment (insufficient cuspal interdigitation of the teeth) assessed on dental casts from 6 months posttreatment by visual inspection and hand-articulating the models - **O**
- Unfavorable growth posttreatment (increase of the ANB and "Wits") - **G**

A relapse of overjet and sagittal molar relationship was seen more often in "early" than in "late" treated subjects (Fig. 22-9). The overjet relapsed in 36% (11/31) of the "early" and in 8% (2/24) of the "late" cases. The sagittal molar relationship relapsed in 29% (9/31) of the "early" and in none of the "late" cases. The comparison of all relapse cases with all stable cases revealed that every "relapse promoting factor" was seen more often in the relapse than in the stable cases. This was true for both the overjet (Fig. 22-10) and the sagittal molar relationship (Fig. 22-11). The most frequent combination of factors was "early" treatment (E), habits (H), treatment in the mixed dentition (M) and occlusal instability (O).

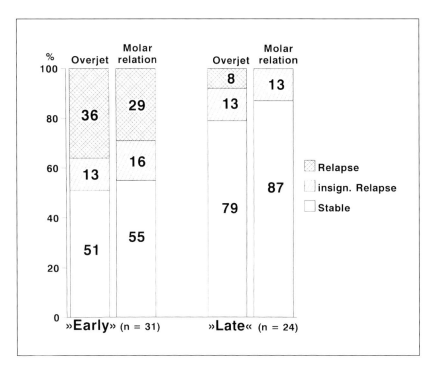

Fig. 22-9 Changes of overjet and sagittal molar relationship. Distribution of "early" and "late" treated Herbst subjects with respect to the long-term treatment result: stable, insignificant relapse and relapse. (*Revised from Pancherz 1994*)

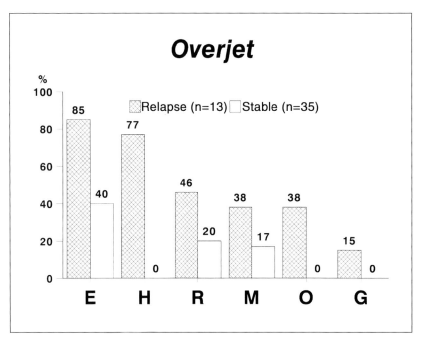

Fig. 22-10 Long-term effects of Herbst treatment on overjet. Distribution of relapse promoting factors in stable and relapse cases: **E** (early treatment), **H** (persisting oral habits), **R** (no posttreatment retention), **M** (mixed dentition treatment), **O** (occlusal instability, **G** (unfavorable growth posttreatment) (*Revised from Pancherz 1994*)

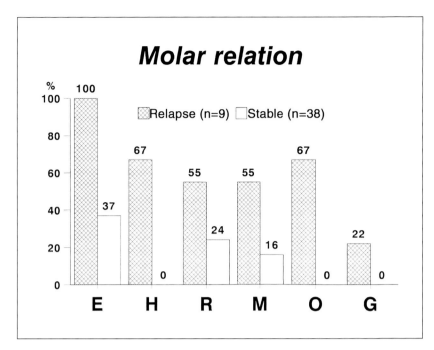

Fig. 22-11 Long-term effects of Herbst treatment on sagittal molar relationship. Distribution of relapse promoting factors in stable and relapse cases: **E** (early treatment), **H** (persisting oral habits), **R** (no posttreatment retention), **M** (mixed dentition treatment), **O** (occlusal instability, **G** (unfavorable growth posttreatment) (*Revised from Pancherz 1994*)

Interpretations of the results

In several Herbst studies (Pancherz 1982, 1991, Pancherz and Hansen 1986, Wieslander 1993), the importance of a stable occlusion for the prevention of a dental and / or skeletal relapse has been noted. If the maxillary and mandibular teeth are locked in a stable Class I cuspal interdigitation, maxillary growth forces and tooth movements are transferred to the mandible or vice versa. Thus, maxillary and mandibular changes may interact as mutually regulating factors. This would mean that a stable occlusion after Herbst, or any orthodontic therapy, could be of greater importance for a long-term stability than the growth period in which the patients are treated. Orthodontic treatment in the mixed dentition does in general not result in a stable cuspal interdigitation and will thus endanger a stable treatment result (Wieslander 1993). This is in accordance with the present findings. Mixed dentition treatment and occlusal instability were seen in 67% and 55%, respectively, of the molar relapse cases, and equally often (38%) in the overjet relapse cases. In none of the stable cases was an occlusal instability diagnosed. Early treatment was the most frequent factor noted in the overjet and molar relapse cases. This does not, however, mean that early treatment per se was responsible for the relapse seen. Instead the reason for the posttreatment relapse was most likely the occlusal instability, as treatment in most of the early cases coincided with treatment in the mixed dentition.

In the same way, the consequences of persisting oral habits, seen in many relapse cases but in none of the stable cases, could be interpreted. The oral habits prevent the teeth occluding properly and will thus result in occlusal instability.

Clinical example

In order to demonstrate the disadvantages of an "early" treatment approach, the case of a girl with a Class II:1 malocclusion that was treated twice with the Herbst appliance is presented.

Case 9-1 (Fig. 22-12)

Herbst treatment was performed at the age of 8 years. At that time the girl was in the early mixed dentition stage and in the Prepeak growth period (MP3-E skeletal maturity stage). Herbst therapy lasted for 6 months and resulted in Class I dental arch relationships. Retention with an activator was performed for 9 months in order to promote settling of the occlusion. However, after retention no stable cuspal interdigitation of the teeth was present as the girl still was in the early mixed dentition stage. At the age of 13 years, a Class II relapse had occurred and the patient was treated for a second time with a Herbst appliance. Then the girl was in the permanent dentition stage and in the Postpeak growth period

(MP3-I skeletal maturity stage). After posttreatment retention with an activator for 6 months, the teeth were in a stable Class I occlusion. At the follow-up examination at the age of 19 years, the result was stable.

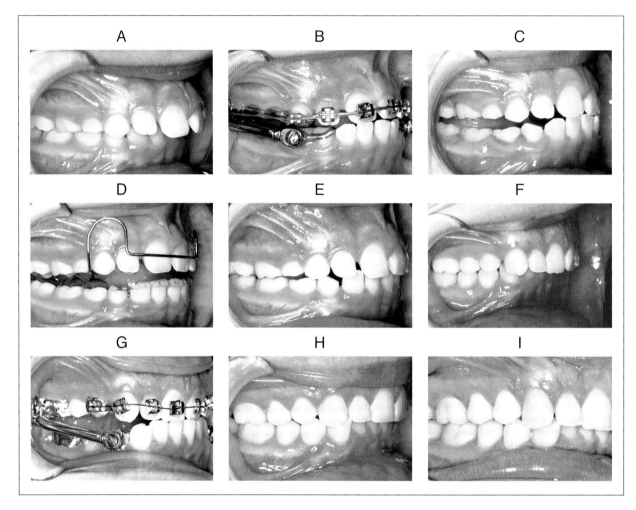

Fig. 22-12 Case 22-1 "Early" Herbst treatment of an 8-year-old girl with a Class II:1 malocclusion. **A**: Before the first period of Herbst treatment. **B**: During treatment. **C**: After 6 months of treatment. **D**: Retention with an activator. **E**: After 9 months of retention. Note the instable cuspal interdigitation of the teeth. **F**: 4 years after retention. Note the Class II relapse. **G**: Second period of Herbst treatment. **H**: 6 months after treatment when the occlusion had settled. Note the stable cuspal interdigitation of the teeth. **I**: 5 years posttreatment. Note the stable result.

Conclusions and clinical implications

When looking for the best period for Herbst appliance treatment, both the dental development and the somatic maturity stages should be taken into consideration.

- The ideal time for Herbst treatment is in the permanent dentition and in the Postpeak growth period.
- This "late" treatment approach will promote occlusal stability after treatment and reduce retention time, as the remaining growth period, which could affect the long-term outcome of therapy negatively, is reduced.
- An "early" treatment approach in the mixed dentition is not recommended. The risk for an occlusal relapse is increased as a stable cuspal interdigitation of the primary teeth is difficult to attain and retention time must thus be prolonged.

References

Ghafari J, Shofer FS, Jacobsson-Hunt U, Markowitz DL, Laster LL. Headgear versus function regulator in the early treatment of Class II, Division 1 malocclusion: A randomized clinical trial. Am J Orthod Dentofac Orthop 1998;113:51.61.

Hägg U, Pancherz H. Dentofacial orthopaedics in relation to chronological age, growth period and skeletal development. An analysis of 72 male patients with Class II division 1 malocclusion treated with the Herbst appliance. Eur J Orthod 1988;10:169-176.

Hägg U, Taranger J. Skeletal stages of the hand and wrist as indicators of the pubertal growth spurt. Acta Odont Scand 1980;38:187-200.

Hägg U, Pancherz H, Taranger J. Pubertal growth and orthodontic treatment. In Carlson DS, Ribbens KA (eds): Craniofacial growth during adolescence. Monograph 20, Craniofacial Growth Series. Center for Human Growth and Development. The University of Michigan 1987.

Hansen K, Pancherz H, Hägg U. Long-term effects of the Herbst appliance in relation to the treatment growth period: a cephalometric study. Eur J Orthod 1991;13:471-481.

Keeling SD, Wheeler TT, King GJ, Garvan CW, Cohen DA, Cabassa S, McGorray SP, Taylor MG. Anteroposterior skeletal and dental changes after early Class II treatment with bionator and headgear. Am J Orthod Dentofac Orthop 1998;113:40-50.

Konik M, Pancherz H, Hansen K. The mechanism of Class II correction in late Herbst treatment. Am J Orthod Dentofac Orthop 1997;112:87-91.

McNamara JA. Functional adaptations in the temporomandibular joint. Dent Clin North Am 1975;19:457-471.

McNamara JA, Carlson DS. Quantitative analysis of temporomandibular joint adaptations to protrusive function. Am J Orthod 1979;76:593-611.

McNamara JA, Hinton RJ, Hoffman DL. Histologic analysis of temporomandibular joint adaptations to protrusive function in young adult rhesus monkeys (Macaca mulatta). Am J Orthod 1982;82:288-298.

O`Brian K, Wright J, Conboy F, Sanjie YW, Mandall N, Chadwick S et al. Effectiveness of early orthodontic treatment with the Twin-block appliance: A multicenter, randomized controlled trial. Part 1: Dental and skeletal effects. Am J Orthod Dentofac Orthop 2003;124:234-243.

Pancherz H. Treatment of Class II malocclusions by jumping the bite with the Herbst appliance. A cephalometric investigation. Am J Orthod 1979;76:423-442.

Pancherz H. The mechanism of Class II correction in Herbst appliance treatment. A cephalometric investigation. Am J Orthod 1982;82:104-113.

Pancherz H. Früh- oder Spätbehandlung mit der Herbst-Apparatur – Stabiität oder Rezidiv? Inf Orthod Orthop 1994;26:437-445.

Pancherz H. The nature of Class II relapse after Herbst treatment: A cephalometric long-term investigation. Am J Orthod Dentofac Orthop 1991;100:220-233.

Pancherz H, Hägg U. Dentofacial orthopedics in relation to somatic maturation. An analysis of 70 consecutive cases treated with the Herbst appliance. Am J Orthod 1985;88:273-287.

Pancherz H, Hansen K. Occlusal changes during and after Herbst treatment: a cephalmetric investigation. Eur J Orthod 1986;8:215-228.

Pancherz H, Littmann C. Somatisch Reife und morphologische Veränderungen des Unterkiefers bei der Herbst-Behandlung. Inf Orthod Kieferorthop 1988;20:455-470.

Pancherz H, Ruf S. The Herbst Appliance: Research based updated clinical possibilities. World J Orthod 2000;1;17-31.

Peterson JE, McNamara JA. Temporomandibular joint adaptations associated with Herbst appliance treatment in juvenile rhesus monkey (Macaca mulatta). Semin Orthod 2003;9:12-25.

Ruf S, Pancherz H. When is he ideal period for Herbst therapy – early or late? Semin Orthod 2003;9:47-56.

Tulloch CJF, Phillips C, Proffit WR. Benefit of early Class II treatment: Progress report of a two-phase randomized clinical trial. Am J Orthod Dentofac Orthop 1998;113:62-76.

Tulloch CJF, Phillips C, Proffit WR. Outcomes in a 2-phase randomized clinical trial of early Class II treatment. Am J Orthod Dentofac Orthop 2004;125:657-667.

von Bremen J, Pancherz H. Efficiency of early and late Class II Division 1 treatment. Am J Orthod Dentofac Orthop 2002; 121:31-37.

Wieslander L. Long-term effects of treatment with the head-gear-Herbst appliance in the early mixed dentition. Stability or relapse? Am J Orthod Dentofac Orthop 1993;104:319-329.

Chapter 23

Treatment of adults – an alternative to orthognathic surgery

Research

Traditionally, the treatment options for an adult with a skeletal Class II malocclusion with mandibular deficiency are: (1) camouflage orthodontics, extracting maxillary premolars in order to allow a retrusion of the upper incisors and to normalize the overjet, thus masking the underlying skeletal problem or (2) orthognathic surgery, repositioning the mandible anteriorly. Recent clinical research has, however, demonstrated, that the Herbst appliance is most effective in adult Class II treatment (Ruf and Pancherz 1999, Pancherz 2000, Pancherz and Ruf 2000, Ruf and Pancherz 2003, 2004, 2006, Marku 2006), and the question arises: To which extent can Herbst treatment be an alternative to orthognathic surgery? Concerning the answer to this question the scientific evidence from two publications will be presented.

The mechanism of Class II correction in surgical orthodontic treatment of adult Class II, division 1 malocclusions (Pancherz et al. 2004)

Orthognathic surgery and dentofacial orthopedics in adult Class II, Division 1 treatment: mandibular sagittal split osteotomy versus Herbst appliance (Ruf and Pancherz 2004)

The dentoskeletal and facial profile changes as well as the mechanism of Class II correction were assessed in treated adult Class II, Division 1 subjects. Twenty-three adults were treated with the Herbst appliance and 46 adults were treated exclusively with a mandibular sagittal split osteotomy (no maxillary surgery,

no genioplasty and no extractions of teeth). In both patient groups treatment was finished with a multi-bracket appliance.

Adulthood in the Herbst subjects was defined by the pretreatment hand-wrist radiographic stages R-IJ (4 subjects) and R-J (19 subjects) according to the method of Hägg and Taranger (1980). Although no skeletal maturity data existed for the surgery subjects, all were considered to have finished their growth. The mean pretreatment age of the Herbst and Surgery subjects was 21.9 years (15.7 - 44.4 years) and 26 years (15.7 - 46.6 years), respectively. The average total treatment time amounted to 1.8 years in the Herbst group and 1.7 years in the Surgery group.

Lateral head films in habitual occlusion from before treatment as well as after all treatment (which means after multibracket appliance treatment following Herbst and Surgery treatment, respectively) were analyzed using standard cephalometrics and the SO-Analysis (see Chapter 6: Herbst research-subjects and methods).

All Surgery and Herbst subjects were treated successfully to Class I dental arch relationships, normal overjet and overbite. The treatment changes of different cephalometric variables are presented in Fig. 23-1. The amount of overjet reduction was largest in the Herbst subjects. This was true both when comparing group averages as well as when looking at the maximum individual overjet reduction. Although Proffit et al. (1992b) stated that orthodontic treatment was likely to fail (even in adolescents in whom growth assists Class II correction) if the overjet exceeds 10 mm, this seems not to be true for Herbst treatment. Average overbite reduction was also larger in the Herbst than in the Surgery group while Class II molar correction was, on average, slightly more pronounced in the Surgery group.

Both Herbst treatment and surgical mandibular advancement resulted in an increase in mandibular prognathism (SNPg) and an improvement in sagittal maxillary/mandibular relationship (ANPg). For natural reasons, however, the changes were larger in the Surgery than in the Herbst subjects. Surprisingly, the mandibular plane angle (ML/NSL) was increased in the Surgery while it was reduced in the Herbst cases. Mainly due to the changes in mandibular position, the hard and soft tissue facial profiles straightened. The treatment changes were larger in the Surgery than in the Herbst patients.

With respect to the SO-Analysis the improvement in sagittal occlusion (overjet, molar relationship) was accomplished by more skeletal than dental changes in the Surgery group, while the opposite was true in the Herbst group (Figs. 23-2 and 23-3). The consistency of success and the predictability of Herbst treatment for occlusal correction was high for both Herbst and Surgery therapy (Fig. 23-4).

For the comparison of the treatment outcome on the skeletofacial morphology in Herbst and surgical treatment, two pairs of subjects (Herbst and Surgery) are presented in Figs. 23-5 and 23-6.

Interpretation of the results

The most profound differences between the Surgery and Herbst subjects was the larger amount of mandibular base advancement (SNPg), with the subsequently larger reduction of the ANPg angle and the skeletal and soft tissue profile convexities in the Surgery group. However, it should be noticed that the differences in SNPg treatment changes, when comparing Surgery and Herbst subjects, amounted to 1.3° only. The corresponding difference in soft tissue profile straightening between the groups was 2.4° (exclusion of the nose in the evaluation). Thus, the clinician will have to ask himself, whether the slightly better improvement in facial esthetics accomplished by orthognathic surgery compared to Herbst treatment is worth the increased costs and risks of the surgical approach. In this context a genioplasty complementary to Herbst treatment should be considered in subjects with a large esthetic treatment demand.

An alternative to Herbst and Surgery could be orthodontic camouflage treatment using upper premolar extractions. This therapy, however, has been reported to decrease the SNPg angle and to lead to a more posterior position of the chin (1-2 mm) (Luecke and Johnston 1992, Proffit et al. 1992a). Thus, when comparing the effects of adult Herbst treatment with camouflage orthodontics and orthognathic surgery, it becomes clear that the indication for adult Herbst treatment, in terms of the amount of mandibular skeletal effects, lies between orthodontic camouflage and orthognathic surgery.

The type of treatment (surgery/camouflage) chosen by Class II patients depends mainly on their self-perception of the facial profile and is not associated with the degree of the dentoskeletal discrepancy existing (Bell et al. 1985, Kiyak et al. 1986). After treatment, the patients are equally satisfied with the profile changes, wether they had undergone surgical or camouflage treatment.

The unexpectedly large amount of dental changes contributing to Class II correction in the Surgery group was the result of the multibracket appliance treatment after surgery as well as the dental compensation of the postsurgical skeletal relapse (Proffit et al. 1996).

The increase of the mandibular plane angle (ML/NSL) in the Surgery subjects, is a negative side effect of mandibular sagittal split therapy and has been reported previously (Proffit et al.1992a). This posterior rotation of the mandible was due to an increase in anterior and a decrease in posterior facial heights. The increase in anterior facial height was most likely a result of the bite raising effect in conjunction with the surgical mandibular advancement procedure. The reduction of the posterior facial height could be explained by the bone remodeling processes at gonion following mandibular surgery (Kohn 1978, Schendel and Epker 1980, Epker and Wessberg 1982, La Blanc et al. 1982, Turvey et al. 1988, Schellhas et al. 1992, Cassidy et al. 1993, Schubert et al. 1999).

The consistency in treatment reaction was insignificantly larger in the Surgery than in the Herbst group for those variables directly or indirectly affected by the amount of mandibular advancement (SNPg, ANPg, hard tissue profile convexity). On the other hand, for the Class II corrective variables (overjet, molar relationship), the opposite was the case. This is in accordance with the findings of Tulloch et al. (1999), who concluded that the success rate of overjet reduction was slightly higher in orthodontic than in surgical treatment, irrespective of age and malocclusion severity. Therefore, the predictability of the overall treatment outcome in terms of consistency of changes was, on average, comparable for the Surgery and Herbst groups.

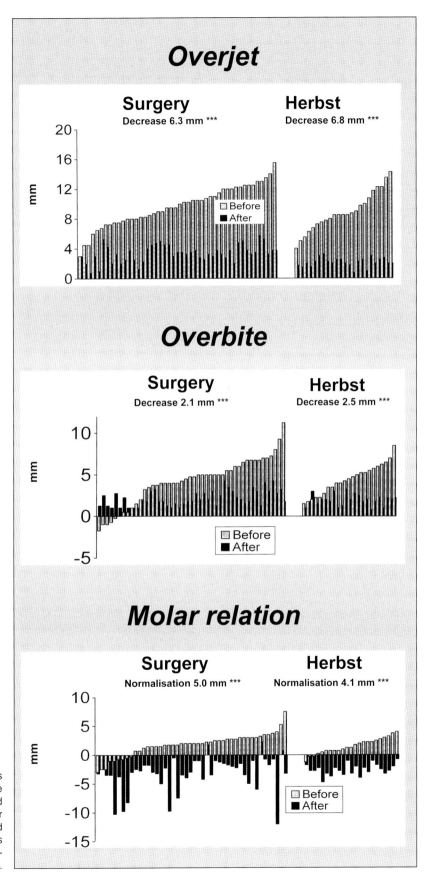

Fig. 23-1 Individual treatment changes of different dental, skeletal and soft tissue variables in 46 Class II:1 adults treated with orthognathic surgery (mandibular sagittal split) in combination with pre- and postsurgical orthodontics and in 23 Class II:1 adults treated with the Herbst appliance followed by multibracket appliances.

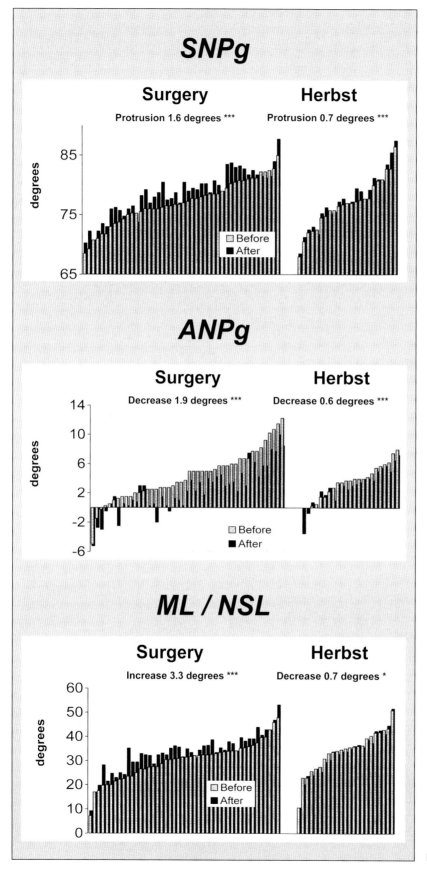

Fig. 23-1 (continued)

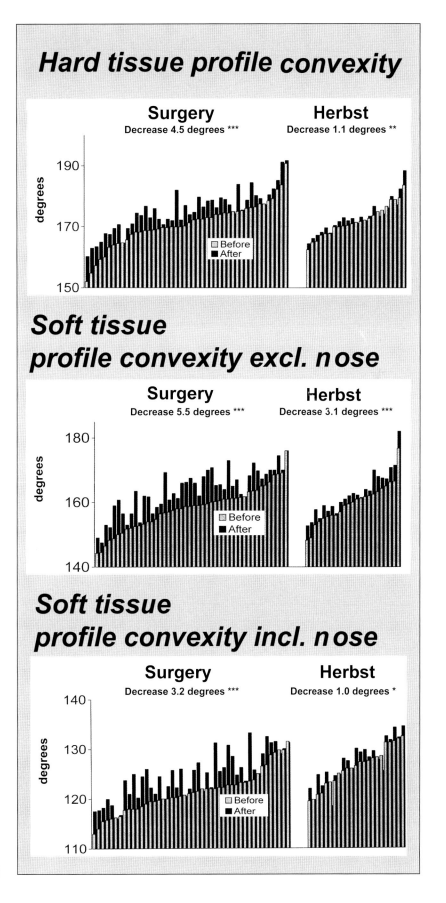

Fig. 23-1 (continued)

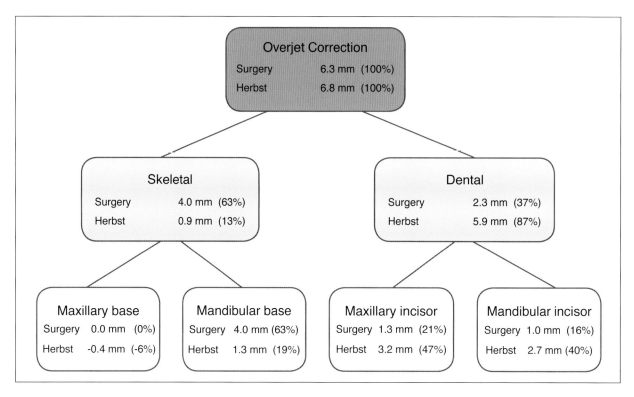

Fig. 23-2 Mechanism of overjet correction in 46 Class II:1 adults treated with orthognathic surgery (mandibular sagittal split) in combination with pre- and postsurgical orthodontics and in 23 Class II:1 adults treated with the Herbst appliance followed by a multibracket appliance. Minus (–) indicates changes that are unfavorable for overjet correction.

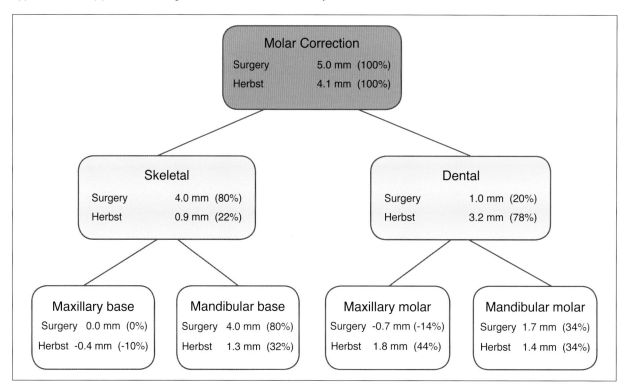

Fig. 23-3 Mechanism of Class II molar correction in 46 Class II:1 adults treated with orthognathic surgery (mandibular sagittal split) in combination with pre- and postsurgical orthodontics and in 23 Class II:1 adults treated with the Herbst appliance followed by a multibracket appliance. Minus (–) sign indicates changes that are unfavorable for Class II molar correction.

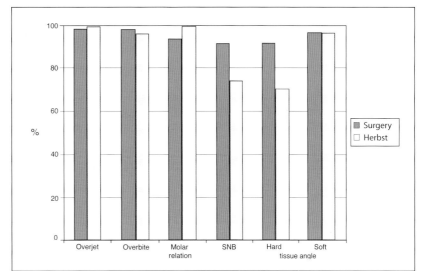

Fig. 23-4 Consistency (%) in dental, skeletal and facial profile treatment changes in 46 Class II:1 adults treated with orthognathic surgery (mandibular sagittal split) in combination with pre- and postsurgical orthodontics and in 23 Class II:1 adults treated with the Herbst appliance followed by a multibracket appliance.

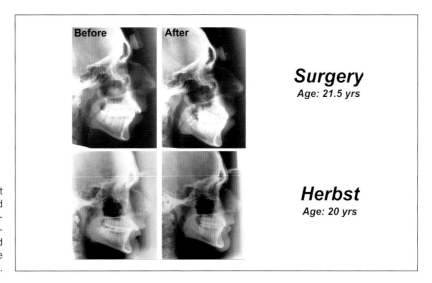

Fig. 23-5 Before and after treatment lateral head films of a 21.5-year-old female, treated with mandibular sagittal split osteotomy followed by postsurgical orthodontics, and a 20-year-old male treated with the Herbst appliance followed by a multibracket appliance.

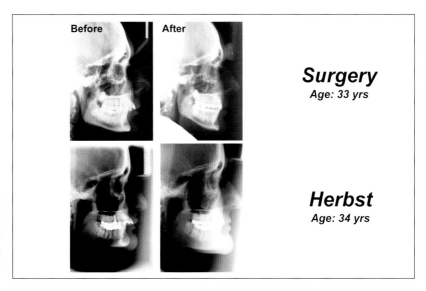

Fig. 23-6 Before and after treatment lateral head films of a 33-year-old female, treated with mandibular sagittal split osteotomy followed by postsurgical orthodontics, and a 34-year-old female treated with the Herbst appliance followed by a multibracket appliance.

Clinical examples

Three adult Class II:1 and one adult Class II:2 subjects treated with the Herbst appliance are presented. All four patients had a normo- or hypodivergent skeletofacial morphology. Herbst therapy was followed by multibracket appliance treatment in all subjects. Long-term posttreatment retention was performed with maxillary and mandibular bonded retainers in combination with an activator (for night time use) in four cases and with an activator alone in one case (Case 23-4). The treatment and posttreatment changes are visualized by the presented head films.

Case: 23-1 (Fig. 23-7)

A 20-year-old male exhibiting a severe Class II:1 malocclusion with an overjet of 11 mm and a deep bite with palatal mucosa impingement. The face was characterized by a retrognathic mandible. The patient had been previously treated for 6 years with removable appliances without any success. Herbst treatment in combination with rapid maxillary expansion (1 month) was performed during a 10-month period. After treatment, overcorrected sagittal relationships and a bilateral open bite existed. The facial profile was straightened. Final tooth alignment and settling of the occlusion was accomplished during 16 months, using a multibracket appliance in combination with Class II elastics. At the time of follow-up, 2 years posttreatment, at the age of 24 years, the treatment result was stable.

Case 23-2 (Fig. 23-8)

A 22-year-old female exhibiting a severe Class II:1 malocclusion with an overjet of 11 mm and a deep bite with traumatic palatal mucosa impingement. The face was characterized by a retrognathic mandible. The patient had been previously treated for 4 years (from 12 to 16 years of age) with fixed and removable appliances and extractions of 4 premolars without any success. She did not want any orthognathic surgery. Herbst treatment was performed during an 11.5-month period. After treatment, overcorrected sagittal dental arch relationships existed and the bite was open bilaterally. The facial profile was improved. Final tooth alignment was accomplished during a 14-month period, using a multibracket appliance. At follow-up, 1.5 years posttreatment, at the age of 25.5 years, the result was stable. The midline deviation existing before treatment prevailed throughout treatment and at follow–up.

Case 23-3 (Fig. 23-9)

A 24.5-year-old male exhibiting a Class II:1 malocclusion with mandibular crowding. The patient had an open bite tendency due to a hyperdivergent skeletofacial morphology (ML/NSL = 40°). Herbst treatment was performed during a period of 10 months. After treatment, overcorrected sagittal arch relationships existed. The facial profile was straigtened. The mandibular crowding problem was dealt with in the subsequent tooth alignment phase, using a multibracket appliance for 21 months. At follow-up, 3 years posttreatment, at the age of 30 years, the treatment result was stable.

Case 23-4 (Fig. 23-10)

A 24-year-old male with a Class II:2 malocclusion, a deep bite and maxillary and mandibular crowding. The patient had a dished-in facial profile with a prominent chin. Herbst treatment was performed during a period of 8 months (after proclination of the maxillary front teeth with a multibracket appliance). After Herbst therapy, corrected sagittal dental arch relationships, but without a secured Class I cuspal interdigitation, existed. Maxillary crowding was relieved due to the headgear effect of the Herbst appliance (see Chapter 9: The headgear effect of the Herbst appliance). The patient had his nose operated on after the removal of the Herbst appliance. Final tooth alignment and settling of the occlusion was accomplished during the 5 months of multibracket appliance treatment. At follow-up, 13 years posttreatment, at the age of 38 years, the result was stable. The facial appearance was more balanced than before treatment.

Conclusion and clinical implications

- The Herbst appliance is a powerful tool for non-surgical, non-extraction treatment of young adult Class II malocclusions. The approximate age for young adulthood is 18-24 years in females and 20-25 years in males.
- With advancing age, the dental contribution to Class II correction and facial profile improvement will dominate increasingly over the skeletal contribution.
- An upper age limit for successful Herbst treatment is difficult to define.
- The Herbst appliance is an alternative to orthognathic surgery in borderline adult skeletal Class II subjects (borderline = those adult skeletal Class II subjects who could have been managed by dentofacial orthopedic means if treatment had been performed during the active growth period).
- If the main wish of the adult Class II patient is a large improvement in facial profile, than orthognathic surgery is a better treatment option than Herbst therapy. However, the clinician and the patient must ask themselves, whether the slightly better improvement in facial esthetics accomplished by orthognathic surgery, compared to Herbst treatment, is worth the increased costs and risks.

References

Bell R, Kiyak HA, Joondeph DR, McNeill RW, Wallen TR. Perceptions of facial profile and their influence on the decision to undergo orthognathic surgery. Am J Orthod 1985;88:323-332.

Cassidy DW, Herbosa EG, Rotskoff KS, Johnston LE. A comparison of surgery and orthodontics in "borderline" adults with Class II, division 1 malocclusions. Am J Orthod Dentofac Orthop 1993;104:455-470.

Epker BN, Wessberg G. Mechanisms of early skeletal relapse following surgical advancement of the mandible. Br J Oral Surg 1982;20:175-182.

Hägg U, Taranger J. Skeletal stages of the hand and wrist as indicators of the pubertal growth spurt. Acta Odont Scand 1980;38:187-200.

Kiyak HA, McNeill RW, West RA, Hohl T, Heaton PJ. Personality characteristics as predictors and sequale of surgical and conventional orthodontics. Am J Orthod 1986;89:383-392.

Kohn MW. Analysis of relapse after mandibular advancement surgery. J Oral Surg 1978;9:676-684.

La Blanc JP, Turvey T, Epker BN, Hill C. Results following simultaneous mobilization of the maxilla and mandible for the correction of dentofacial deformities. Oral Surg Oral Med Oral Pathol 1982;54: 07-612.

Luecke PE, Johnston LE. The effect of maxillary first premolar extraction and incisor retraction on mandibular position: testing the central dogma of "functional orthodontics". Am J Orthod Dentofac Orthop 1992;101:4-12.

Marku K. Die Klasse II/2 Behandlung bei Postadoleszenten und jungen Erwachsenen mit der Herbst-/Multibracket-Apparatur. Diss. med. dent. (Thesis), Giessen 2006.

Pancherz H. Dentofacial orthopedics or orthognathic surgery: is it a matter of age? Am J Orthod Dentofac Orthop 2000;117:571-574.

Pancherz H, Ruf S. The Herbst appliance: research based clinical possibilities. World J Orthod 2000;1:17-31.

Pancherz H, Ruf S, Erbe C, Hansen K. The mechanism of Class II correction in surgical orthodontic treatment of adult Class II, Division 1 malocclusions. Angle Orthod 2004;74:800-809.

Proffit WR, Turvey T, Phillips C. Orthognathic surgery: a hierarchy of stability. Int J Adult Orthod Orthognath Surg 1996;11:191-204.

Proffit WR, Phillips C, Douvartzidis N. A comparison of outcomes of orthodontic and surgical-orthodontic treatment of Class II malocclusion in adults. Am J Orthod Dentofac Orthop 1992a;101:556-565.

Proffit WR, Phillips C, Tulloch JFC, Medland PH. Surgical versus orthodontic correction of skeletal Class II malocclusion in adolescents: effects and indications. Int J Adult Orthod Orthognath Surg 1992b;7:209-220.

Ruf S, Pancherz H. Dentoskeletal effects and facial profile changes in young adults treated with the Herbst appliance. Angle Orthod 1999;69:239-246.

Ruf S, Pancherz H. When is the ideal period for Herbst therapy – early or late? Semin Orthod 2003;9:47-56.

Ruf S, Pancherz H. Orthognathic surgery and dentofacial orthopedics in adult Class II, Division 1 treatment: mandibular sagittal split osteotomy versus Herbst appliance. Am J Orthod Dentofac Orthop 2004;126:140-152.

Ruf S, Pancherz H. Herbst/multibracket appliance treatment of Class II, Division 1 malocclusions in early and late adulthood. A prospective cephalometric study of consecutively treated subjects. Eur J Orthod 2006; 28:352-360.

Schellhas KP, Piper MA, Bessette RW, Wilkes CH. Mandibular retrusion, temporomandibular joint derangement, and orthognathic surgery planning. Plast Reconstr Surg 1992;90:218-229.

Schendel SA, Epker BN. Results after mandibular advancement surgery: an analysis of 87 cases. J Oral Surg 1980;38:255-282.

Schubert P, Bailey LTJ, White RP, Proffit WR. Long-term cephalometric changes in untreated adults compared to those treated with orthognathic surgery. Int J Adult Orthod Orthognath Surg 1999;14:91-99.

Tulloch JFC, Lenz BE, Phillips C. Surgical versus orthodontic correction for Class II patients: Age and severity in treatment planning and treatment outcome. Sem Orthod 1999;5:231-240.

Turvey T, Phillips C, Laytown HS, Proffit WR. Simultaneous superior repositioning of the maxilla and mandibular advancement. A report on stability. Am J Orthod Dentofac Orthop 1988;94:372-383.

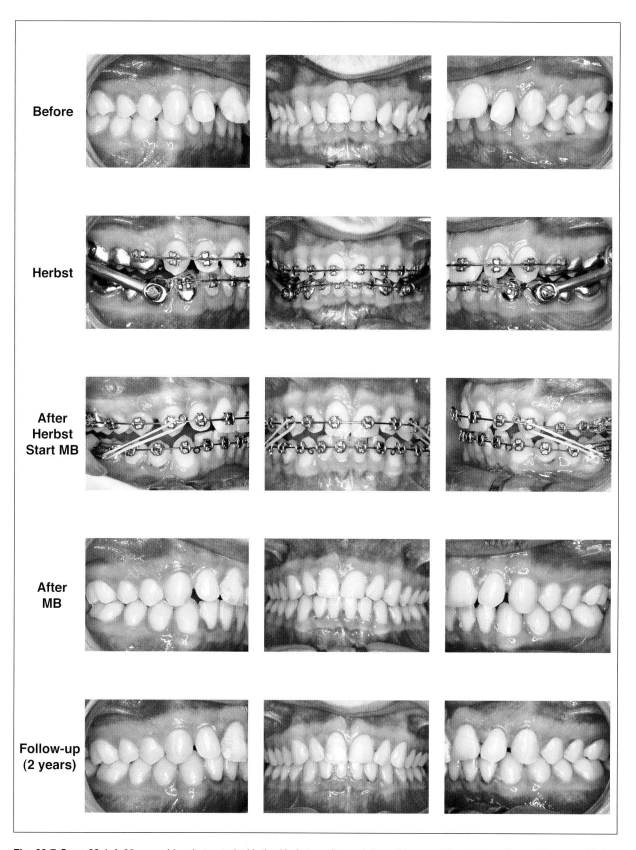

Fig. 23-7 Case 23-1 A 20-year-old male treated with the Herbst appliance followed by a multibracket appliance (the same Herbst subject as in Fig. 23-5).

| Before | After Herbst / MB | Follow-up (2 years) |

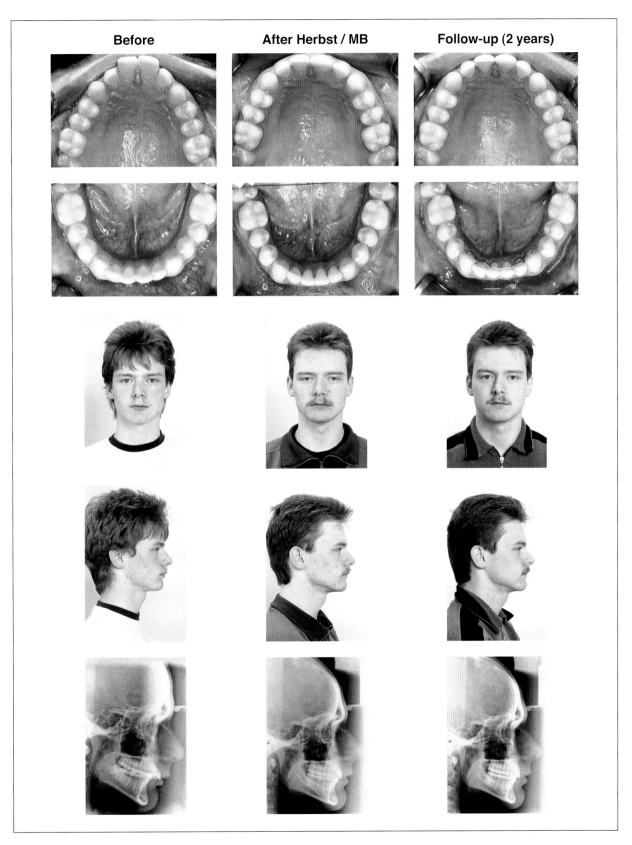

Fig. 23-7 Case 23-1 (continued)

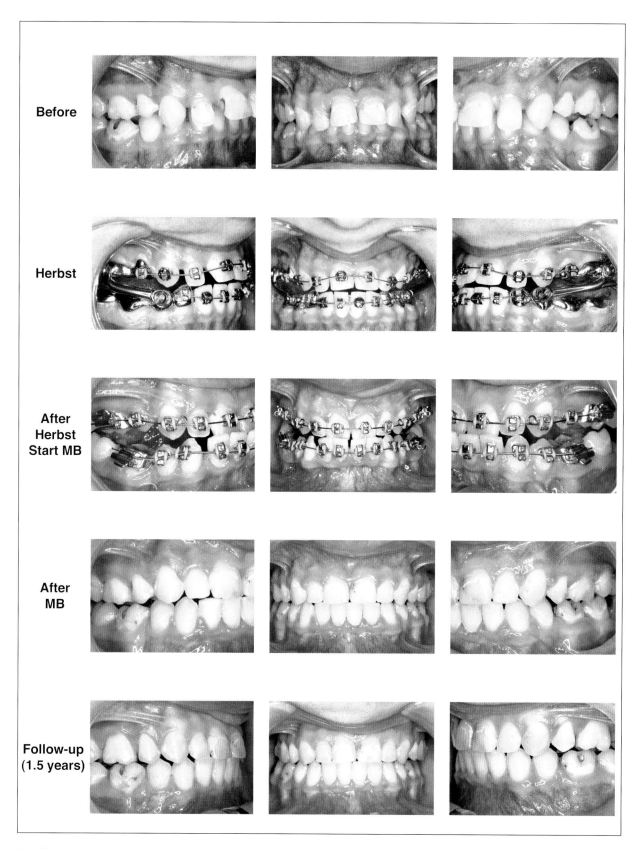

Fig. 23-8 Case 23-2 A 22-year-old female treated with the Herbst appliance followed by a multibracket appliance.

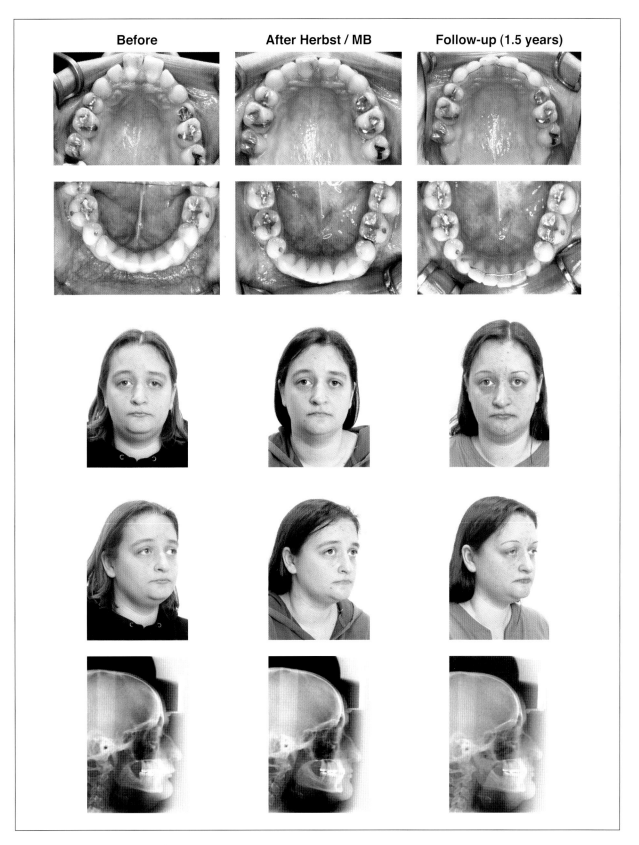

Fig. 23-8 Case 23-2 (continued)

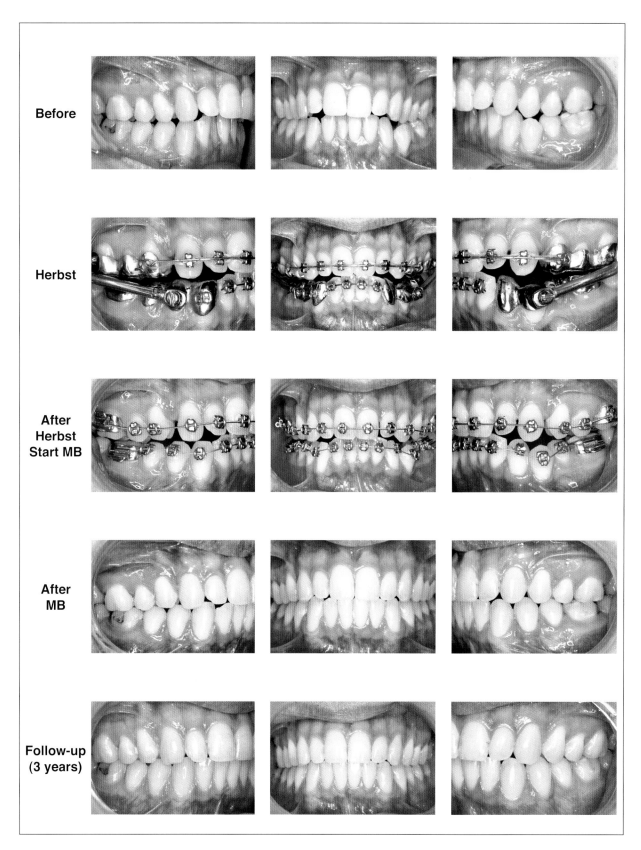

Before

Herbst

After Herbst Start MB

After MB

Follow-up (3 years)

Fig. 23-9 Case 23-3 A 24.5-year-old male treated with the Herbst appliance followed by a multibracket appliance.

Before	After Herbst / MB	Follow-up (3 years)

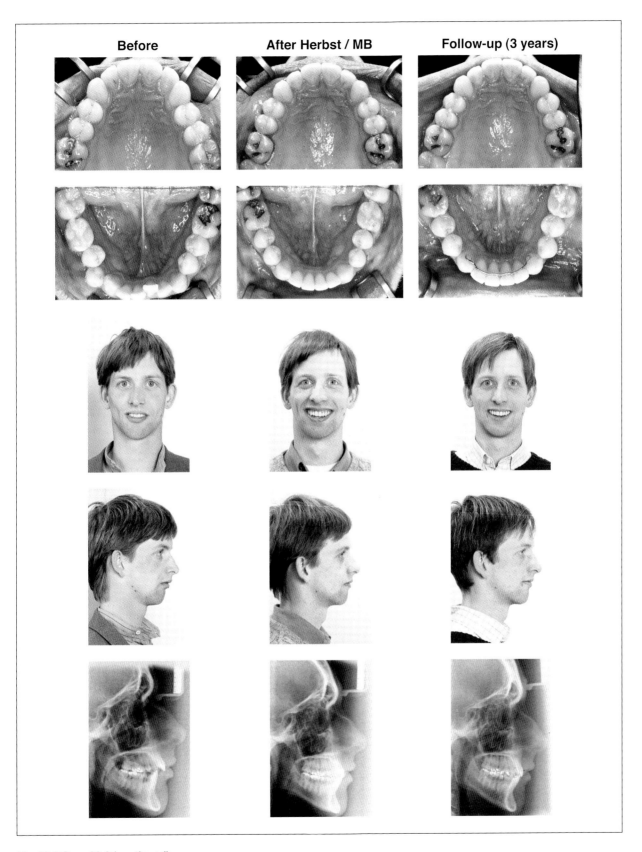

Fig. 23-9 Case 23-3 (continued)

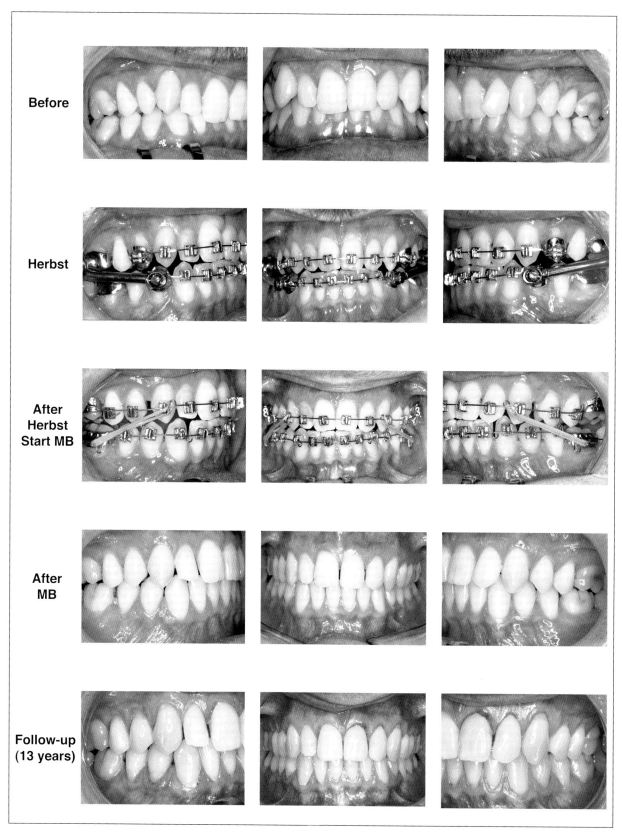

Before

Herbst

After Herbst Start MB

After MB

Follow-up (13 years)

Fig. 23-10 Case 23-4 A 24-year-old male treated with the Herbst appliance followed by a multibracket appliance.

Before	After Herbst / MB	Follow-up (13 years)

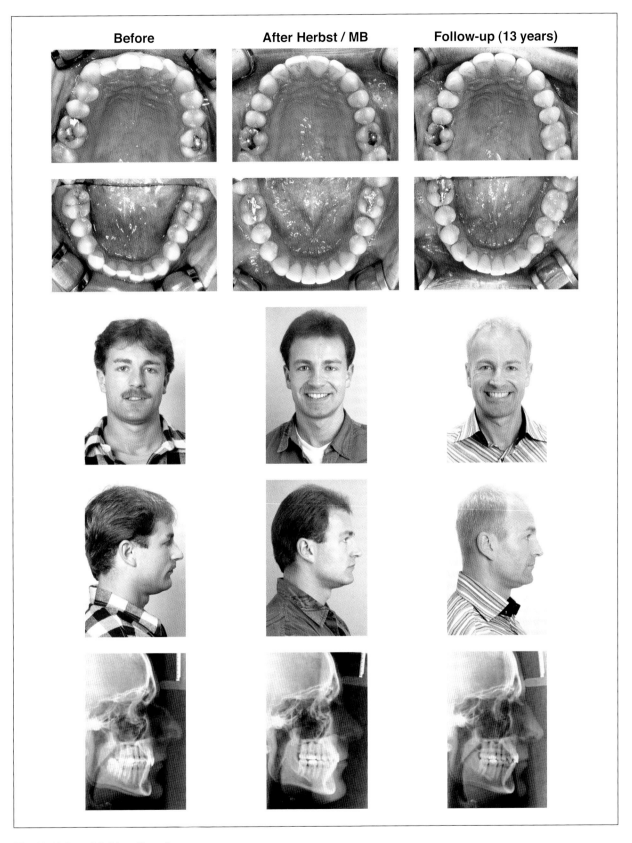

Fig. 23-10 Case 23-4 (continued)

Chapter 24

Complications

There are four basic types of Herbst appliances: (1) banded Herbst, (2) cast splint Herbst, (3) acrylic splint Herbst and (4) integrated Herbst (a Herbst telescope mechanism attached to the existing multibracket appliance).

As all patients (except one) presented in this book are treated with either the banded or the cast splint Herbst appliance, the discussion about complications will be confined to these two types of appliances.

Two main groups of complications during Herbst treatment will be addressed: (1) complications related to the appliance, and (2) complications related to the patient.

Research

In three publications on the rate of complications, related to the appliance, a comparison of the banded and cast splint Herbst appliance (Hägg et al. 2002, Sanden et al. 2004) as well as of a standard and reduced cast splint Herbst appliance (Schiöth et al. 2007) was performed. The most frequent complication found in these studies was loosening of bands and splints followed by breakages of the appliance. However, in a survey in which 425 German orthodontists were questioned about the prevalence of complications with the banded and cast splint Herbst appliances (Thiebes 2006) the results revealed breakages of the appliance to occur more often than loosening.

In this chapter, the scientific evidence on complications related to Herbst treatment will be addressed at by reviewing the studies of Sanden et al. (2004) and Schioth et al. (2007).

Complications during Herbst treatment (Sanden et al. 2004)

An assessment on the complication prevalence was performed by analysing 316 consecutively treated Herbst patients, of which 134 (82 males and 52 females) were treated with a banded Herbst and 182 (93 males and 89 females) with a cast splint Herbst appliance. The average treatment time for both types of appliances was 7 months.

For the banded Herbst appliance, two forms of mandibular anchorage were used, incorporating a different number of teeth: partial anchorage (Fig. 24-1) and total anchorage (Fig. 24-2). Maxillary anchorage was the same (partial anchorage) for both forms of mandibular anchorage.

For the cast splint Herbst appliance, cobalt chromium splints covering the teeth in the maxillary and mandibular lateral segments were used for anchorage (Fig. 24-3). Sectional arch wires were connected to the maxillary front teeth (regular measure) and to the mandibular front teeth (occasional measure).

Zinc phosphoric cement (less often) and brown copper cement (more often) were used to attach the banded appliances to the teeth. Glass ionomer cement was utilized to attach the cast splint appliances to the dentition.

When comparing males and females as well as partial and total anchorage of the banded Herbst design, no significant differences in complications (type and frequency) existed. Therefore, the males and females and the two anchorage forms were pooled in the final calculations.

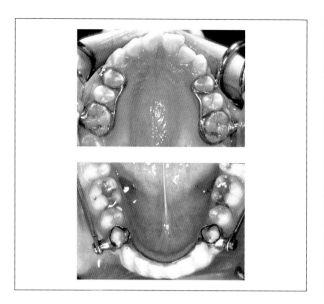

Fig. 24-1 Banded Herbst appliance with partial mandibular anchorage.

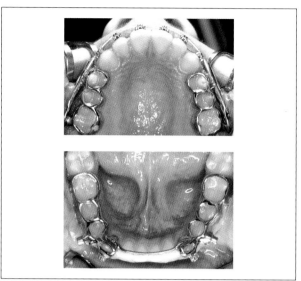

Fig. 24-3 Cast splint Herbst appliance.

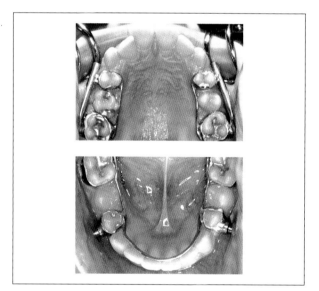

Fig. 24-2 Banded Herbst appliance with total mandibular anchorage.

Of the 134 banded Herbst patients, 33%, and of the 182 cast splint Herbst patients 40%, showed no complications during treatment. The remaining 67% of the banded and 60% of the cast splint Herbst patients experienced complications (Fig. 24-4). Of all complications (Fig. 24-5), loosening of bands (64%) and splints (94%) dominated. Breakages of bands (30%), splints (2%) and telescopes (6% in the banded Herbst and 4% in the cast splint Herbst) were seen less often. Of the 90 banded and 110 cast splint Herbst patients who had complications, 55% experienced one to three problems, 29% four to six problems and 26% seven or more problems (Fig. 24-6).

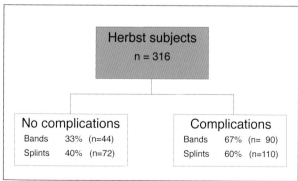

Fig. 24-4 Prevalence of complications in 316 subjects treat-ed with the Herbst appliances (134 subjects with the banded and 182 subjects with the cast splint Herbst appliance).

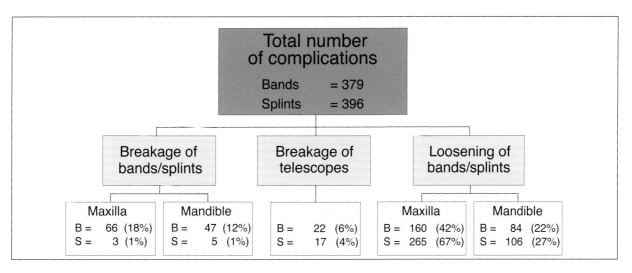

Fig. 24-5 Frequency and type of complications in 90 complication subjects treated with the banded (B) Herbst appliance and in 110 complication subjects treated with the cast splint (S) Herbst appliance . (*Revised from Sanden et al. 2004*)

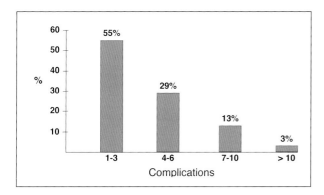

Fig. 24-6 Distribution (in %) of 200 Herbst subjects with complications in relation to the number of problems experienced in each patient.

Interpretation of the results

In general, loosening and breakage of bands and splints are caused by biting and chewing forces transmitted to the anchorage units by the telescopic parts. In reducing the lateral component of force transmission, an adequate capacity of lateral jaw movement (Fig. 24-7) is important and is enhanced by widening the axle openings of the plunger and tube (Fig. 24-8). The forces acting on the bands and splints can possibly also be reduced by advancing the mandible in steps rather than all at once. Research in this area is needed, however.

The most common complication in both types of Herbst appliances was loosening of bands and splints, with maxillary problems seen twice as often as mandibular problems.

The splints loosened more often than did the bands, which could be due to differences in the retention of the two appliances. The splints did not cover the interproximal areas and were extended to the anatomic equator of the teeth only. The bands, on the other hand, covered the interproximal tooth surfaces and were extended as far as or past the gingival margin. In the mandibular molar area the bands and splints loosened by lever arm forces working on them. They were lifted of the teeth (Figs. 24-9 and 24-10).

The influence of the type of cement on the retention of the appliances seemed not to be of decisive importance. However, no scientific comparison has been conducted between the modern glass ionomer cement and the older copper cement. To reduce the incidence of splint loosening in problematic cases, we, in our department in Giessen, use a light-cured glass ionomer cement in combination with tooth surface etching.

Bands broke considerably more often than splints. This is not surprising as the splints are much thicker than the 0.15 to 0.18 mm band material used. Furthermore, the bands are weakened by the soldering procedure, when the axles are attached to the bands.

Due to the forces acting on the upper and lower anchorage teeth, the majority of band breakages were seen mesiobuccally at the maxillary first molar bands (Fig. 24-11) and distobuccally at the mandibular first premolar bands (Fig. 24-11). The few cast splint breakages noted were caused by the casting material being too thin (Fig. 24-12).

Telescope breakage was an uncommon finding. This problem tends to occur in patients who can open their mouths so wide that the tube and plunger nearly disengage from each other. The patients then panic, closing the mouth so forcefully that the plunger gets stuck in the tube opening (Fig. 24-13 A) and causes either the tube to split (Fig. 24-13 B) or the tube to break in the pivoting area (Fig. 24-14). Furthermore, due to the large forces transmitted to the telescoping axles, they can break or disengage from their points of attachment on the bands and splints (Fig. 24-15). In preventing these problems patient education is important, as is ensuring that the plunger is long enough.

Further considerations in appliance construction to avoid problems with loose or broken bands or splints are discussed in Chapter 3: Design, construction and clinical management of the Herbst appliance.

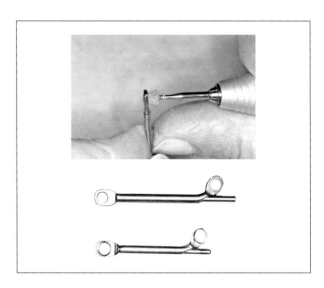

Fig. 24-8 Widening of plunger and tube axle openings to enhance mandibular lateral movement range.

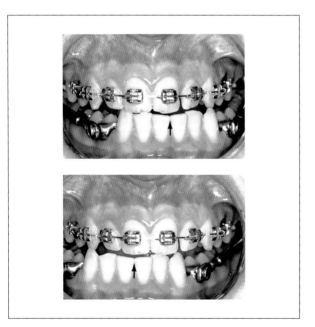

Fig. 24-7 Adequate lateral movement capacity of the Herbst appliance.

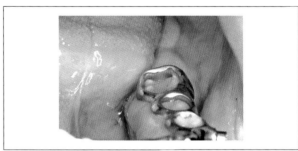

Fig. 24-9 Loosening of mandibular splint from the molar and second premolar. By lever arm forces the splint was lifted off the teeth.

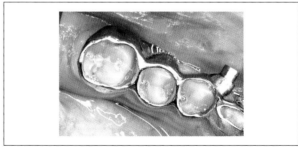

Fig. 24-10 Loosening of mandibular splint from the molar. By lever arm forces the splint was lifted off the tooth. The problem, in this patient, was unobserved for several months and led to space opening between the molar and second premolar, as the teeth in front of the molar were driven anteriorly by the Herbst appliance. Thus, in case of recementation, the splint will never fit on the molar.

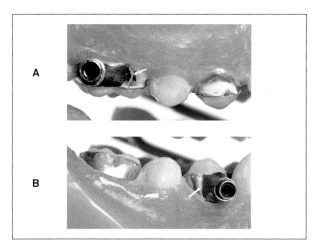

Fig. 24-11 Common band breakage **A**: Mesiobuccally at maxillary first molar. **B**: Distobuccally at mandibular first premolar.

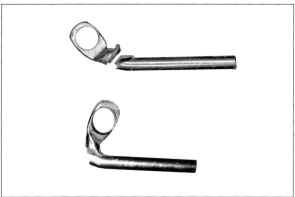

Fig. 24-14 Tube breakage.

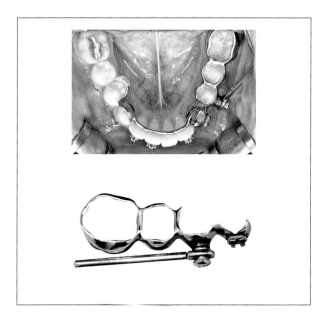

Fig. 24-12 Mandibular cast splint breakage.

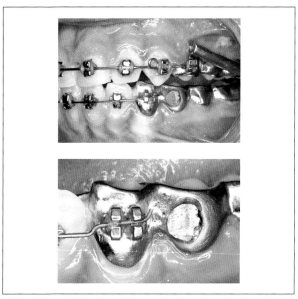

Fig. 24-15 Mandibular premolar axle breakage.

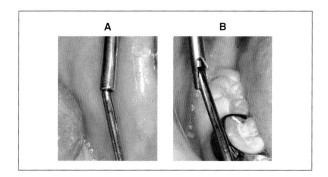

Fig. 24-13 Plunger stuck in tube opening (A). Tube splitting (B).

Complications during Herbst treatment with reduced mandibular casted splints. A prospective multicenter clinical trial (Schiöth et al. 2007)

As the efficiency of mandibular anchorage in Herbst treatment using the banded type of appliance seems to be independent of the number of teeth involved (Pancherz and Hansen 1988, Weschler and Pancherz 2005) (see Chapter 19: Anchorage problems), a reduced mandibular cast splint anchorage form (reduced splints) would be expected to be as efficient as the extended cast splint form generally used (standard splints). The advantage of reduced splints would be, provided the complication rate is not increased, that they are easier and cheaper to construct.

In a prospective two-center study (Giessen, Germany and Berne, Switzerland) the complication prevalence of a reduced mandibular cast splint (RS) Herbst appliance, with the splints extending from the canine to the second premolar (Fig. 24-16) was compared to a standard mandibular cast splint (SS) Herbst appliance, with the splints extending from the canine to the first or second permanent molar (Fig. 24-17).

Fifty consecutive Herbst patients treated with reduced mandibular splints (RS) were compared with the previously presented group of 182 consecutive Herbst patients (Sanden et al. 2004), treated with standard mandibular splints (SS). The average treatment time amounted to 8 months in the RS group and 7 months in the SS group.

Despite the slightly longer treatment time in the RS group, the overall prevalence of complications did not differ significantly between the groups and amounted to 58% of the patients in the RS group and 60% of the patients in the SS group (Fig. 24-18). The most frequent type of complication in both groups (Fig. 24-19) was loosening of splints in the maxilla, which occurred in 55% of the RS and 67% of the SS patients, followed by loosening of the splints in the mandible (Fig. 24-19), which occurred in 32% of the RS and in 27% of the SS subjects. Breakages of maxillary and mandibular splints occurred very seldom in both groups (0-3%). Telescope breakages were seen twice as much in the RS group (10%) compared to the SS group (4%). Of the 29 RS subjects and 110 SS subjects who had problems, one to three complications occurred in 80% of the RS and in 56% of the SS subjects, four to six complications in 10% of the RS and in 31% of the SS subjects. Seven complications or more were experienced by 10% of the RS and by 13% of the SS subjects (Fig. 24-20).

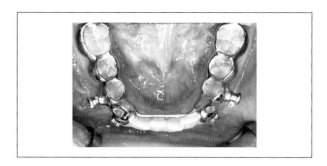

Fig. 24-17 Standard mandibular Splint (SS).

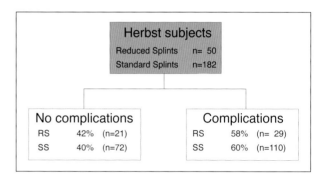

Fig. 24-18 Prevalence of complications in reduced mandibular splint (RS) and standard mandibular splint (SS) Herbst appliances.

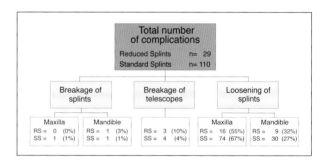

Fig. 24-19 Frequency and type of complications in 29 complication subjects treated with the reduced mandibular splint (RS) Herbst appliance and in 110 complication subjects treated with the standard mandibular splint (SS) Herbst appliance.

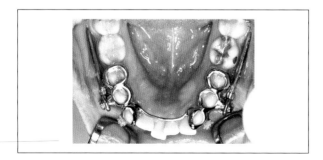

Fig. 24-16 Reduced mandibular Splint (RS).

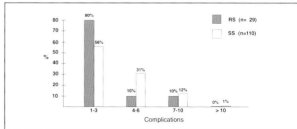

Fig. 24-20 Distribution (in %) of 29 RS and 110 SS Herbst subjects with complications in relation to the number of problems experienced in each patient.

Interpretation of the results

When comparing the two Herbst groups, maxillary splint loosening was more frequent (12% more) in the SS group and mandibular splint loosening was more frequent (5% more) in the RS group. The slightly higher prevalence of mandibular splint loosening in the RS group could possibly be due to the smaller retentive surface for the cement (less teeth involved) in comparison to that of the SS group splints. However, why the prevalence of maxillary splint loosening was lower in the RS group cannot be explained by the changes in mandibular splint design. The prevalence of telescope breakages was relatively low, however, it was twice as high in the RS compared to the SS group. A possible explanation could be that the telescopic parts were adjusted differently in the RS (patients treated in Berne) and SS (patients treated in Giessen) groups. Perhaps the pivot openings of the telescopic parts in the RS group were not extended as much as in the SS group, thus not allowing full lateral movements of the mandible, which consequently would put larger strains on the telescopes.

The frequency of patients experiencing 4 complications or more was higher in the SS group and the frequency of patients with less problems (1 to 3 complications) was higher in the RS group (Fig. 24-20). However, with respect to the prevalence and type of complications during Herbst treatment, the two forms of splints, RS and SS, were comparable.

An additional problem, not addressed in the above investigations, is the loss of premolar brackets, spot welded on the maxillary bands and splints (Fig. 24-21). This is an annoying complication, as a bracket loss will make it impossible to properly use a sectional arch wire, connecting the premolar bands or splints to the front teeth. This is necessary for the prevention of space opening between the maxillary canines and first premolars (see Chapter 9: The headgear effect of the Herbst appliance).

Complications related to the patient

Problems in this category are seen only occasionally during Herbst treatment. These complications are possible to prevent. The most obvious patient related complications are listed below:

• Loss of the screw, attaching the tube on the maxillary molar axle. This complication can be prevented by applying cement in the thread of the screw hole. This is an advantageous measure, as the tube part of the telescope mechanism usually can be left untouched during the course of therapy.

• Plunger and tube disengagement (Fig. 24-22). This is not a serious complication. It happens upon wide mouth opening when the plunger is too short in relation to the tube. By a long maxillary-mandibular inter-axle distance when constructing the appliance (see Chapter 3: Design, construction and clinical management of the Herbst appliance) or a change to a longer plunger, the problem could be omitted. However, if a plunger disengagement still occurs, it is easy for the patient to reassemble the telescopic parts. Patient instruction is needed, however.

• Ulcerations of the soft tissues due to appliance impingement (Figs. 24-23 A to D).

• Tooth fractures upon removal of the bands or splints by the use of a band removing pliers (Fig. 24-24). If difficulties are encountered during the removal procedure it is advisable to split the bands or splints beforehand (Fig. 24-25).

Finally, in the literature four additional complications have been discussed in connection with Herbst treatment. Three of the complications are said to be due to an appliance overload on the anchorage teeth and tooth-supporting soft and hard tissue structures: (1) gingival recessions, (2) marginal bone loss and (3) root resorptions. The fourth complication concerns TMJ problems, which are supposed to result from keeping the mandible continuously in a protruded position by the telescope mechanism. However, none of the four stated problems have been verified scientifically. They are discussed more extensively in Chapter 20: Effects on anchorage teeth and tooth-supporting structures, and in Chapter 16: Effects on TMJ function.

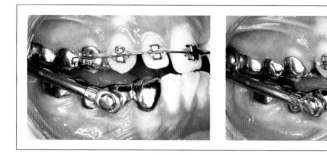

Fig. 24-21 Bracket loss on the right maxillary first premolar.

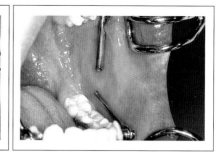

Fig. 24-22 Plunger and tube disengagement upon wide mouth opening.

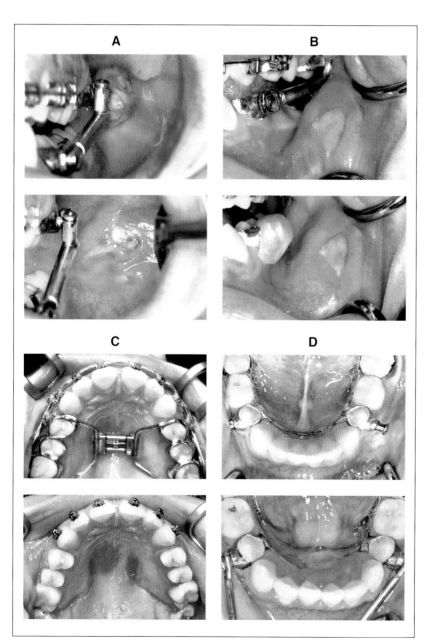

A **B**

C **D**

Fig. 24-23 Ulcerations of the soft tissues. **A**: Plunger impingement distally. Note, a double-joint Herbst appliance was used. **B**: Screw impingement. Protection wax was used to facilitate healing. **C**: Rapid palatal expander impingement. **D**: Lingual pelott impingement.

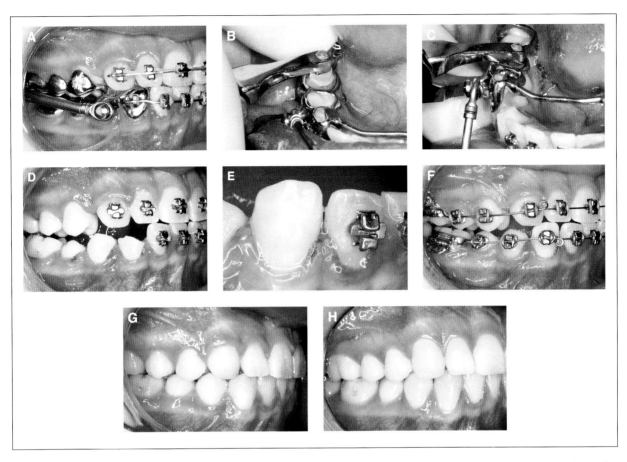

Fig. 24-24 Canine cusp fracture, upon removal of a mandibular cast splint. **A**: At the end of the Herbst treatment phase, before splint removal. **B**: At splint removal with band removing pliers. **C**: After splint removal. Note, the mandibular canine is fractured with the cusp tip still in the splint. **D**: After splint removal. Note, the fractured mandibular canine. **E**: Bonding of the fractured cusp on the canine. **F**: Start of multibracket treatment phase. Note, the bracket bonded on the damaged canine. **G**: After treatment. **H**: 5 years posttreatment.

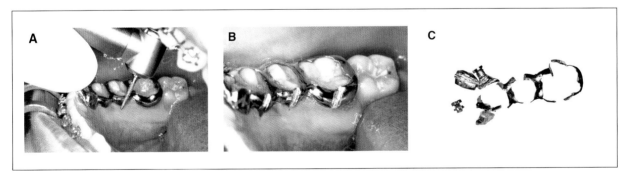

Fig. 24-25 Splitting of mandibular splint into pieces in order to facilitate removal from the teeth.

Conclusions and clinical implications

In Herbst treatment several types of complications can be encountered.

Appliance related complications:
- These problems occur rather often and are time consuming to handle, especially when using the banded type of Herbst appliance.
- In the investigation of Sanden et al. (2004), complications occurred in 67% of the banded and in 60% of the cast splint Herbst subjects. No complications were seen in 33% of the banded and in 40% of the cast splint Herbst cases. (1) Loosening and breakages of bands and splints were the most common complications. (2) Bands broke more often than splints. (3) Splints loosened more often than bands. (4) Maxillary problems were seen twice as often as mandibular problems.
- In the investigation of Schiöth et al. (2007), complication prevalence was similar when using reduced mandibular splints (extending from the canine to the second premolar) and standard mandibular splints (extending from the canine to the permanent first or second molar).

Patient related complications:
- These problems are seen only occasionally and are easy to handle.
- Loosening of axle-screws, plunger and tube disengagement and ulcerations of the soft tissues are problems to be considered.

Recommendations:
- Despite the fact that the overall frequency of complications was the same in the banded and cast splint Herbst appliance (Sanden et al. 2004), the use of a cast splint appliance is to be preferred as it saves both clinical and laboratory service time (Hägg et al. 2002).
- Although the prevalence of complication is comparable when using reduced and standard mandibular splints, the former has the advantage of that it is easier to fabricate and the costs are less.

References

Hägg U, Tse EIK, Rabie ABM, Robinson W. A comparison of splinted and banded Herbst appliances: treatment changes and complications. Austr Orthod J 2002;18:76-81.

Pancherz H, Hansen K. Mandibular anchorage in Herbst treatment. Eur J Orthod 1988;10:149-164.

Sanden E, Pancherz H, Hansen K. Complications during Herbst treatment. J Clin Orthod 2004;38:130-133.

Schiöth T, von Bremen J, Pancherz H, Ruf, S. Complications during Herbst appliance treatment with reduced mandibular casted splints. A prospective, clinical multicenter study. J Orofac Orthop 2007;68:302-326

Thiebes RE. Bekanntheitsgrad und Verwendung der Herbst Apparatur in der deutschen Kieferorthopädie. Diss. med. dent. (Thesis), Giessen 2006.

Weschler D, Pancherz H. Efficiency of three mandibular anchorage forms in Herbst treatment: a cephalometric investigation. Angle Orthod 2005;75:23-27.

Chapter 25

Relapse and Retention

Research

At the end of Herbst treatment, overcorrected sagittal dental arch relationships with an incomplete cuspal interdigitation are a common finding (Pancherz 1979,1981,1982,1985, Pancherz and Hansen 1986). As a result of recovering tooth movements, however, the occlusion generally settles into a Class I relationship within a period of 6 months after therapy (Pancherz and Hansen 1986). On a long-term follow-up basis, a Class I dental arch relationship seems to be maintained by a stable cuspal interdigitation of the maxillary and mandibular teeth, while relapses occur in cases with unstable occlusal conditions (Pancherz 1981, 1994, Wieslander 1993). In the publication of Pancherz (1991), the mechanism of the Class II relapse after Herbst therapy has been analyzed. The amount of and the interrelationship between skeletal and dental components contributing to the relapse have been assessed.

The nature of Class relapse after Herbst appliance treatment: a cephalometric long-term investigation (Pancherz 1991)

At the time of examination, a total amount of 118 patients with Class II:1 malocclusions were treated at the Department of Orthodontics, University of Lund, Sweden. Herbst therapy resulted in Class I dental arch relationships in all 118 cases. From this patient group, 45 subjects, followed for at least 5 years (5 to 10 years) after treatment were used as target sample for this investigation (Fig. 25-1). The patients were divided into three groups with respect to stability or

relapse in sagittal dental arch relationships, decided on the changes occurring during the period from 6 months posttreatment (after settling of the occlusion) to 5-10 years posttreatment:

Stable (S) – overjet unchanged or reduced and molar relationship in Class I (n=14).

Insignificant relapse – overjet increased ≤ 1 mm and / or molar relationship in Class I or in Class II (= a deviation of less than one-half cusp width from normal relationship) (n=16).

Relapse (R) – overjet increased > 1 mm and / or molar relationship in Class I or in Class II (Class II = a deviation of one-half cusp width or more from normal relationship) (n=15).

In the analysis of the nature of occlusal relapse after Herbst treatment, a comparison was made between the stable (S) and the relapse (R) group. The insignificant relapse group was excluded from the study. With respect to appliance design, a partial anchorage form was used in 36% (5/14) and a total anchorage form in 64% (9/14) of the subjects in the stable group. In the relapse group the corresponding figures were 53% (8/15) and 47% (7/15), respectively. Posttreatment retention was performed in 60% (9/15) of the stable cases and in 53% (8/15) of the relapse cases. The rest of the subjects in both groups had no retainers. Lateral head films in habitual occlusion from before treatment, after 7 months of Herbst treatment, 6 months posttreatment when the occlusion had settled (Pancherz and Hansen 1986) and 5 to 10 years posttreatment were evaluated using the SO-Analysis (see Chapter 6: Herbst research - subjects and methods). The amount of skeletal and dental changes contributing to the alteration in overjet and

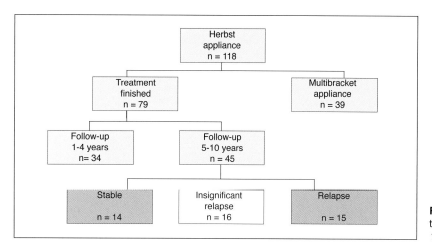

Fig. 25-1 Outline of the patient selection procedure. (*Revised from Pancherz 1991*)

sagittal molar relationship in the stable (S) and the relapse (R) subjects are shown in Figs. 25-2 to 25-4.

Treatment period (T) changes

At the end of 7 months of Herbst treatment, when the appliance was removed, there was a Class I or overcorrected Class I dental arch relationship in all stable and in all relapse patients investigated. The improvement in overjet and sagittal molar relationship was statistically comparable in the two groups (Fig. 25-4) and resulted from both skeletal and dental changes (Figs. 25-2 and 25-3).

Early posttreatment period (P1) changes

During the period from after treatment to 6 months posttreatment the occlusion settled into a Class I relationship in all subjects in both the stable and relapse groups. The amount of recovery in overjet and sagittal molar relationship was statistically comparable in the two groups (Fig. 25-4) and was mainly the result of recovering maxillary and mandibular tooth movements (Figs. 25-2 and 25-3).

Late posttreatment period (P2) changes

Due to the method of patient selection, sagittal dental arch relationships were unchanged or had even become improved in the stable group, whereas a rebound had occurred in the relapse group. During the period from 6 months posttreatment to an average of 6 years posttreatment, the relapse in overjet and sagittal molar relationship resulted mainly from maxillary dental changes: the maxillary incisors and molars moved significantly more anteriorly in the relapse group than in the stable group (Fig. 25-4). Growth did not, as might have been expected, contribute to the occlusal relapse seen. The interrela-

tion between maxillary and mandibular posttreatment growth was favorable and, on average, the same (mandibular growth exceeding maxillary growth by 2.8 mm) in both groups (Figs. 25-2 and 25-3).

Interpretation of the results

The SO-Analysis used is confined to horizontal changes only. Although vertical growth development is an important factor in successful Class II therapy, it is the horizontal component in jaw growth and tooth movements that is decisive for the final treatment outcome.

The target sample could be considered to be composed of consecutively treated cases (Fig. 25-1). The subjects in the two examination groups were evenly distributed with respect to appliance design (anchorage system) and posttreatment management procedures (retention / nonretention). At the end of the observation period (5-10 years posttreatment, growth was finished (Hägg and Taranger 1980) in all cases except one in the relapse group. Furthermore, the subjects in the two examination groups responded equally to therapy and were also comparable with respect to the changes in the early posttreatment period (P1) (Figs. 25-2 to 25-4). During the second posttreatment period (P2), however, relapsing dental changes especially in the maxilla (anterior movements of the incisors and molars) were more pronounced in the relapse group than in the stable group (Figs. 25-2 to 25-4). Posttreatment growth did not contribute to the occlusal relapse.

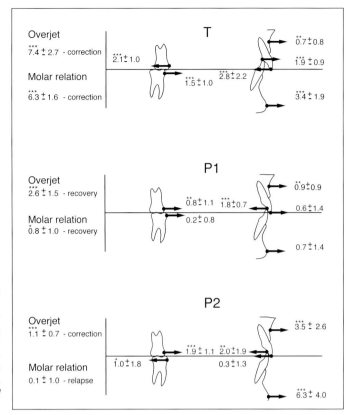

Fig. 25-2 Skeletal and dental changes (mm) contributing to alterations in overjet and sagittal molar relationships. SO-Analysis in 14 Class II:1 subjects exhibiting **stability (group S)** in sagittal dental arch relationships in the late posttreatment period (P2). Registrations (Mean and SD) during the treatment period (T), early posttreatment period (P1) and late postteatment period (P2). * Indicates significance at 5% level; ** Indicates significance at 1% level; *** Indicates significance at 0.1% level. (*Revised from Pancherz 1991*)

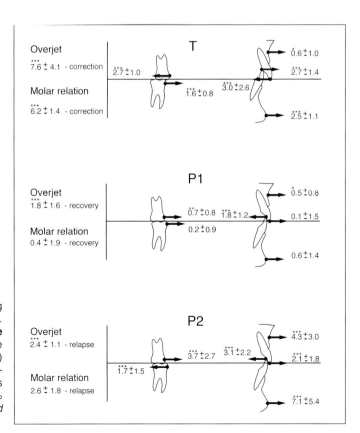

Fig. 25-3 Skeletal and dental changes (mm) contributing to alterations in overjet and sagittal molar relationships. SO-Analysis in 15 Class II:1 subjects exhibiting **relapse (group R)** in sagittal dental arch relationships in the late posttreatment period (P2). Registrations (Mean and SD) during the treatment period (T), early posttreatment period (P1) and late postteatment period (P2). * Indicates significance at 5% level; ** Indicates significance at 1% level; *** Indicates significance at 0.1% level. (*Revised from Pancherz 1991*)

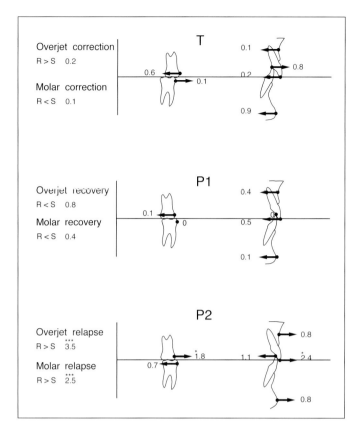

Overjet correction
R > S   0.2

Molar correction
R < S   0.1

T   0.1   0.8   0.6   0.1   0.2   0.2   0.9

Overjet recovery
R < S   0.8

Molar recovery
R < S   0.4

P1   0.4   0.1   0   0.5   0.1

Overjet relapse
R > S   3.5 ***

Molar relapse
R > S   2.5 ***

P2   0.8   1.8   0.7   1.1   2.4   0.8

Fig. 25-4 Differences between the relapse (R) and stable (S) groups (R minus S) with respect to skeletal and dental changes (mm) contributing to alterations in overjet and sagittal molar relationships. Registrations (Mean) during the treatment period (T), early posttreatment period (P1) and late posttreatment period (P2). * Indicates significance at 5% level; *** Indicates significance at 0.1% level. (*Revised from Pancherz 1991*)

When the patients were examined clinically and with the aid of their dental casts, two relapse promoting factors were observed, which could explain the differences in adverse tooth movement seen in the two groups: (1) a lip-tongue dysfunction habit at the end of the total observation period was noted in 64% (9/15) of the relapse cases but in none of the stable cases and (2) an unstable Class I cuspal interdigitation (registered by visual inspection of the dental casts 6 months posttreatment) existed in 57% (8/15) of the relapse cases but in only 13% (2/16) of the stable cases. Thus, it could be hypothesized that the main cause of the Class II relapse seen in the Herbst patients was a persisting lip-tongue dysfunction habit and an unstable occlusion after treatment.

It could be expected that the subjects who wore retainers after Herbst therapy would show fewer dental relapses than subjects without retainers. However, no differences between retention and nonretention cases were seen. This was true for both the stable group and relapse group. Furthermore, the retainers were used only for 1 to 2 years, which most likely was too short a period for long-term interarch stability, especially in cases with unstable occlusal conditions after treatment.

Clinical example

From the group of 15 relapse subjects a 13.1-year-old boy (Case 25-1), whose Class II:1 malocclusion relapsed completely, will be presented (Fig. 25-5A and B). This was the most severe relapse case of all patients analyzed.

The boy was treated with the Herbst appliance for 6 months. A partial maxillary and mandibular anchorage system was used (see Chapter 3: Design, construction and clinical management of the Herbst appliance). At the end of treatment overcorrected Class I dental arch relationships existed. Within 6 months posttreatment the occlusion settled into Class I. No retention was performed after Herbst therapy. At the follow-up examination when the patient was 20.5 years old (6.9 years posttreatment), a full Class II molar relationship and an increased overjet was present. At the clinical examination of the patient, a lip-tongue dysfunction habit at speech and swallowing was noted and was thought to be the main cause of the occlusal relapse. In detail the following dentoskeletal changes were registered in Case 25-1.

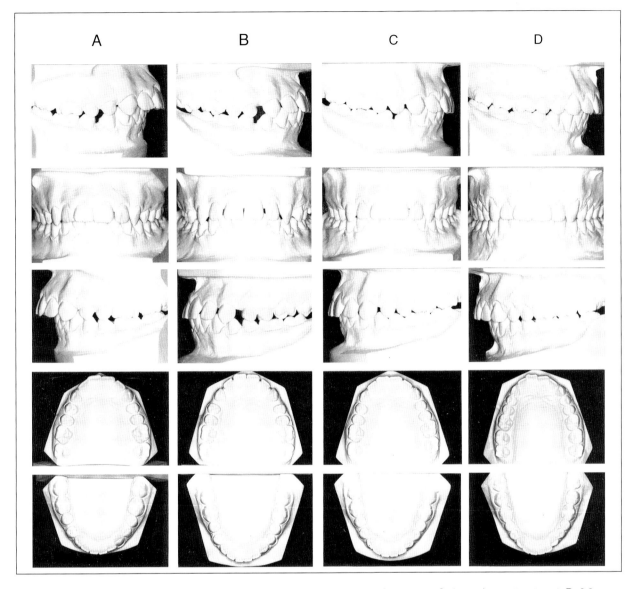

Fig. 25-5A Case 25-1 Plaster casts. **A**, Before treatment. **B**, After 6 months of treatment. **C**, 6 months posttreatment. **D**, 6.9 years posttreatment. (*Revised from Pancherz 1991*)

Treatment period (T) changes

During the 6 months of treatment, the overjet was reduced by 6 mm and the sagittal molar relationship was improved by 8 mm (Fig. 25-5B). Overjet reduction was accomplished by a favorable mandibular/maxillary growth difference of 3.5 mm, a 0.5 mm palatal movement of the maxillary incisors and a 2.0 mm labial movement of the mandibular incisors. Improvement in molar relationship was a result of a 4.5 mm distal movement of the maxillary molars in addition to the favorable difference in mandibular/maxillary growth.

Early posttreatment period (P1) changes

During the first 6 months after Herbst treatment when the occlusion had settled the overjet rebounded by 1.5 mm and the sagittal molar relationship by 2.0 mm (Fig. 25-5B). These changes were a result of recovering maxillary and mandibular tooth movements. The difference in mandibular/maxillary was favorable (sagittal mandibular growth exceeding maxillary growth by 1.5 mm) and counteracted the occlusal changes.

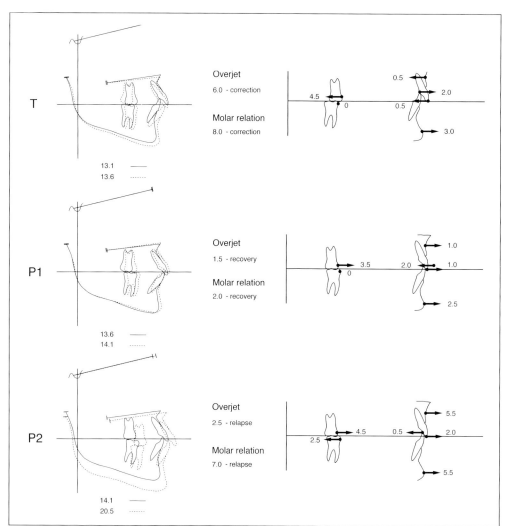

Fig. 25-5B Case 10-1 Superimposed cephalometric tracings (left column) and SO-Analysis (right column). T, Treatment period of 6 months. P1, Early posttreatment period of 6 months. P2, Late posttreatment period of 6.4 years. (*Revised from Pancherz 1991*)

Late posttreatment period (P2) changes
During the following 6.4 years after Herbst treatment the overjet relapsed by 2.5 mm and the sagittal molar relationship by 7 mm (Fig. 25-5B). Overjet relapse was a result of a 2.0 mm labial movement of the maxillary incisors and a 0.5 mm lingual movement of the mandibular incisors. Molar relapse was a result of a 4.5 mm mesial movement of the maxillary molars and a 2.5 mm distal movement of the mandibular molars. Sagittal growth was equally large in both the mandible and the maxilla and thus, did not contribute to the occlusal relapse.

Retention after Herbst treatment

The following annotations made and recommendations given on retention after Herbst therapy are based only on clinical experience, and not on scientific evidence.

The improvement in sagittal molar and incisor relationship accomplished during Herbst therapy is mainly a result of an increase in mandibular growth, distal tooth movements in the maxilla and mesial tooth movements in the mandible (Figs. 25-2 and 25-3). A posttreatment relapse seems in the first place to result from maxillary and mandibular dental changes (Fig. 25-4). A stable functional occlusion after treatment will counteract this relapse (Pancherz 1994). As treatment generally leads to overcorrected sagittal dental arch relationships with an incomplete cuspal interdigitation (Pancherz and Hansen 1986), a period of "active" retention until the occlusion has settled will thus be necessary.

The Andresen activator (night time use only) has been found to be a most suitable "active" retention device (Fig. 25-6) after Herbst treatment. The appliance holds the teeth in the desired position and makes interocclusal adjustments possible.

Although the unharmonious muscle contraction pattern seen in Class II:1 malocclusions (Pancherz 1980) is normalized during Herbst treatment (Pancherz and Anehus-Pancherz 1980), the musculature would most likely need a longer time for permanent adaptation than the Herbst treatment time of 6 to 8 months. Again, an activator seems to be the appliance of choice for the training and accommodation of the musculature to the new mandibular position. A musculature in harmony with the dentofacial structures is certainly of utmost importance for a stable treatment result.

The length of an activator retention is dependent on the age and growth period of the patient (Wieslander 1993) as well as on the severity of the Class II malocclusion. Therefore, activator retention is recommended to be performed for at least 2 years in adolescent patients and 3 to 4 years in post-adolescent / young adult patients. In severe Class II malocclusions (with a Class II molar relationship >1 premolar width and / or an overjet of more than 12 mm with or without a very deep bite) it would be advisable to increase the retention time additionally. As the mandibular incisor region is a sensible area prone to crowding it would be good practice always to combine the activator with a mandibular cuspid-to-cuspid retainer (Fig. 25-7).

When Herbst treatment is followed by a multibracket (MB) treatment period, then the retention regime could be changed as a stable occlusion should have been attained during the MB phase. Thus, instead of an activator, a maxillary plate (Fig. 25-8) in combination with a mandibular cuspid-to-cuspid retainer could be used. The plate is used full-time the first 6 months posttreatment, thereafter only nighttime.

In severe Class II malocclusions and in postadolescent / young adult patients, it could be advantageous to retain the treatment result with a maxillary plate during daytime and an activator during nighttime.

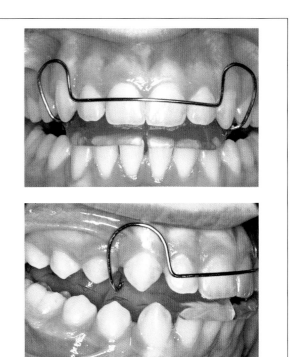

Fig. 25-6 Activator for "active" retention after Herbst treatment.

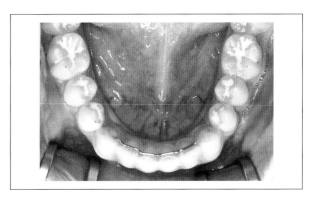

Fig. 25-7 Mandibular cuspid-to-cuspid retainer.

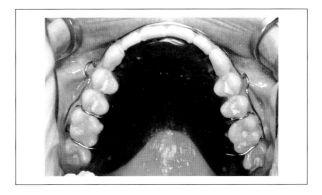

Fig. 25-8 Maxillary retention plate.

Conclusions and clinical implications

- A Class II relapse after Herbst treatment is mainly a result of dental changes.
- A persisting lip-tongue dysfunction habit and an incomplete cuspal interdigitation of the teeth posttreatment are considered to be the main relapse promoting factors.
- An unfavorable maxillary/mandiblar growth pattern will play a minor role in the development of a Class II relapse.
- For the prevention of a postreatment relapse, a solid Class I occlusion after treatment is of utmost importance.
- "Active" retention with an activator and a mandibular cuspid-to-cuspid retainer is recommended.
- Long-term retention seems indicated in patients with severe Class II malocclusions, especially in those treated at late age.

References

Hägg U, Taranger J. Skeletal stages of the hand and wrist as indicators of the pubertal growth spurt. Acta Odont Scand 1980;38:187-200.

Pancherz H. Treatment of Class II malocclusions by jumping the bite with the Herbst appliance. A cephalometric investigation. Am J Orthod 1979;76:423-442.

Pancherz H. Activity of the temporal and masseter muscles in Class II, Division 1 malocclusions. Am J Orthod 1980;77:679-688.

Pancherz H. The effect of continuous bite jumping on the dentofacial complex: a follow-up study after Herbst appliance treatment of Class II malocclusions. Eur J Orthod 1981;3:49-60.

Pancherz H. The mechanism of Class II correction in Herbst appliance treatment. a cephalometric investigation. Am J Orthod 1982;82:104-113.

Pancherz H. The Herbst appliance – Its biologic effects and clinical use. Am J Orthod 1985;87:1-20.

Pancherz H. The nature of Class II relapse after Herbst treatment: A cephalometric long-term investigation. Am J Orthod Dentofac Orthop 1991;100:220-233.

Pancherz H. Früh- oder Spätbehandlung mit der Herbs-Apparatur – Stabiität oder Rezidiv? Inf Orthod Orthop 1994;26:437-445.

Pancherz H, Anehus-Pancherz M. Muscle activity in Class II, Division 1 malocclusions treated by bite jumping with the Herbst appliance. Am J Orthod 1980;78:321-329.

Pancherz H, Hansen K. Occlusal changes during and after Herbst treatment: a cephalmetric investigation. Eur J Orthod 1986;8:215-228.

Wieslander L. Long-term effects of treatment with the headgear-Herbst appliance in the early mixed dentition. Stability or relapse? Am J Orthod Dentofac Orthop 1993;104:319-329.

Chapter 26

Concluding remarks

The Herbst appliance is the most thoroughly analyzed functional appliance in orthodontics / dentofacial orthopedics, and its mode of action is predominantly evidence based. The following should be considered in the clinical use of the Herbst appliance.

1. The Herbst appliance is most effective in the treatment of Class II:1 and Class II:2 malocclusions.
   - Depending on the age of the patient, Class II correction is accomplished by varying amounts of maxillary and mandibular dental and mandibular skeletal changes. In adolescents, a relative contribution of 50% to 70% dental and 30% to 50% skeletal changes could be expected. In older subjects the skeletal part is reduced while the dental part is increased.
   - Maxillary dental changes result in a distalization of the molars. This headgear effect is most useful in both Class II correction and in space gain for crowded canines and incisors.
   - Mandibular dental changes result in a proclination of the incisors. These tooth movements are basically a result of anchorage loss and difficult to control. In Class II:1 subjects, incisor proclination is mostly unwanted but in Class II:2 cases it is advantageous for a stable inter-incisor support, counteracting an overbite relapse posttreatment.

2. With respect to treatment timing, a late approach in the permanent dentition and during the postadolescent growth period is to be preferred as this will favour a stable cuspal interdigitation after therapy and reduce retention time and relapse. On the other hand, early Herbst treatment in the mixed dentition is not recommended, as a stable occlusion is difficult to attain, thus increasing the risk for relapse. Therefore, in early Herbst treatment, posttreatment retention will be crucial.

3. Hyperdivergent and retrognathic Class II subjects are good Herbst patients. There is no contraindication for their treatment. They react readily to therapy. However, the risk of a posttreatment occlusal relapse is larger in hyperdivergent (high-angle) than in hypodivergent (low-angle) subjects due to the prevailing unfavorable growth pattern in the hyperdivergent patients. A stable cuspal interdigitation of the teeth will, however, counteract this relapse.

4. The Herbst appliance has not been found to have any harmful effects on the:
   - TMJ (does not induce TMD);
   - anchorage teeth (does not cause root resorptions);
   - tooth-supporting structures (does not cause marginal bone loss);
   - gingival structures (does not cause gingival recessions due to proclination of the mandibular incisors).

5. Herbst treatment in young adults (20 to 30 years of age) is generally most successful. Class II correction is mainly accomplished by dental changes (80% to 90%), while mandibular skeletal changes (condylar and glenoid fossa modeling) contribute to a minor degree (10% to 20%).

Paradigm shift in Class II therapy

The current and widely accepted concept of non-syndrome skeletal Class II treatment follows (Fig. 26-1).

- Growth modification in children and adolescents using various types of removable functional appliances (e.g. activator, bionator, Fränkel) and/or headgear.
- Camouflage orthodontics in postadolescents and adults by the extraction of teeth and the use of fixed multibracket appliances.
- Orthognathic surgery in adults (e.g. sagittal mandibular split osteotomy).

Due to the results from our clinical research in adult Herbst patients and from the experimental research in adult animals (Herbst appliances in monkeys and protrusion splints in rats), we propose a new concept for the treatment of non-syndrome skeletal Class II malocclusions (Fig. 26-2):

- Growth modification / skeletal tissue adaptation in children, adolescents, postadolescents and young adults. In the children and in the mixed dentition adolescents, treatment should be performed with removable functional appliances. The Herbst appliance is indicated in the permanent dentition adolescents, the postadolescents and the adults.
- Camouflage orthodontics in mature adults by the extraction of teeth and the use of fixed multibracket appliances.
- Orthognathic surgery in mature adults (e.g. sagittal mandibular split osteotomy).

Strategy in modern Class II therapy

To make Class II treatment as effective as possible, the following strategy is recommended.

- If an early approach is indicated (e.g. prevention of incisor trauma), treatment is initiated in the mixed dentition by using a removable functional appliance but not the Herbst appliance.
- If, however, the treatment response by this early approach is slow and insufficient or the patient does not cooperate, a break in treatment should be made.
- Then, in the permanent dentition / postadolescent growth period the Herbst appliance is indicated as part of a two- or three-step treatment approach.

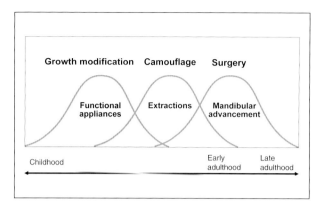

Fig. 26-1 The current concept of Class II treatment Frequency distribution of the treatment options: growth modification, camouflage orthodontics and orthognathic surgery in relation to growth development. The illustration is a visual expression of a theory and not based on quantitative scientific data.

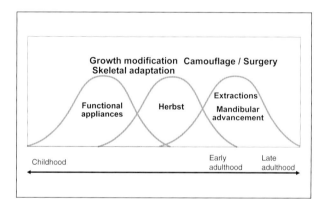

Fig. 26-2 The new concept of Class II treatment Frequency distribution of the treatment options: growth modification / skeletal tissue adaptation, camouflage orthodontics and orthognathic surgery in relation to growth development. The illustration is a visual expression of a theory and not based on quantitative scientific data.

Contents Index